GRAY'S

Clinical Photographic Dissector of the Human Body

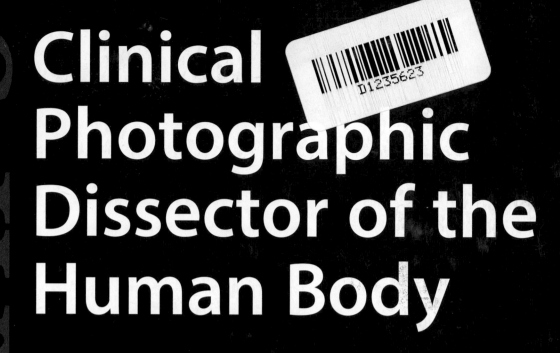

Marios Loukas, MD, PhD
Professor and Chair
Department of Anatomical Sciences
Dean of Research, School of Medicine
St. George's University
Grenada, West Indies

Brion Benninger, MD, MSc
Professor, Vice Chair, Co-Course Director
Department of Medical Anatomical Sciences
Department of Family Medicine
COMP-Northwest and College of Dental Medicine
Western University of Health Sciences
Lebanon, Oregon;
Samaritan Orthopaedic Residency Program Faculty
Samaritan General Surgery Residency Program Faculty
Corvallis, Oregon;
Department of Surgery
Department of Orthopedics and Rehabilitation
Department of Oral Maxillofacial Surgery
Oregon Health and Science University
Portland, Oregon

R. Shane Tubbs, PhD
Editor-in-Chief, *Clinical Anatomy*
Pediatric Neurosurgery
Children's Hospital
Birmingham, Alabama

ELSEVIER
SAUNDERS

1600 John F. Kennedy Blvd.
Ste. 1800
Philadelphia, PA 19103-2899

GRAY'S CLINICAL PHOTOGRAPHIC DISSECTOR
OF THE HUMAN BODY

ISBN: 978-1-4377-2417-2

ISBN: 978-1-4377-2417-2

Content Strategy Director: Madelene Hyde
Content Development Specialist: Christine Abshire
Publishing Services Manager: Patricia Tannian
Senior Project Manager: John Casey
Design Direction: Steven Stave

I would like to dedicate this book to my brilliant and wonderful wife, Joanna, who has been the bright star of my life. Her continuous support, dedication, love, and affection give me the energy and courage to fulfill all our dreams.

ML

I would like to dedicate this novel text to my lovely wife, Alison, and inquisitive son, Jack, who make each day worthwhile, my clinical and anatomy mentors—Gerald Tresidder, Sir Harold Ellis, and Sir Peter Bell, and to my students and current colleagues—Paul Aversano, Paula Crone, John Pham, Robyn Dreibelbis, William Merbs, Leon Assail, Brian Bell, Lynn Loriaux, Peter Sullivan, Richard Mullins, and Donald Trunkey

BB

I would like to thank my wife, Susan, and son, Isaiah, for their support and patience during the writing of this book. All that I do, I do for them. I also want to dedicate this book in memory of my brother-in-law, Nelson Jones, whose intellect, engagement of others, and curiosity about life have been examples for me.

RST

PREFACE

Time allotted for anatomical education continues to be whittled down in most curricula. Therefore, instructors of courses that continue to dissect the human cadaver must utilize all available time wisely. Traditionally, in most dissection courses students begin their dissections with the aid of a dissector and follow step-by-step instructions of how to dismantle the human form to identify various structures. Such guides, in general, are written much like recipes. However, such instructions for the most part do not provide students with the same step-by-step visual instructions of what to expect during their exploration of the human body, and if they do, these are most likely schematic drawings that often look nothing like the actual anatomical structures. It is this deficit in available dissectors on the market that compelled us to put together a collection of dissection photographs with accompanying text to better assist the student of anatomy. It is our hope that being able to see what students are expected to find during their dissection, from superficial to deep, will allow them to be more efficient not only in their learning experience but also with their time.

Marios Loukas
Brion Benninger
R. Shane Tubbs

ACKNOWLEDGMENTS

This dissection book is the work not only of the authors but also of numerous scientific and clinical friends and colleagues who have been so generous with their knowledge and given significant feedback and help. This book would not have been possible were it not for the contributions of the colleagues and friends listed below.

A very special group of medical students, members of the Student Clinical Research Society in the Department of Anatomical Sciences at St. George's University, helped enormously with the completion of this project through their comments and criticism.

Theofanis Kollias
Elizabeth Hogan
Frank Scali

We would also like to thank the following colleagues for their technical expertise in dissections and their enormous help with this project:

Alysia Tucker, MD
Kathleen Bubb, MD
Ewarld Marshall, MD
William Merbs (PhD candidate)
Michael Snosek (PhD candidate)
Benjamin Turner (PhD candidate)

The following St. George's University alumni and current research fellows of the Department of Anatomical Sciences have been great friends and colleagues. Their continuous support, comments, criticism, and enthusiasm have contributed enormously to the completion of this project.

Denzil Etienne, MD
Alana John, MD
Mitchell Muhlman, MD
Stephen Osiro, MD
Andrew Walters, MD

The following individuals from the Department of Anatomical Sciences at St. George's University have also been very helpful with their comments and criticisms:

Feisal Brahim, PhD
Danny Burns, MD, PhD
Cathleen Bubb, MD
Brian Curry, PhD
Francis Fakoya, MBBS, PhD
Rachel George, MD
Robert Hage, MD, PhD
Robert Jordan, PhD
Ewarld Marshall, MD
Vish Rao, PhD
Alana Wade, MD

We are also grateful to the following members of St. George's University for their photographic and technical expertise:

Joanna Loukas (photography and design)
Rayn Jacobs (design)
Carlson Dominique (laboratory technician)
Rodon Marast (laboratory technician)
Christopher Belgrave (laboratory technician)

The following great friends have been very instrumental over the years with their enthusiasm, continuous support, and most important, mentoring in the completion of this and many other projects:

Allen Pensick, PhD
Peter Abrahams, MD
Gene Colborn, PhD
Vid Persaud, MD, PhD
Mohammadali M. Shoja, MD
W. Jerry Oakes, MD

The authors would also like to thank Shivayogi Bhusnurmath, MD, and Bhati Bhusnurmath, MD, for their important comments on the pathological specimens.

Finally, the authors would also like to give a very special thank you to Dr. George Salter for his generous efforts in reviewing this book.

REVIEWERS

Argentina
Susana Biasutto, PhD
Professor, Anatomical Institute
National University of Cordoba
Cordoba, Argentina

Australia
Fiona Stewart, PhD
Associate Professor, School of Rural Medicine
University of New England
Armidale, NSW, Australia

Austria
Andreas H. Weiglein, MD
Vice Chair, Institute of Anatomy
Medical University Graz
Graz, Austria

Canada
Vid Persaud, MD, PhD, DSc, FRCPath (Lond.)
Professor Emeritus and Former Head
Department of Human Anatomy and Cell Science
University of Manitoba
Winnipeg, Manitoba, Canada

China
Changman Zhou, MD, PhD
Professor, Department of Anatomy and Embryology
Peking University Health Science Center
Beijing, China

Czech Republic
J Stingl, PhD
3rd Faculty of Medicine, Department of Anatomy
Charles University
Prague, Czech Republic

France
Fabrice DuParc, MD, PhD
Professor of Anatomy
Department of Medicine and Pharmacy
University of Rouen
Rouen, France

Germany
Reinhard Putz, MD
Professor, Institute of Anatomy
Ludwig-Maximilians-University Munich
Munich, Germany

India
SD Joshi, MBBS, MS
Dean, SAIMS Medical College
Indore, India

Iran
Mohammadali M. Shoja, MD
Medical Philosophy and History Research Center
Tabriz University of Medical Sciences
Tabriz, Iran

Italy
Raffaele De Caro, MD
Full Professor, Director of Institute of Human
Anatomy
University of Padova
Padova, Italy

Japan
Tatsuo Sato, MD, PhD
President
Tokyo Ariake University of Medicine and Health
Sciences
Tokyo, Japan

New Zealand
Helen Nicholson, BSc (Hons), MBChB, MD (Bristol)
Professor and Dean
Otago School of Medical Sciences
University of Otago
Otago, New Zealand

Mark Stringer, BSc (Hons), MBBS, MS (Lond), MRCP
(UK)
Professor, Department of Anatomy
Otago School of Medical Sciences
University of Otago
Otago, New Zealand

Poland
Jerzy Gielecki, MD, PhD
Dean for English Division
University of Varmia and Masuria
Olsztyn, Poland

Anna Zurada, MD, PhD
Medical Faculty
Department of Anatomy
University of Varmia and Masuria
Olsztyn, Poland

Saudi Arabia
Abdullah M. Aldahmash
Chairman of Anatomy and Director of Stem
Cell Unit
College of Medicine
King Saud University
Riyadh, Saudi Arabia

South Africa
Dr. Albert van Schoor, PhD
Senior Lecturer, Department of Anatomy
University of Pretoria
Johannesburg, South Africa

Turkey
Nihal Apaydin, MD
Associate Professor, Department of Anatomy
Ankara University
Ankara, Turkey

United Kingdom
Bernard Moxham, BDS, PhD, FHEA, FSB
Professor of Anatomy and Head of Teaching in
Biosciences
President of the International Federation of
Associations of Anatomists (IFAA)
Cardiff School of Biosciences
Cardiff, UK

Jonathan Spratt, MA(Cantab), FRCS (Eng), FRCS
(Glasg), FRCR
Consultant Clinical Radiologist
University of North Durham
Durham, UK

United States of America
Anthony V. D'Antoni, DC, PhD
Associate Professor and Director of Anatomy
Division of Pre-clinical Sciences
New York College of Podiatric Medicine
New York, NY, USA

Camille DiLullo, PhD
Professor, Department of Anatomy
Philadelphia College of Osteopathic Medicine
Philadelphia, Pennsylvania, USA

Anthony Olinger, PhD
Assistant Professor
Department of Anatomy
Kansas City University of Medicine and Biosciences
Kansas City, Missouri, USA

David J Porta, PhD
Professor, Department of Biology
Bellarmine University
Louisville, Kentucky, USA

Kyle E. Rarey, PhD
Professor, Departments of Anatomy & Cell Biology
and Otolaryngology
University of Florida College of Medicine
Gainesville, Florida, USA

George Salter, Jr., PhD
Professor Emeritus of Anatomy
University of Alabama at Birmingham
Birmingham, Alabama, USA

Carol EH Scott-Conner, MD, PhD
Professor, Division of Surgical Oncology and
Endocrine Surgery
Department of Surgery
University of Iowa Carver College of Medicine
Iowa City, Iowa, USA

Joel Vilensky, PhD
Professor, Department of Anatomy and Cell Biology
School of Medicine
Indiana University
Fort Wayne, Indiana, USA

CONTENTS

NOTE: This dissection guide is cross-referenced to the following atlases: Netter, Atlas of Human Anatomy, 5e (***Netter***); McMinn's Clinical Atlas of Human Anatomy, 6e (***McMinn***); and Gray's Atlas of Anatomy (***Gray's Atlas***). Page references from each atlas are provided at the beginning of Chapters 2 through 29 to give you the opportunity to study the relevant anatomy in depth to aid in your dissection.

DISSECTION LABORATORY MATERIALS, TOOLS, AND TECHNIQUES

Using the appropriate dissection laboratory materials and tools is essential in making the dissection of a cadaver as rewarding as possible. Many experienced dissectors have their favorite tool. The following list of materials and dissection tools allows dissectors to care for their cadaveric donor while acquiring the experience and knowledge of a successful dissection. Although not comprehensive, this list provides the appropriate tools to dissect a cadaveric donor in the anatomy teaching laboratory.

MATERIALS AND TOOLS

Cadaver Materials

BLOCKS. Plastic or wooden blocks of different shapes and sizes (6-18 inches) can be used to position the cadaver (Fig. 1-1).

STANDS. Removable stands that either bridge or attach to dissection tables are useful for holding dissection guides, texts, and atlases for dissection.

PLASTIC SHEETS. Plastic sheets can be used to cover the cadaver, which comes with a shroud and a cotton sheet. This helps maintain moisture within the cadaver, to prevent drying and to allow dissection of appropriately hydrated tissue.

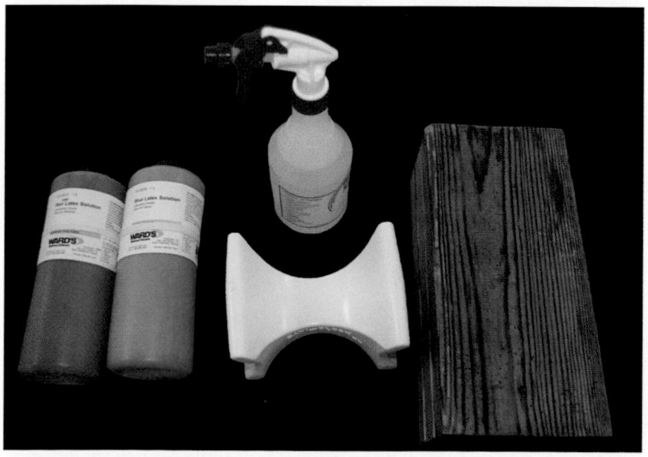

COTTON SHEETS. Surgical green or blue sheets covering a plastic sheet help preserve the cadaver and create a professional working environment.

SPRAY BOTTLE. An individual plastic spray bottle (1 quart) at each cadaver station allows dissectors to maintain good-quality tissue (Fig. 1-1). An alternative is a 2- to 3-gallon pressure spray unit shared among the dissection laboratory stations.

HOLDING CONTAINER. The plastic, 5- to 10-gallon container with a spigot stores cadaver hydration solution.

CADAVER HYDRATING SOLUTION. Several types of mixtures are available to hydrate and maintain cadaver tissue. The authors use a solution with 3000 mL of propylene glycol, 500 mL of ethyl alcohol, and 300 mL of fabric softener, in a 10-gallon holding unit, with the remainder filled with water.

CADAVER BAG. The bag helps to maintain hydration and care of the cadaver (Fig. 1-2).

FIGURE 1-1. Red and blue latex wrap (to keep cadaver moist); spray bottle; plastic and wooden blocks.

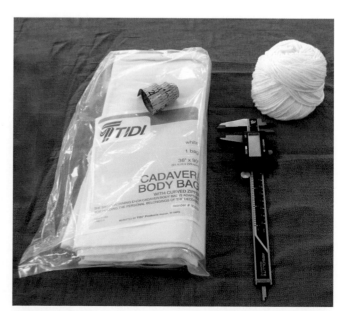

FIGURE 1-2. Cadaver bag and cloth measuring tape; ball of string and digital calipers.

Dissector Materials

DISPOSABLE SHOE COVERS. Shoe covers protect shoes worn in the laboratory during dissection and can be disposed of on exiting, ensuring cleanliness inside and outside the laboratory (Fig. 1-3). Closed-toed shoes should be worn in the dissecting laboratory.

GLOVES. Gloves vary in the type of synthetic material used; both powdered gloves and powder-free gloves are available (Fig. 1-4). Offer both types to protect dissectors with different skin sensitivities. *Double gloving* helps to prevent contact with cadaver embalming fluids to which the dermis might be sensitive.

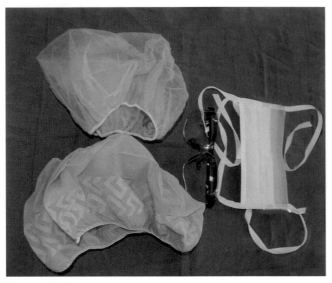

FIGURE 1-3. Disposable hair and shoe covers; mask with eye shield; goggles.

SCRUBS. Comfortable clothing can also be worn with scrubs, ideally under a lab coat.

GOGGLES. Protective safety goggles or glasses should be worn at all times during dissection (see Fig. 1-3).

FACE SHIELDS. Shields can be worn when using bone saws or when excessive fluids are present (see Fig. 1-3).

Dissection Tools

SKIN MARKER PEN. Marking pens can be helpful tools for tracing out the incision before dissection. Markers can also be used to highlight surface anatomy (Fig. 1-5).

SCALPEL HANDLES AND BLADES. Metal scalpel blades are relatively standardized. Many different blade shapes are available; however, dissectors should experiment to determine which best suits them and the targets to be dissected. The authors prefer larger blades for their students. Scalpels are primarily used to make skin incisions but can also be used to reflect the dermis and areas with dense connective tissue.

DISPOSABLE SCALPELS. Disposable scalpels have an advantage because the blade is already secured to the handle. Have a disposable sharps bin in the laboratory (see Fig. 1-5).

SHARPS BIN OR CONTAINER. For safety compliance, all dissection laboratories should have a sharps bin to dispose of scalpel blades, disposable scalpels, pins, and needles.

SCISSORS. Both 5-inch and 7-inch straight and curved scissors may be used. It is important that the scissors used for each dissection are appropriate in size

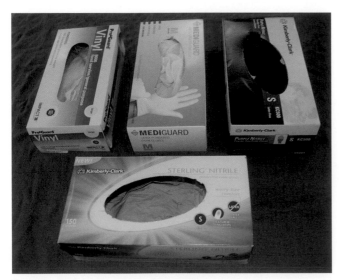

FIGURE 1-4. Laboratory gloves differentiated by powder and powder free, latex and latex free.

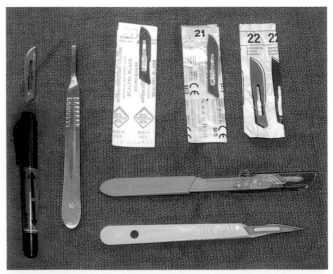

FIGURE 1-5. Various scalpel blades and handles (metal and disposable scalpels). An example of a skin marker that can be used for outlining skin incisions is shown.

(Fig. 1-6). Generally, head and neck dissection can be conducted with a 5-inch scissor. The remainder of the body can be dissected with 7-inch scissors. The classic dissection technique is a *reverse dissection*. Straight and curved scissors tend to be user specific.

HEMOSTAT CLAMPS. Both corrugated and smooth, 5-inch and 7-inch hemostat clamps are available (Fig. 1-7). The corrugated type can be used to clamp onto the edge of skin incisions to aid in flap removal. Smooth clamps can be used to hold onto delicate structures during dissection. Hemostat clamps can be used when retracting tissue over relatively long dissection periods.

NEEDLE HOLDERS. The needle holder allows the user to secure and remove scalpel blades (see Fig. 1-7).

FORCEPS. Toothed and nontoothed forceps are 5 inches and greater than 5 inches long. Toothed forceps enable the dissector to grip tissue without it sliding out of the hands. Nontoothed forceps allow the dissector to control delicate tissues during meticulous dissection (see Fig. 1-7).

SPATULA PROBE/POINTER. Instruments that have a probe or tip on one end and spatula on the other can be used to highlight dissected structures. The spatula can aid blunt dissection (see Fig. 1-7).

T-PINS. T-pins (1½-2 inches) are useful in securing structures away from the desired dissection region. T-pins can also be used when setting up laboratory examinations (see Fig. 1-7).

CHISEL (OSTEOTOME). Narrow-blade and broad-blade chisels are important for performing osteotomies and can help dissect between the occipital condyles and various vertebrae (Fig. 1-8). Chisels can be used to break up a bone surface to view the soft tissue deep to it (e.g., anterior cranial fossa).

RUBBER MALLET. A mallet is used when striking the chisel to crack surface areas such as when performing osteotomies (see Fig. 1-8).

ELECTRIC STRYKER SAW. Used when cutting bone, the Stryker saw has a safety mechanism that prevents the blade from cutting the user's skin and soft tissue.

HANDSAW. A simple bone saw can be used to customize various dissections and amputations for plastination (see Fig. 1-8). A handsaw is important for hemipelvectomy dissections.

CLOTH MEASURING TAPE. A cloth tape can be invaluable when measuring distances from landmarks of surface anatomy (see Fig. 1-2).

FIRST-AID KIT. In a dissection laboratory, nicks and pricks are inevitable, so an up-to-date first-aid kit is essential. It should contain adhesive strips (e.g., Band-Aids), cleansing solutions (e.g., hydrogen peroxide), gauze rolls/pads, and eyewash solution.

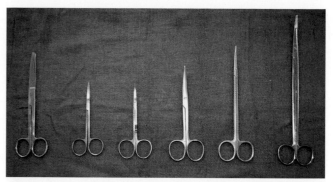

FIGURE 1-6. Various scissors differentiated by length and blade type (straight or curved, pointed or blunted): 6-inch Deaver, straight fine scissor, curved fine scissor, 5-inch Mayo, 7-inch Metzenbaum, 9-inch Metzenbaum.

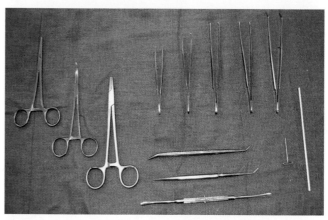

FIGURE 1-7. *Left,* Hemostat or artery clamps (straight and curved). *Upper,* Needle holder; various forceps differentiated by length, toothed and nontoothed. *Lower,* Probes and dissectors. *Right,* T-pin and orange stick.

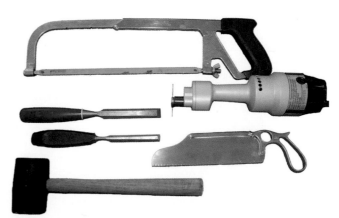

FIGURE 1-8. Handsaws (long and short) for bone; electric Stryker bone saw; chisel (broad and narrow blades); rubber mallet.

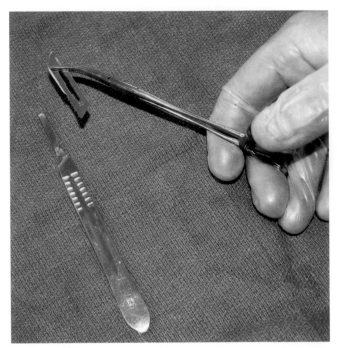

FIGURE 1-9. Placing or replacing scalpel blades onto a scalpel handle. Use hemostat or needle holder to grip the scalpel blade. Line up the base angle of the blade with the tip-of-handle angle.

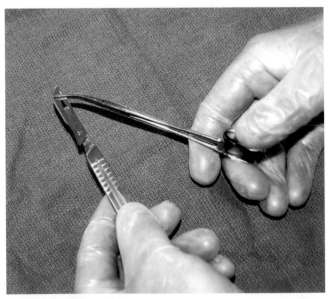

FIGURE 1-10. Placing the blade onto the scalpel handle tip. Generally, a clicking sound confirms the blade is secured correctly.

DISSECTION TECHNIQUES

Using the proper technique during dissection is important when developing good dissection skills. Initially, holding the instruments correctly and practicing the techniques may not feel natural. The authors believe that cadaver dissection techniques should reflect the techniques used during surgical procedures. Learning to hold forceps and scissors is fundamental during dissection. These techniques can also be used in the operating room and certain office settings during interventional procedures.

Scalpel

The technique for placing a blade onto a scalpel handle requires a hemostat to hold the blade and then place it onto the handle while holding the forceps (Figs. 1-9 and 1-10). When cutting with the blade, use the tip and the first centimeter of the blade. Direct the scalpel using smooth, sweeping motions (Fig. 1-11). Avoid "sawing" and "woodpecker" techniques. Dull blades that require "pushing" the scalpel are dangerous; therefore, maintain a sharp blade at all times.

Forceps

Hold the forceps as you would hold a pencil, with a pincer grip. The classic mistake is holding the forceps in the palm of the hand as if grasping. The forceps is held vertically and perpendicularly to the target tissue to allow a 360-degree window of use (Fig. 1-12).

Scissors

The appropriate technique when dissecting with scissors is called *reverse dissection* (Fig. 1-13). This requires the user to keep the scissor blades closed when entering into the tissue to be dissected, then opening the blades to create a splaying of the tissue. This results in natural separation of tissue structures and planes. Cut only tissue that is fully exposed, so that the desired tissue can be preserved.

Buttonhole Maneuver

A buttonhole maneuver is helpful when dissecting a flap of dermis. Create a 2-cm parallel incision along the original skin incision, 2 to 3 cm (~1 inch) from the edge. Repeat this, generally near the corners of the skin flap. Place your index finger into the parallel incision, and retract the skin flap with appropriate tension that would allow either blunt dissection or a sharp edge to cut the apex of the flap (Figs. 1-14 and 1-15).

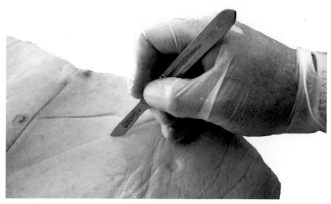

FIGURE 1-11. Using the scalpel tip to create skin incisions. Note the grip of the scalpel provides side-to-side and back-to-front blade stability.

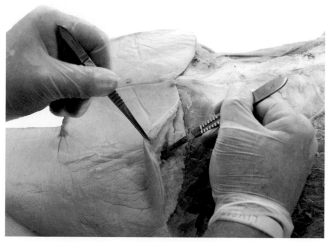

FIGURE 1-12. Holding toothed forceps with a 360-degree view, and using the scalpel tip between tissue layers while maintaining tension of superficial tissue layer.

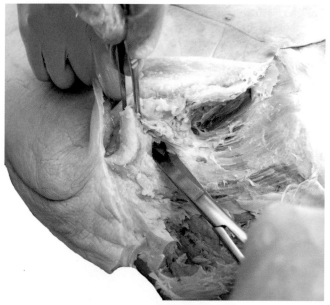

FIGURE 1-13. Blunt dissection introduces the scissor tips into the tissue, and then reverse-dissection opens the tissue planes.

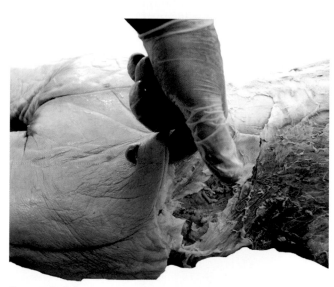

FIGURE 1-14. The buttonhole maneuver is helpful when dissecting large skin flaps and provides appropriate tension to expedite dissection. Place your fingertip(s) into the parallel incision and retract with appropriate tension.

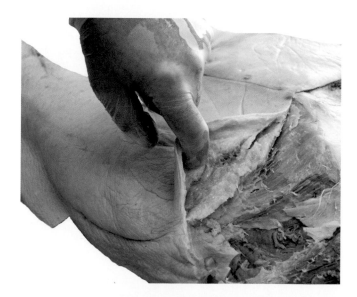

FIGURE 1-15. The buttonhole maneuver for retraction of the skin allows adequate visualization of the underlying tissue for further dissection.

Surface Fracturing Technique

The surface fracturing technique requires placing the broad blade of a chisel parallel to the bone and with as much of the blade along the bone. Strike the chisel head with a mallet using a technique that does *not* follow through once the head is struck. The objective is to direct the energy through the blade onto the bony surface, causing multiple fractured segments while protecting the soft tissue beneath the bone (e.g., fracturing anterior cranial fossa plate before superior orbit dissection) (Fig. 1-16).

Direct Fracturing Technique

The direct fracturing technique can be performed using a narrow-bladed chisel or by tilting a broad-bladed chisel so that a direct point touches the bone to be fractured. Strike the chisel head with the mallet as if driving a nail. This technique will fracture through a specific part of outer layer of bone (Fig. 1-17).

Prying Technique

The prying technique requires placing the blade of a chisel into the gap created by a handsaw or electric saw. Once in the gap, rotate the chisel blade using a circular motion of the wrist while gripping the chisel to pry the two bony edges apart. Prying is especially useful when performing a craniotomy (see Chapter 23).

Stryker Saw

The technique for using the electric bone saw is performed by placing the blade directly perpendicular to the bone. Place enough pressure onto the bony surface until the blade has gone through the thickness of the bone. Once through the bone, remove the blade, and assess whether the prying technique is required.

Stryker Saw Scoring

The scoring technique requires using a Stryker electric saw blade to score the surface of the bone region to be removed. Often an "x" pattern of scoring can weaken the bony cortex. Once the scoring is completed, use the surface fracturing technique. This will allow fracture of the cortex and removal of bony fragments without damaging soft tissue beneath the cortex (e.g., removing outer cortex of mandibular ramus; see Chapter 22).

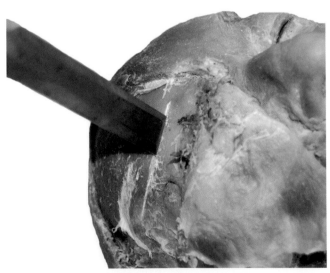

FIGURE 1-16. Place chisel blade flat and parallel on the desired bone surface. The surface fracturing technique generally results in multiple fragments protecting the deep tissue.

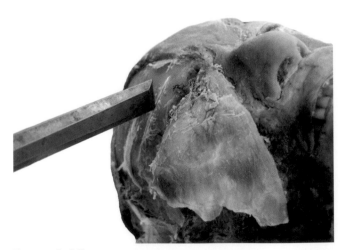

FIGURE 1-17. Place chisel blade at an angle on the desired bone surface. The direct fracturing technique will create a specific fracture at the point of the chisel blade.

SPECIALIZED MATERIALS TO HIGHLIGHT STRUCTURES

LATEX SOLUTIONS. Use latex solutions as an injection to highlight vessels, especially small vessels that may not be easily dissectible.

NEEDLE AND SYRINGE. Multiple syringe sizes and needle sizes are used to inject latex or dye into spaces (Fig. 1-18). Injection of the globe (eyeball) with water may also be useful to obtain lifelike qualities.

SUTURE MATERIAL. Multiple sizes of suture material to reattach dissected structures can be useful when demonstrating superficial and deep structures after dissection (Fig. 1-18).

RETRACTORS. Types include (1) single-handled manual retractor for dynamic traction and (2) self-retractor or spreader, used to retract two sides simultaneously, allowing the dissector to practice surgical procedures without needing others to retract structures manually (Fig. 1-18).

FOOD COLORING. Mix with a solution to inject into the body, to fill up potential spaces and to highlight others.

ELECTRONIC DIGITAL CALIPERS. Use to measure specific length, size, and shape of anatomic structures (see Fig. 1-2).

PLASTINATION. The plastination technique preserves dissected regions or structures to be used as *prosected material,* with a life span of 6 months to 20 years, depending on technique, body part, and frequency of use.

RONGEUR AND RIB CUTTERS. These can be used to cut through small to medium-sized bones and to customize cut ends of all bone sizes (Fig. 1-19).

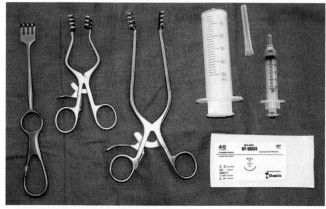

FIGURE 1-18. *Left to right,* Static retractor (Volkmann); dynamic self-retaining retractors (Weitlaner); syringes (50 mL and 5 mL); suture material.

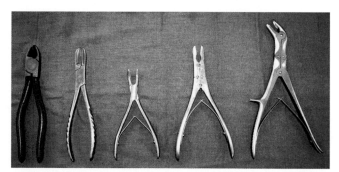

FIGURE 1-19. *Left to right,* Metal wire cutters (2), bone cutter (Liston), 5-inch bone-cutter forceps, 7-inch bone-cutter rongeur (Stille).

MUSCLES OF THE BACK AND SCAPULA

Netter: 149–154, 168–171, 248, 411, 413–415

McMinn: 94–98, 110–115, 117–121, 138–141, 148

Gray's Atlas: 20–32, 36–42, 364–367

Note: This dissection guide is cross-referenced to the following atlases: Netter, Atlas of Human Anatomy, 5e (*Netter*); McMinn's Clinical Atlas of Human Anatomy, 6e (*McMinn*); and Gray's Atlas of Anatomy (*Gray's Atlas*). Page references from each atlas are provided at the beginning of Chapter 2 through 29 to give you the opportunity to study the relevant anatomy in depth to aid in your dissection.

BEFORE YOU BEGIN

Make sure that you have palpated the following anatomic landmarks on yourself and classmates:

- Superior nuchal line
- External occipital protuberance
- Mastoid process
- Spine of the 7th cervical vertebra (C7, vertebra prominens)
- Spines of the thoracic and lumbar vertebrae, the sacrum, and the coccyx

- Medial and lateral parts of the clavicles
- Iliac crests
- Trapezius muscle
- Latissimus dorsi muscle
- Deltoid muscle
- Triceps brachii muscle

Before each dissection, palpate the region for bony landmarks.

With a marker, draw the following lines on the skin of the cadaver (Figs. 2-1 and 2-2):

1. From the external occipital protuberance, down the midline of the back to the sacrum.
2. Laterally, from the external occipital protuberance to the mastoid process on each side of the cadaver.
3. Laterally, from the spine of the vertebra prominens to the acromion process of each shoulder.
4. Superiorly from the sacrum, curving obliquely over the iliac crests to the midaxillary line on each side of the body; that is, to a point about halfway around the upper edge of each iliac crest.

Incise the skin along the lines just described, and reflect it laterally.

Start the reflection of the skin from the point where the incisions for the midline and from the shoulders meet. Retract the skin carefully (with toothed forceps), leaving the fat (superficial fascia) intact (Figs. 2-3 and 2-4).

> **DISSECTION TIP:** Place absorptive cloths at the inferolateral spaces of the iliac crest. Excessive amounts of embalming fluid often accumulate at this location.

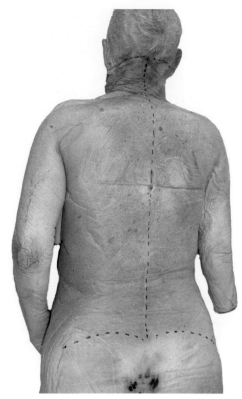

FIGURE 2-1. Skin markings for incision lines: neck and back.

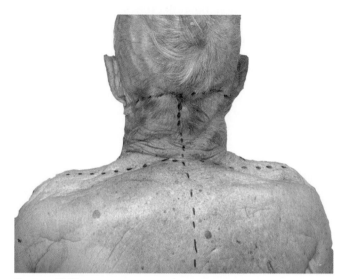

FIGURE 2-2. Skin dissection incision lines: neck and shoulders.

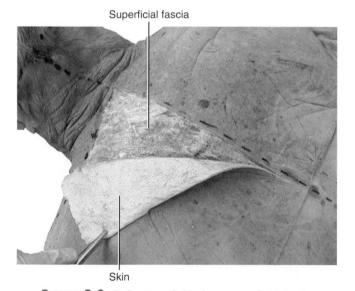

Superficial fascia

Skin

FIGURE 2-3. Reflection of skin from superficial fascia.

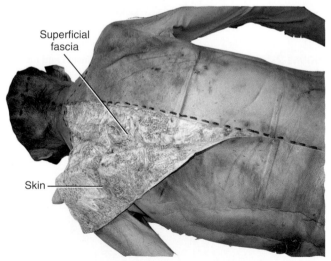

Superficial fascia

Skin

FIGURE 2-4. Further reflection of skin of back.

Start the separation of the superficial fascia from the underlying deep fascia in the midline, by identifying a small part of the trapezius muscle. Carefully scrape off the superficial fascia from the top of the muscle with your scalpel (Fig. 2-5).

On one side of the body, the dissectors should first reflect only the skin, leaving the superficial fascia (tela subcutanea) in place. The superficial fascia of that side will then be reflected separately. On the other side of the body, the skin and superficial fascia can be reflected together (Fig. 2-6). Care must be taken in this latter approach to avoid damage to the underlying muscles, especially the trapezius and latissimus dorsi muscles and their aponeuroses. Identify these before the skin and fascia are reflected more than a few centimeters.

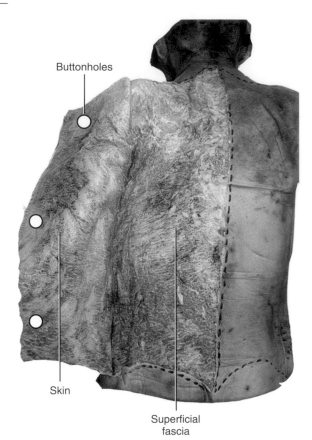

FIGURE 2-7. Complete reflection of skin from superficial fascia.

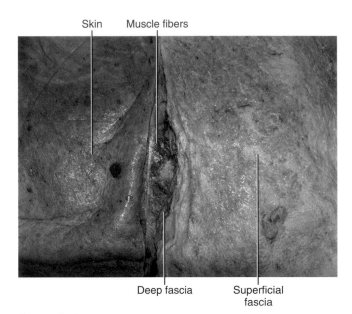

FIGURE 2-5. Deep skin incisions showing deep fascia and muscle fibers.

✎ *DISSECTION TIP:* Make necessary "buttonholes" in the skin to facilitate the dissection (Fig. 2-7), as indicated in Chapter 1.

Take precautions to avoid cutting too deeply with the scalpel. In some cadavers, the superficial fascia is quite thin, and more deeply situated structures can be easily cut and destroyed (Figs. 2-8 and 2-10).

☞ *DISSECTION TIP:* As the superficial fascia is reflected, watch for the passage of neurovascular bundles from the deep fascia into the deep surface of the superficial fascia (see Figs. 2-22 and 2-23). Save short segments of several of these for later demonstration and review.

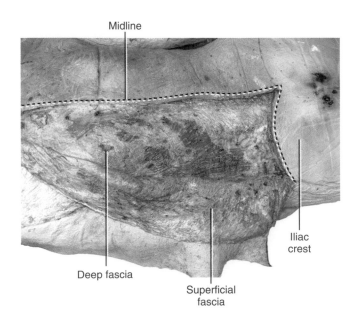

FIGURE 2-6. Reflection of skin and superficial fascia.

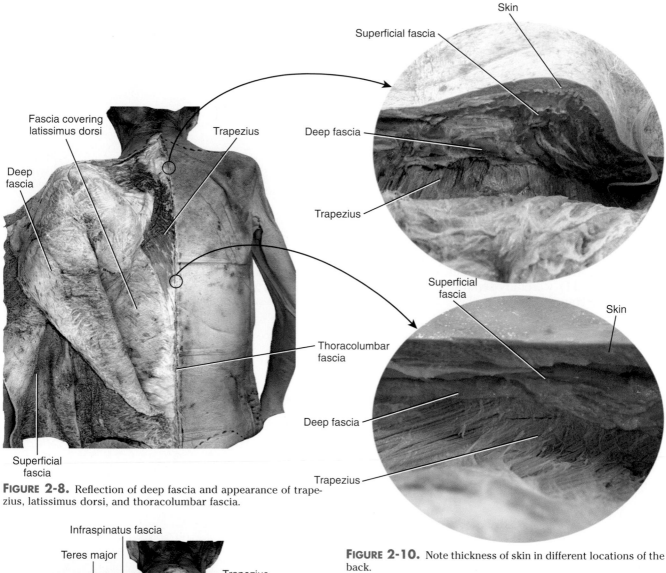

FIGURE 2-8. Reflection of deep fascia and appearance of trapezius, latissimus dorsi, and thoracolumbar fascia.

FIGURE 2-10. Note thickness of skin in different locations of the back.

Remove enough deep fascia to clarify the borders of the two most superficial extrinsic muscles of the back, the trapezius and latissimus dorsi (Fig. 2-9).

> ☝ *DISSECTION TIP:* Note the diamond-shaped aponeurotic area of the trapezius, at the upper middle thoracic region. The skin, superficial fascia, and deep fascia are relatively thin here. This is in contrast to the lateral lumbar region, where the subcutaneous fat is usually increased (Figs. 2-8 and 2-10).

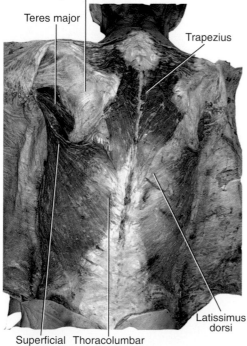

FIGURE 2-9. Complete reflection of deep fascia and identification of superficial structures of back.

The infraspinatus fascia covers the infraspinatus muscle and is attached to the margins of the infraspinous fossa. The fascia is continuous with the deltoid fascia along the posterior border of the deltoid muscle (Fig. 2-11). Carefully separate the deep fascia covering the trapezius muscle (Figs. 2-12 and 2-13).

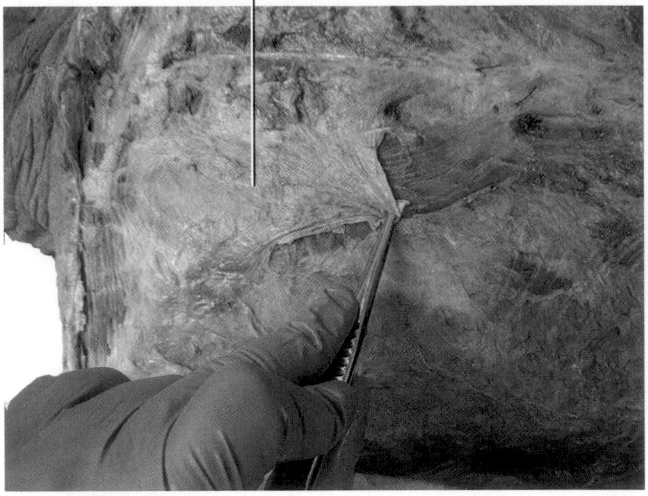

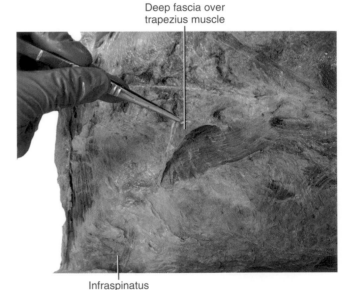

FIGURE 2-12. Careful separation of deep fascia covering superficial muscles of back.

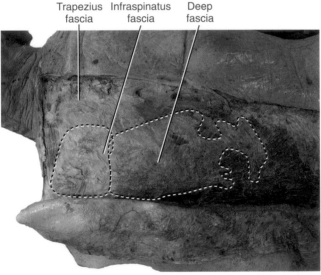

FIGURE 2-11. Complete reflection of skin and superficial fascia from this area. Observe deep fascia over trapezius muscle and infraspinatus fascia over infraspinatus muscle *(dotted lines).*

FIGURE 2-13. Careful separation of deep fascia covering trapezius muscle.

Completely remove superficial fascia and expose the muscles of the back (Figs. 2-14 and 2-15).

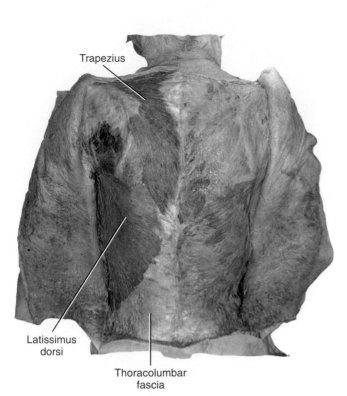

FIGURE 2-14. Complete removal of superficial fascia over trapezius, latissimus dorsi, and posterior layer of thoracolumbar fascia on left side of cadaver. Deep fascia and some adipose tissue have been left intact on right side.

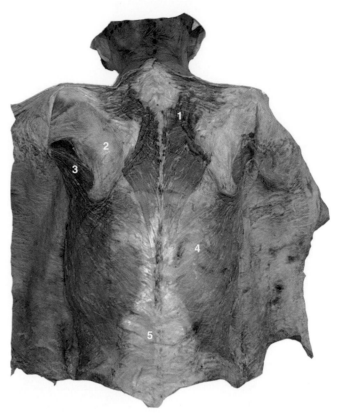

FIGURE 2-15. Complete exposure of superficial muscles of the back: *1,* trapezius; *2,* infraspinatus fascia; *3,* teres major; *4,* latissimus dorsi; *5,* thoracolumbar fascia.

To detach the trapezius from its origin, first make a small vertical cut through the lower part of the trapezius at the 12th thoracic vertebra (T12) level as it attaches to the midline. Continue the incision to the external occipital protuberance (Figs. 2-16 to 2-18). Define and loosen the trapezius with your fingers or with scissors before you proceed further upward along the midline.

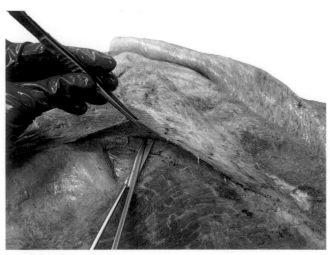

FIGURE 2-17. Dissection of lateral trapezius muscle facilitated by a separation technique using dissecting scissors.

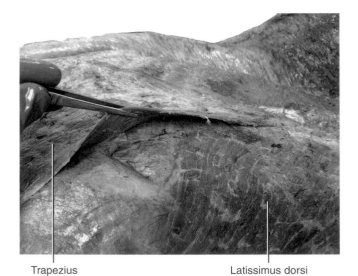

Trapezius   Latissimus dorsi

FIGURE 2-16. Dissection of left lateral trapezius muscle.

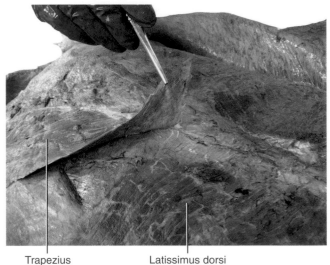

Trapezius   Latissimus dorsi

FIGURE 2-18. Beginning of reflection of trapezius muscle, cutting it along its origin from the midline.

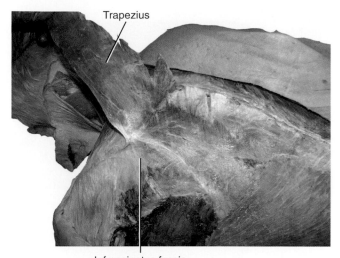

FIGURE 2-19. Separation of connective tissue on the deep surface of trapezius.

Detach the trapezius from its origin on the superior nuchal line and the external occipital protuberance, and sever the fibers that arise from the spines and associated ligaments of the cervical and thoracic vertebrae. Reflect the trapezius laterally toward its insertion onto the scapula (Figs. 2-19 to 2-21). On the deep surface of the trapezius, near the superior angle of the scapula, look for the nerve that supplies the trapezius, the spinal accessory nerve. Also note the artery that supplies it, the ascending branch of the transverse cervical artery.

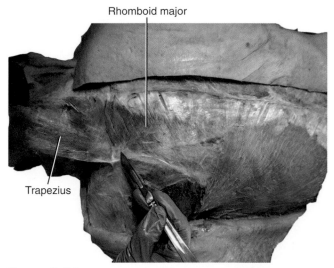

FIGURE 2-20. Separation of the connective tissue on the deep surface of trapezius.

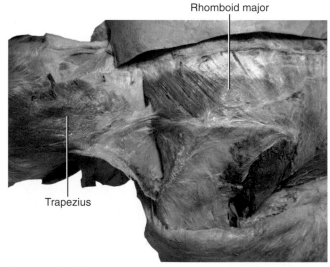

FIGURE 2-21. Separation of connective tissue on the deep surface of trapezius.

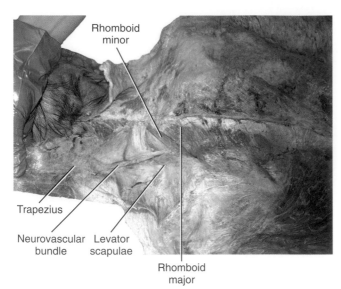

FIGURE 2-22. Complete reflection of trapezius and appearance of the underlying levator scapulae and rhomboid muscles.

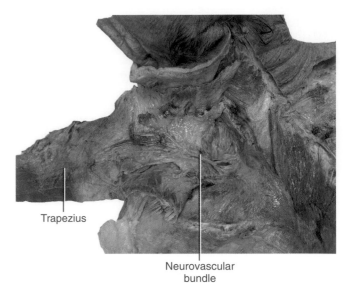

FIGURE 2-23. Careful dissection is essential to identify the spinal accessory nerve.

Identify the levator scapulae, rhomboid minor and major muscles, and neurovascular bundle (Figs. 2-22 and 2-23). Clean the fascia from these muscles so that their fibers can be seen clearly.

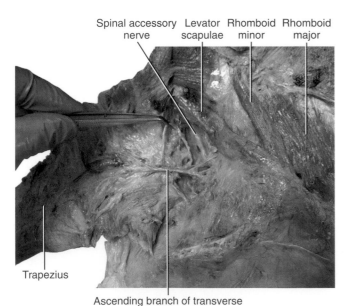

FIGURE 2-24. Identification of spinal accessory nerve, emerging deep from medial side at midpoint of levator scapulae muscle.

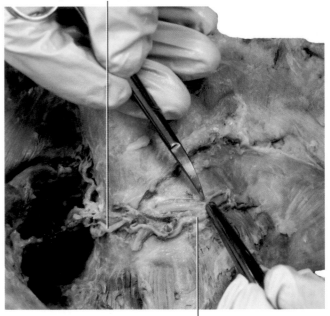

FIGURE 2-25. Careful separation of neurovascular bundle to identify spinal accessory nerve, ascending branch of transverse cervical artery, and tributaries of transverse cervical vein.

🖊 *DISSECTION TIP:* Identify the levator scapulae muscle and gently retract it medially. At the midpoint of the levator, you will see the spinal accessory nerve exit and run on the internal surface of the trapezius muscle (Figs. 2-24 to 2-27).

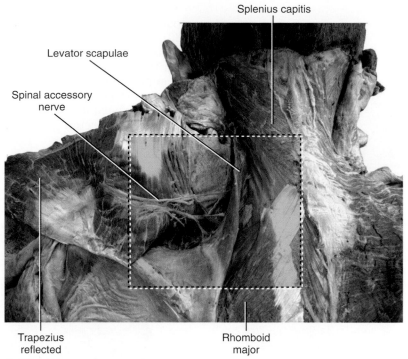

FIGURE 2-26. After careful dissection of connective tissue, trapezius muscle is reflected and the spinal accessory nerve identified.

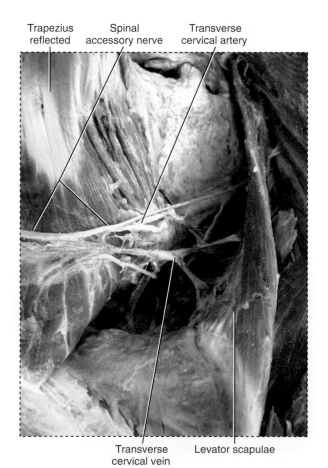

FIGURE 2-27. Trapezius muscle is reflected and the spinal accessory nerve identified.

While cleaning away the fascia that overlies the most cephalic portion of the trapezius (Figs. 2-28 to 2-30), look for the greater occipital nerve. This nerve can usually be found approximately 1 inch (2.5 cm) from the midline of the neck and 1 inch inferior to the superior nuchal line, as the nerve pierces the trapezius (Figs. 2-31 to 2-33). Also at this location, locate the occipital artery, and preserve it as the trapezius is reflected.

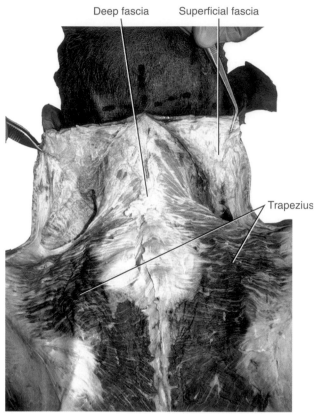

Deep fascia   Superficial fascia

Trapezius

FIGURE 2-28. Exposure of superior part of trapezius with portions of deep fascia still covering uppermost portion.

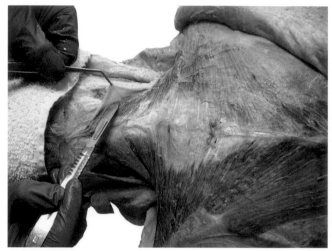

FIGURE 2-29. Exposure of superior part of trapezius deep fascia covering its upper portion.

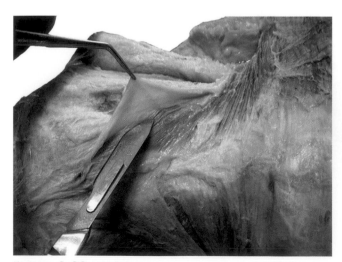

FIGURE 2-30. Careful exposure of superior part of trapezius muscle by reflecting deep fascia.

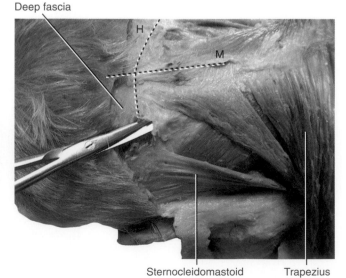

Deep fascia

H

M

Sternocleidomastoid   Trapezius

FIGURE 2-31. After identifying the greater occipital nerve, separate and remove the deep fascia; *M,* midline; *H,* horizontal line.

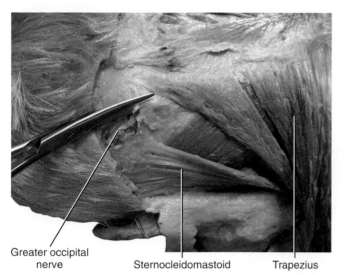

FIGURE 2-32. Carefully cut the deep fascia to trace the greater occipital nerve deeply toward the suboccipital triangle.

Greater occipital nerve

Sternocleidomastoid   Trapezius

Greater occipital nerve

FIGURE 2-33. Deep fascia is cut, and the greater occipital nerve and occipital artery are visible.

Occipital artery   Trapezius

🖐 *DISSECTION TIP:* Usually the deep fascia over the trapezius muscle below the superior nuchal line is very thick and difficult to cut until the 7th cervical vertebra (C7) level. Pay special attention to the dissection process. Intermingled with the deep fascia over this area is the 3rd occipital nerve; try to expose and save it (Fig. 2-34).

Reflection of the trapezius and latissimus dorsi muscles exposes underlying intermediate extrinsic muscles of the back (Fig. 2-35).

🖐 *DISSECTION TIP:* To identify the greater occipital nerve, draw a horizontal imaginary line from the external occipital protuberance to the mastoid process. At 3 cm lateral to the occipital protuberance on the imaginary line, remove the deep fascia to identify this nerve (Figs. 2-31 to 2-33).

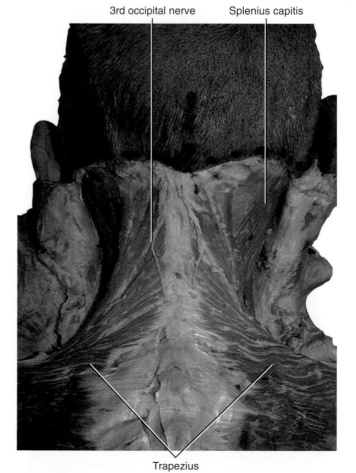

3rd occipital nerve   Splenius capitis

Trapezius

FIGURE 2-34. Complete exposure and detachment of the superior part of the trapezius from the deep fascia. Observe the 3rd occipital nerve and the splenius capitis muscle.

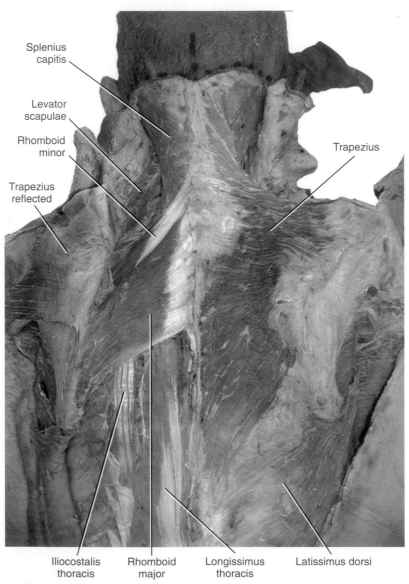

Splenius
capitis

Levator
scapulae

Rhomboid
minor

Trapezius
reflected

Trapezius

Iliocostalis
thoracis

Rhomboid
major

Longissimus
thoracis

Latissimus dorsi

FIGURE 2-35. Trapezius and latissimus dorsi muscles are reflected. Underlying intermediate extrinsic muscles of the back are exposed.

DISSECTION TIP: In about 50% of the specimens, the dorsal scapular artery is absent and the deep branch of the transverse cervical artery replaces it. The dorsal scapular artery typically arises from the 3rd part of the subclavian artery and runs posteriorly through the brachial plexus.

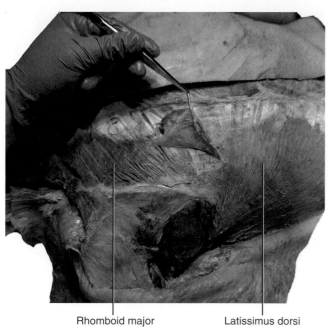

Rhomboid major　　　　Latissimus dorsi

FIGURE 2-36. Carefully expose deep fascia over the rhomboid major and minor muscles.

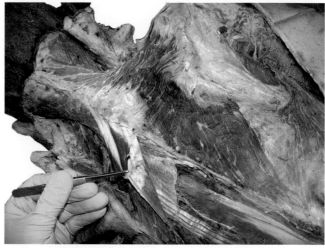

FIGURE 2-37. After the trapezius is exposed, reflect the rhomboid major and minor muscles carefully to expose the serratus posterior superior.

In some specimens the line of cleavage between the rhomboid muscles may be unclear (Figs. 2-36 and 2-37). Cut the rhomboid major and minor muscles at their origins from the midline of the lower cervical and upper thoracic vertebrae.

Turn the rhomboid muscles toward their insertion onto the medial border of the scapula. Deep to the rhomboids, identify the serratus posterior superior muscle, which inserts onto the ribs rather than onto the scapula. This fact will assist you in its identification. Sever the fibers of origin of the serratus posterior inferior muscle, and reflect it toward its insertion (Fig. 2-37).

Transect the rhomboid muscles at their vertebral origin. On their deep surface, try to identify the dorsal scapular nerve and dorsal scapular artery (Fig. 2-38). The dorsal scapular nerve innervates the rhomboid and levator scapulae muscles (in addition to branches from C3 and C4). The dorsal scapular nerve arises from C5, one of the two nerves that arise directly from the roots of the brachial plexus.

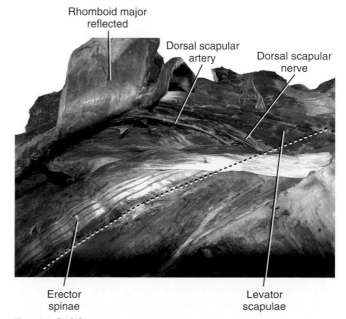

Rhomboid major
reflected

Dorsal scapular
artery

Dorsal scapular
nerve

Erector
spinae

Levator
scapulae

FIGURE 2-38. View of deep surface of scapula illustrating dorsal scapular artery and nerve running at medial border of scapula.

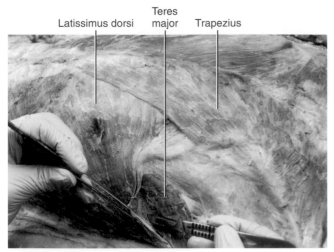

FIGURE 2-39. Careful separation of teres major from upper border of latissimus dorsi muscle.

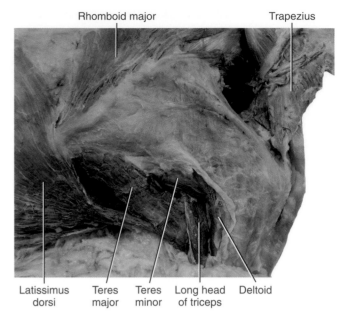

FIGURE 2-41. Infraspinatous fascia is removed over long head of triceps brachii and a portion of teres minor and deltoid muscles.

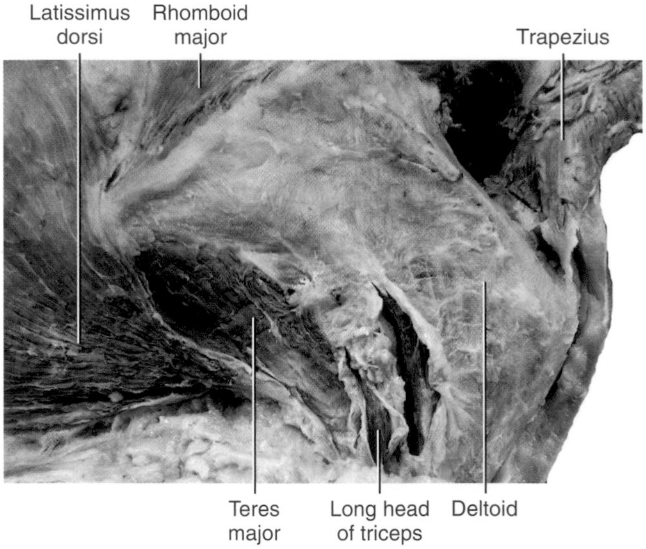

Identify and clean the teres major muscle. Then, beginning superiorly, reflect the infraspinatus fascia to expose the long head of triceps and deltoid muscles (Figs. 2-42 and 2-43).

FIGURE 2-40. View of deltoscapular region. Long head of triceps brachii and deltoid muscles are exposed after careful separation from infraspinatus fascia.

> ☝ *DISSECTION TIP:* The fibers of the teres minor muscle run more or less parallel to the fibers of the teres major and are medial to the long head of the triceps brachii and deltoid muscles.

Using toothed forceps, scalpel, and scissors, reflect the posterior border of the deltoid laterally, dividing its attachment onto the spine and acromion process (Fig. 2-39). Continue reflecting the muscle laterally and posteriorly until the surgical neck of the humerus is visible, but leave the deltoid muscle attached to the deltoid tuberosity, the insertion of the muscle (Fig. 2-40). The infraspinatus fascia is attached to the scapula around the boundaries of the attachments of the infraspinatus, teres minor and major, long head of triceps brachii, and deltoid muscles (Fig. 2-41).

Detach the deltoid muscle from its scapular attachments using a scalpel, and reflect it laterally (Fig. 2-44). Identify the axillary nerve as it appears posterior to the surgical neck of the humerus (Fig. 2-45). The nerve is accompanied by the posterior circumflex humeral artery, a branch of the third portion of the axillary artery. The axillary nerve and posterior circumflex humeral artery appear in the field by emerging through the quadrangular space.

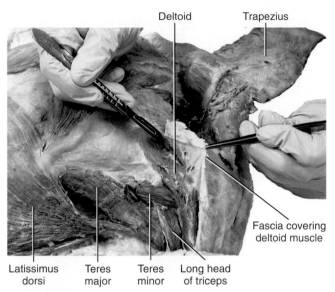

FIGURE 2-42. With scalpel, carefully detach deep fascia covering deltoid muscle.

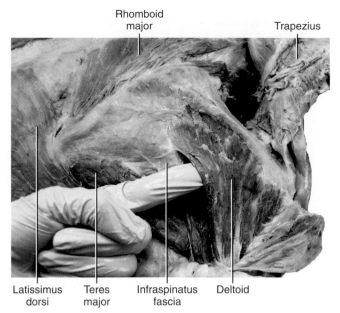

FIGURE 2-44. Insert your index finger under deltoid muscle, and with a scalpel, detach its attachments to scapula.

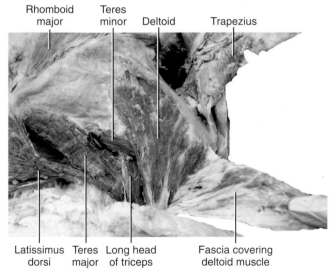

FIGURE 2-43. Deep fascia covering deltoid muscle is reflected, exposing deltoid muscle with its attachments onto spine of scapula.

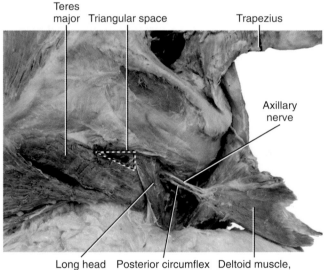

FIGURE 2-45. View of internal surface of reflected deltoid muscle with posterior circumflex humeral artery and axillary nerve exposed. Note dotted lines between teres major and minor and long head of triceps, forming the triangular space.

Identify the *triangular space* between the teres minor, teres major, and the long head of the triceps, in order to find the scapular circumflex artery (Fig. 2-45).

DISSECTION TIP: Thoroughly clean the axillary nerve and the posterior circumflex humeral vessels at their entrance into the deltoid muscle behind the surgical neck of the humerus. Protect these as you clean connective tissue away from the muscles that help form the boundaries of the quadrangular space. The axillary nerve typically branches off to several smaller branches and is usually superior to the posterior circumflex humeral artery.

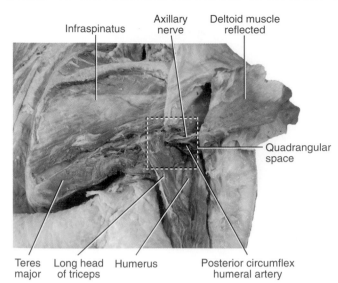

FIGURE 2-46. View of internal surface of reflected deltoid muscle with posterior circumflex humeral artery and axillary nerve exposed. Note dotted lines showing the quadrangular space.

Identify the *quadrangular space* containing the axillary nerve and posterior circumflex humeral artery, bordered posteriorly by the teres major and minor muscles, long head of triceps brachii and surgical neck of the humerus (Fig. 2-46).

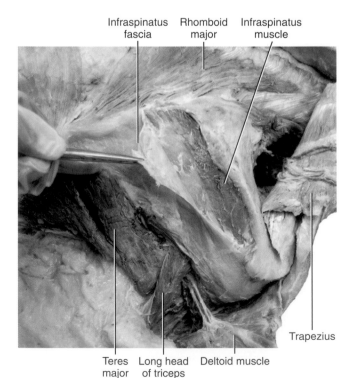

FIGURE 2-47. With a scalpel, carefully detach deep fascia (infraspinatus fascia) covering infraspinatus muscle.

The supraspinatus and infraspinatus fasciae are attached to the scapula around the boundaries of the attachments of the supraspinatus and infraspinatus muscles, respectively. Identify the medial border of the infraspinatus muscle, and reflect it laterally from the infraspinous fossa toward its humeral insertion (Figs. 2-47 to 2-50). Identify and clean the supraspinatus muscle; then, beginning medially, reflect the muscle laterally from the supraspinous fossa far enough to expose the suprascapular nerve and artery (Figs. 2-51 and 2-52).

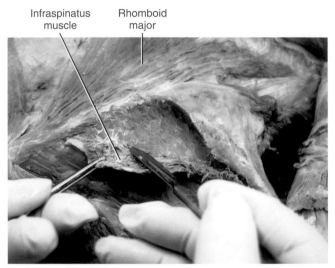

FIGURE 2-48. With scalpel, carefully detach infraspinatus muscle from infraspinous fossa.

> ✋ *DISSECTION TIP:* Carefully separate the connective tissue over the neurovascular bundle to expose the suprascapular artery, nerve, and vein (see Fig. 2-50). The scapular circumflex artery is typically located at the midpoint of the lateral border of the scapula.

Trace the suprascapular artery from its origin to its crossing of the superior transverse scapular ligament to enter the supraspinous fossa, deep to the supraspinatus muscle (Fig. 2-52). Note the passage of the suprascapular nerve and vessels around the greater scapular notch, where they enter the infraspinatus muscle.

Note the triangular space and the scapular circumflex artery within it, giving branches to the overlying skin of the area before turning around the lateral border of the scapula and passing deep to the infraspinatus muscle. The scapular circumflex artery originates from the subscapular artery, one of the three branches of the third part of the axillary artery, and has rich anastomoses with the suprascapular artery (see Fig. 2-50). This arrangement allows strong collateral arterial supply to develop between the subclavian artery and the third part of the axillary artery in the event of occlusion of the more proximal portions of the axillary artery.

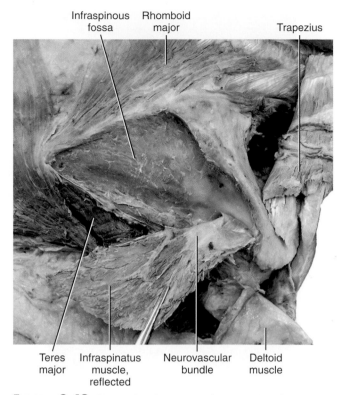

Infraspinous fossa   Rhomboid major   Trapezius

Teres major   Infraspinatus muscle, reflected   Neurovascular bundle   Deltoid muscle

FIGURE 2-49. View of infraspinous fossa with infraspinatus muscle reflected. Note the neurovascular bundle covered with connective tissue, which contains the suprascapular artery, vein, and nerve.

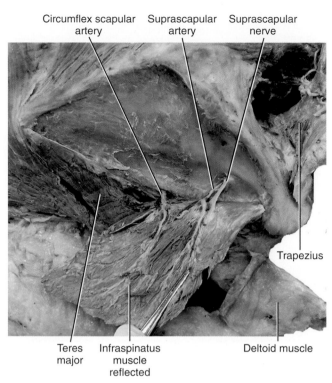

Circumflex scapular artery   Suprascapular artery   Suprascapular nerve

Trapezius

Teres major   Infraspinatus muscle reflected   Deltoid muscle

FIGURE 2-50. Connective tissue is dissected out, exposing the suprascapular artery, vein, and nerve, as well as the scapular circumflex artery.

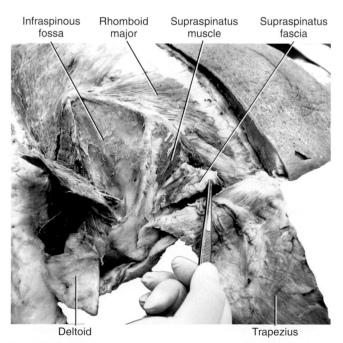

Infraspinous fossa   Rhomboid major   Supraspinatus muscle   Supraspinatus fascia

Deltoid   Trapezius

FIGURE 2-51. Supraspinatus fascia is reflected and the supraspinatus muscle exposed.

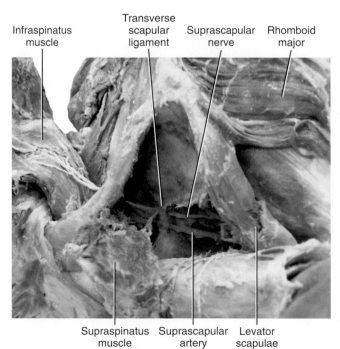

Infraspinatus muscle   Transverse scapular ligament   Suprascapular nerve   Rhomboid major

Supraspinatus muscle   Suprascapular artery   Levator scapulae

FIGURE 2-52. View of internal surface of the supraspinous fossa. Notice suprascapular artery passing over superior transverse scapular ligament and suprascapular nerve underneath it.

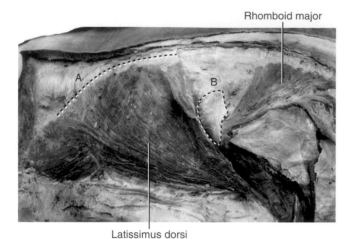

FIGURE 2-53. Dotted line *A* shows location of incision through aponeurosis of latissimus dorsi muscle. Dotted line *B* shows area of connective/adipose tissue covering serratus anterior muscle.

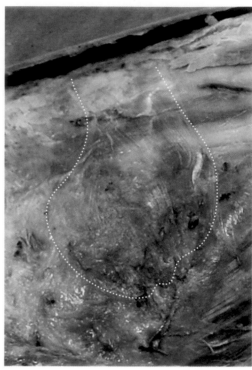

FIGURE 2-55. Dotted lines show borders of serratus posterior inferior muscle.

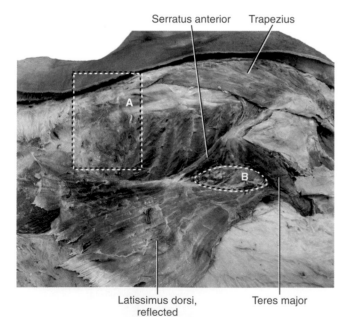

FIGURE 2-54. Latissimus dorsi muscle is reflected, and dotted outline *A* shows serratus posterior inferior muscle. Connective/adipose tissue of Figure 2-53 is removed and serratus anterior muscle exposed. Dotted line *B* shows second area of connective/adipose tissue between serratus anterior and latissimus dorsi muscles.

Make an incision through the aponeurosis of the latissimus dorsi muscle about ½ inch (1.25 cm) from the midline of the back, and cut its attachments to the crest of the ilium. Reflect the latissimus dorsi muscle superiorly and laterally (Fig. 2-53).

> ✋ *DISSECTION TIP:* If you do not exercise care, you will reflect the serratus posterior inferior muscle with the latissimus dorsi. The key to their separation lies in the recognition that although the serratus posterior inferior arises in common with part of the latissimus dorsi, the serratus inserts onto the lower ribs. These fibers can be observed as they diverge from those of the latissimus to pass to their insertion (Figs. 2-54 and 2-55). Cut the origin of the serratus posterior inferior muscle and reflect it toward its insertion.

Pay special attention when removing the connective/adipose tissue between the latissimus dorsi, serratus anterior, and teres major muscles so as not to injure the thoracodorsal artery and vein (Figs. 2-56 and 2-57).

Make a longitudinal incision through the lumbar part of the thoracolumbar fascia near the midline. Then, by cutting its attachments to the underlying musculature, reflect this thick fascia/aponeurosis combination laterally far enough to expose the erector spinae muscle layer (Figs. 2-58 and 2-59).

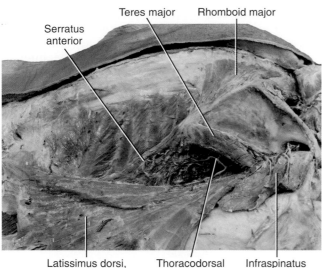

FIGURE 2-56. View of the internal surface of the scapula and dorsal scapular artery traveling at the medial border of the scapula.

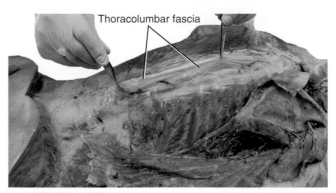

FIGURE 2-58. Reflection of thoracolumbar fascia.

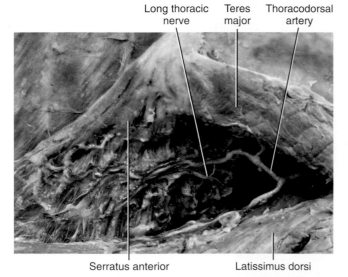

FIGURE 2-57. Close-up view of space between teres major, serratus anterior, and latissimus dorsi muscles (area *B* in Fig. 2-54). Note the thoracodorsal artery and long thoracic nerve supplying the serratus anterior muscle.

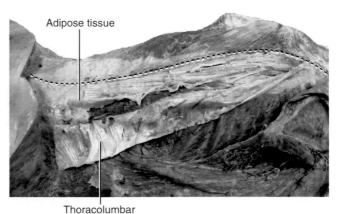

FIGURE 2-59. Thoracolumbar fascia is reflected, and erector spinae muscles are exposed. Note adipose tissue overlying erector spinae. Dotted line represents longitudinal incision of thoracolumbar fascia from the midline.

DISSECTION TIP: The reflection of the thoracolumbar fascia will be performed in the lumbar region only. For the thoracic region, it is unnecessary because the fascia is much thinner there. In this specimen, the fascia in the thoracic region was thick enough to be reflected (Fig. 2-58).

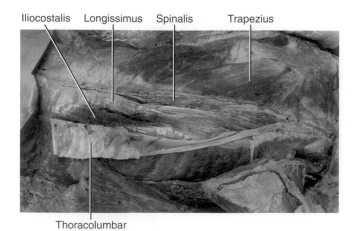

Iliocostalis Longissimus Spinalis Trapezius

Thoracolumbar
fascia

FIGURE 2-60. The thoracolumbar fascia is reflected, and the erector spinae muscles are exposed.

Identify and separate the three longitudinally oriented columns of the erector spinae muscle: the spinalis, longissimus, and iliocostalis (Figs. 2-60 and 2-61). The spinalis is the more medial muscle; the longissimus is the longest muscle, extending to the neck; and the iliocostalis is the most lateral of the three muscles, attaching the iliac crest to the ribs. To expose the deeper musculature, remove a block of the erector spinae muscles several inches long from the lower thoracic and upper lumbar region, and identify the transversospinalis musculature (Fig. 2-62). The transversospinalis muscles include the semispinalis, multifidus, and rotators.

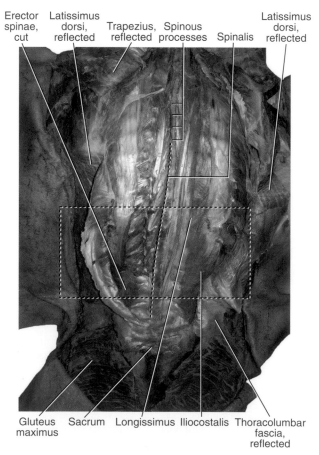

Erector   Latissimus   Latissimus
spinae,   dorsi,   Trapezius, Spinous   dorsi,
cut   reflected   reflected processes   Spinalis   reflected

Gluteus   Sacrum   Longissimus Iliocostalis Thoracolumbar
maximus   fascia,
                                                reflected

FIGURE 2-61. The thoracolumbar fascia is reflected laterally, and the erector spinae muscles (spinalis, longissimus, iliocostalis) are exposed on the right. On the left, the erector spinae muscles are cut to expose the deeper muscles of back.

Latissimus dorsi,
reflected   Multifidus   Spinous
process

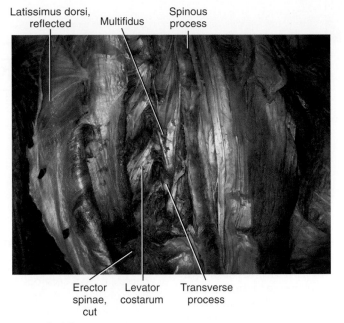

Erector   Levator   Transverse
spinae,   costarum   process
cut

FIGURE 2-62. Multifidus and intertransverse muscles are exposed.

LABORATORY IDENTIFICATION CHECKLIST

Osteology
☐ Skull and vertebrae
☐ Superior nuchal line
☐ External occipital
protuberance
☐ Mastoid process
☐ Vertebra prominens (C7)
☐ Spines of thoracic and lumbar
vertebrae, sacrum, and coccyx

Clavicle
☐ Medial and lateral ends, shaft,
and curvatures

Scapula
☐ Acromion process (tip of
shoulder)
☐ Spine of scapula
☐ Medial or vertebral border
☐ Superior border
☐ Suprascapular notch
☐ Inferior angle
☐ Superior angle
☐ Lateral or axillary border
☐ Coracoid process

Other
☐ Iliac crests

Muscles
☐ Trapezius
☐ Latissimus dorsi
☐ Serratus posterior inferior
☐ Serratus posterior superior
☐ Levator scapulae
☐ Rhomboid minor
☐ Rhomboid major
☐ Deltoid
☐ Triceps brachii, long head
☐ Supraspinatus
☐ Infraspinatus
☐ Teres major
☐ Teres minor
☐ Spinalis
☐ Longissimus
☐ Iliocostalis
☐ Transversospinalis
☐ Semispinalis
☐ Splenius capitis
☐ Erector spinae

Nerves
☐ Greater occipital
☐ Spinal accessory
☐ Dorsal scapular
☐ Suprascapular
☐ Axillary

Fasciae
☐ Thoracolumbar
☐ Supraspinatus/infraspinatus

Ligament
☐ Superior transverse scapular

Arteries
☐ Occipital
☐ Suprascapular
☐ Scapular circumflex
☐ Transverse cervical
☐ Dorsal scapular
☐ Posterior circumflex humeral

Vein
☐ Transverse cervical

CHAPTER 3

SUBOCCIPITAL TRIANGLE AND SPINAL CORD

Netter: 155–156, 162–166, 169–172

McMinn: 104–109

Gray's Atlas: 43–49

Make a midline skin incision from the spinous process of the 7th cervical vertebra (C7) to the external occipital protuberance (Fig. 3-1). At the level of the external occipital protuberance, make a horizontal skin incision connecting the right and left mastoid processes. Reflect the skin and the subcutaneous fat as one layer. Beneath the subcutaneous tissue a connective tissue layer covers the upper portion of the trapezius muscle (Fig. 3-2); dissect away this layer and expose the trapezius (Fig. 3-3).

While cleaning out the fascia that overlies the most cephalic portion of the trapezius muscle (see Figs. 2-29 and 2-30), look for the greater occipital nerve (Fig. 3-4). The greater occipital nerve can usually be found about 1 inch (2.5 cm) from the midline of the neck and 1 inch inferior to the superior nuchal line, as this nerve pierces the trapezius muscle (see Figs. 2-31 to 2-33). Also at this location, locate the occipital artery and preserve it as the trapezius is reflected.

> ☝ *DISSECTION TIP:* Usually, the deep fascia over the trapezius muscle, below the superior nuchal line, is thick and difficult to cut until the C7 level. About 1 cm lateral to the midline, the 3rd occipital nerve (medial branch of dorsal ramus of C3 spinal nerve) is seen along the nuchal ligament (ligamentum nuchae) intermingled with the deep fascia over this area (Figs. 3-3 and 3-4). Generally, the 3rd occipital nerve is very small and is often cut during routine dissections.

Carefully reflect the trapezius muscle from its cranial and cervical attachments (Figs. 3-5 to 3-7). The small amount of connective tissue between the trapezius and splenius capitis muscles can be cleaned out (Fig. 3-8). At the lateral border of the splenius capitis, identify the lesser occipital nerve (see Fig. 3-7).

> ☝ *DISSECTION TIP:* The trapezius is thin at its cephalic and cervical attachments (see Fig. 3-6). Be extremely careful during its reflection. While reflecting the trapezius up from its distal end, keep the scalpel blade facing downward toward the vertebrae, not upward, to prevent damage to the muscle.

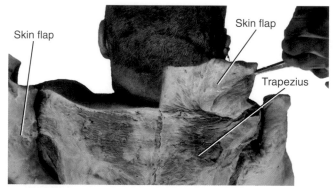

FIGURE 3-1. Once the overlying skin is reflected, the deeper lying trapezius muscle is seen.

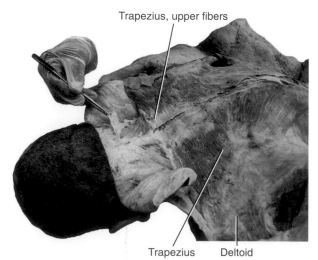

FIGURE 3-2. Reflected skin and fascia revealing upper, middle, and lower fibers of the trapezius muscle.

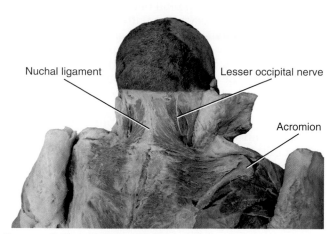

FIGURE 3-3. Superficial upper back and suboccipital regions: upper, middle, and lower fibers of trapezius muscle and nuchal ligament (ligamentum nuchae).

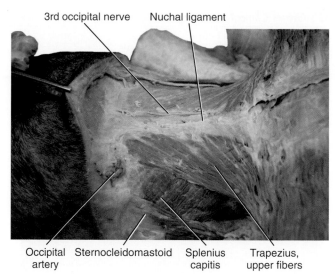

FIGURE 3-4. Structures superficial to suboccipital triangle: nuchal ligament, trapezius (upper fibers), spanius capitis, sternocleidomastoid, 3rd occipital nerve, and occipital artery.

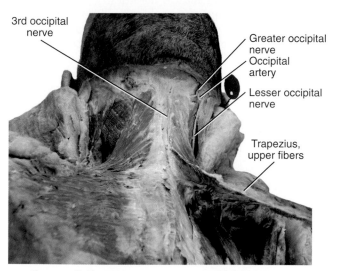

FIGURE 3-5. Initial reflection of the trapezius muscle.

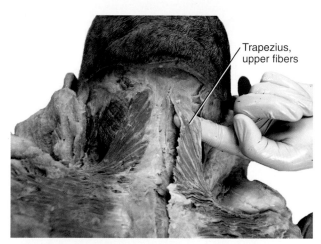

FIGURE 3-6. Elevation of upper fibers of the trapezius muscle reflected away from the nuchal ligament.

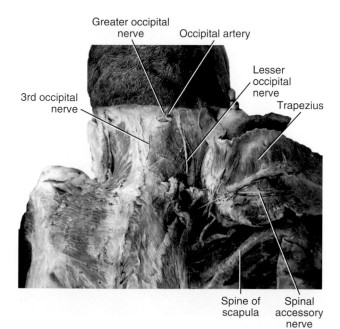

FIGURE 3-7. Posterolateral view of superficial suboccipital region with reflected trapezius muscle and its associated neurovascular bundle pasted on its undersurface.

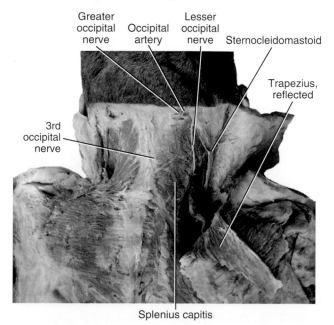

FIGURE 3-8. Superficial suboccipital region with the trapezius muscle reflected to expose the splenius capitis muscle. All connective tissue has been cleaned away.

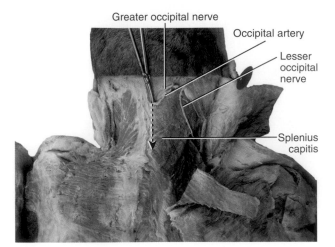

FIGURE 3-9. Insert the scissors deep to the splenius capitis muscle at the midline and continue the incision inferiorly along the nuchal ligament.

Identify the greater occipital nerve and the 3rd occipital nerve, and preserve them after reflecting the trapezius away from its cranial and cervical attachments (Fig. 3-9). Identify the splenius capitis and splenius cervicis muscles; divide them at their origins from the spines of the cervical and upper thoracic vertebrae, and reflect them laterally, exposing the semispinalis capitis muscle (Figs. 3-10 and 3-11). Cut the attachment of the semispinalis capitis muscle from the skull and the ligamentum nuchae to reveal the suboccipital triangle. Preserve the greater occipital and lesser occipital nerves as the semispinalis muscle is reflected.

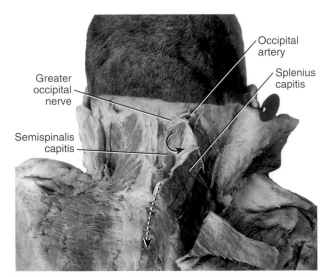

FIGURE 3-10. Reflect splenius capitis laterally, and continue incision toward 1st thoracic vertebra (T1) level.

> ☝ *DISSECTION TIP:* Make one small cut on the semispinalis capitis muscle medial to the greater and lesser occipital nerves (Fig 3-12). In this way, the semispinalis capitis muscle can be easily reflected laterally without disturbing the course of the nerves (Fig 3-13). Trace the occipital nerves down through the underlying fat and tough connective tissue, clearing away the connective tissue using the "separating scissors technique" (Fig 3-14). Even after the semispinalis capitis muscle is reflected, generally, the boundaries or contents of the suboccipital triangle will not be immediately apparent, being hidden by overlying tough connective tissue. Remove these tissues carefully (Figs 3-15 and 3-16). Place the tip of your finger into the suboccipital triangle to locate the posterior arch of the atlas using palpation.

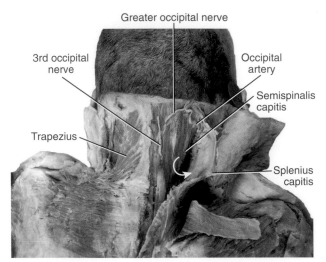

FIGURE 3-11. Complete reflection of the splenius capitis muscle laterally.

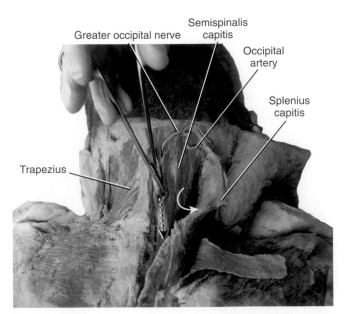

FIGURE 3-12. Make an incision into the semispinalis capitis muscle near the midline down to approximately the T1 level. Preserve the greater and 3rd occipital nerves.

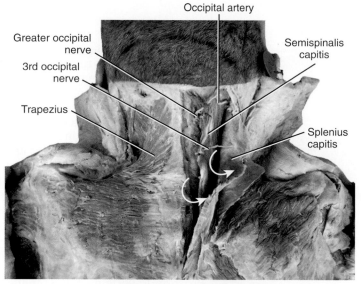

FIGURE **3-13.** Reflected trapezius, splenius capitis, and semispinalis capitis muscles.

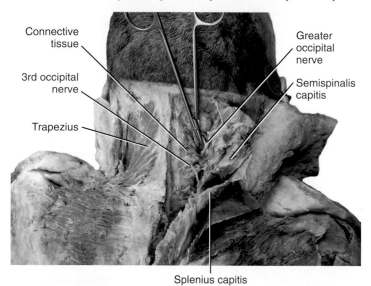

FIGURE **3-14.** Remove fat and connective tissues from around the greater and 3rd occipital nerves. Use the separation technique with your scissors.

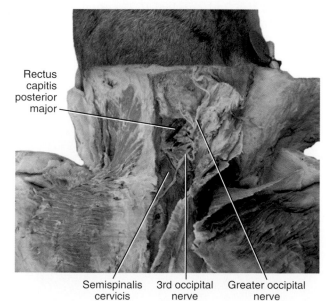

FIGURE **3-15.** Dissection of suboccipital triangle demonstrating the rectus capitis posterior major muscle and greater and 3rd occipital nerves. Remove all fat and connective tissue.

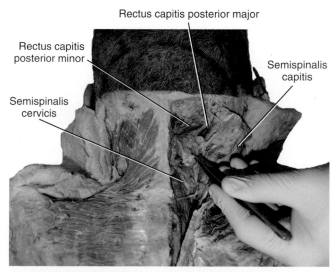

FIGURE **3-16.** Dissection of suboccipital triangle revealing surrounding muscles, including the rectus capitis posterior major and minor and semispinalis capitis muscles.

Rectus capitis posterior minor   3rd occipital nerve   Greater occipital nerve   Occipital artery

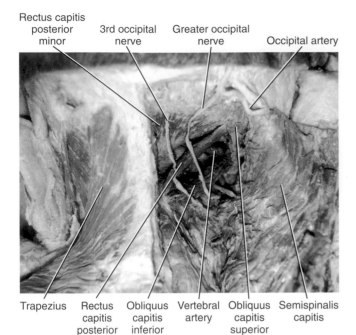

Trapezius   Rectus capitis posterior major   Obliquus capitis inferior   Vertebral artery   Obliquus capitis superior   Semispinalis capitis

FIGURE 3-17. Dissection of the suboccipital triangle highlighting borders and contents.

Trapezius   Rectus capitis posterior minor   Suboccipital nerve   Obliquus capitis superior   Occipital artery   Greater occipital nerve

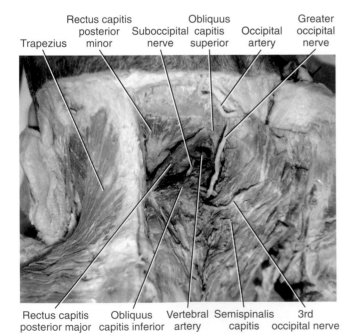

Rectus capitis posterior major   Obliquus capitis inferior   Vertebral artery   Semispinalis capitis   3rd occipital nerve

FIGURE 3-18. Suboccipital triangle borders (rectus capitis posterior major, superior and inferior capitis oblique muscles) and contents (vertebral artery, suboccipital nerve).

After removal of the tough connective tissue, identify the muscles that form the sides of the suboccipital triangle: inferior capitis oblique, superior capitis oblique, and rectus capitis posterior major (Fig 3-17). Typically, the rectus capitis posterior major is found superficial to the rectus capitis posterior minor. Although the rectus capitis posterior minor is considered a "suboccipital" muscle, it does not contribute to the margins of the suboccipital triangle.

Expose the posterior arch of the atlas, and identify a tough connective tissue layer joining the posterior arch of the atlas to the skull, the posterior atlanto-occipital membrane. Clean the loose connective tissue away from the arch and expose the vertebral artery, which lies in the sulcus of the posterior arch of the atlas. Between the sulcus of the posterior arch and the vertebral artery, identify the suboccipital nerve, which innervates the suboccipital muscles and overlying semispinalis capitis muscle (Fig. 3-18).

> ✎ *DISSECTION TIP:* Use fine scissors and take your time to expose and clearly demonstrate the vertebral artery. Besides the tough connective tissue over the vertebral artery, a rich venous plexus is also present. Clean away the connective tissue and venous plexus. You will only see the posterior wall of the vertebral artery.

Using a scalpel, cut the rectus capitis posterior major and inferior capitis oblique muscles from the spinous process of the axis, and reflect them laterally (Fig. 3-19). Note the exit of the greater occipital nerve emerging from tough connective tissue (Fig. 3-20). Remove this connective tissue surrounding the greater occipital nerve, and expose its exit from the dura mater (Fig 3-21). Retract the rectus capitis posterior minor superiorly, and expose the dorsal root ganglion of the 2nd cervical (C2) spinal nerve (Fig. 3-22). In the lumbar region, identify the multifidus and erector spinae muscles.

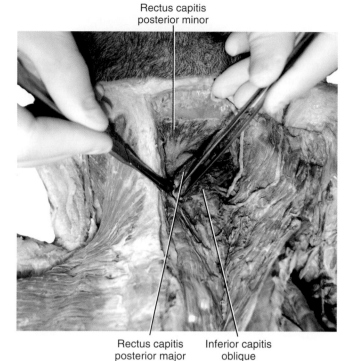

Rectus capitis posterior minor

Rectus capitis posterior major   Inferior capitis oblique

Figure 3-19. Dissection of suboccipital triangle, reflecting rectus capitis posterior major and inferior capitis oblique muscles laterally.

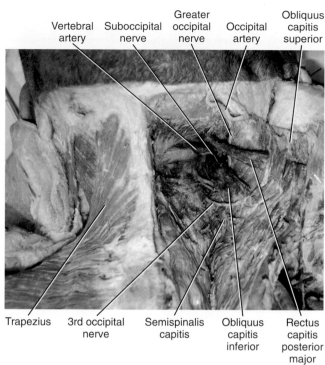

Vertebral artery   Suboccipital nerve   Greater occipital nerve   Occipital artery   Obliquus capitis superior

Trapezius   3rd occipital nerve   Semispinalis capitis   Obliquus capitis inferior   Rectus capitis posterior major

FIGURE 3-20. Dissection of suboccipital triangle illustrating the inferior capitis oblique and rectus capitis posterior major muscles, and revealing suboccipital nerve and vertebral artery.

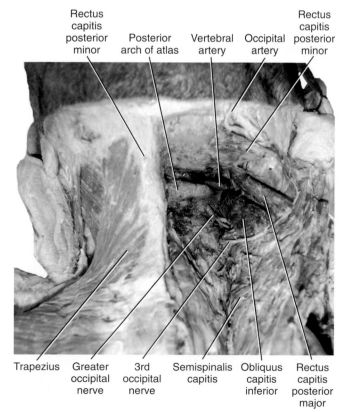

Rectus capitis posterior minor   Posterior arch of atlas   Vertebral artery   Occipital artery   Rectus capitis posterior minor

Trapezius   Greater occipital nerve   3rd occipital nerve   Semispinalis capitis   Obliquus capitis inferior   Rectus capitis posterior major

FIGURE 3-21. Dissection of suboccipital triangle, with reflected rectus capitis posterior minor exposing tectorial membrane and posterior arch of atlas.

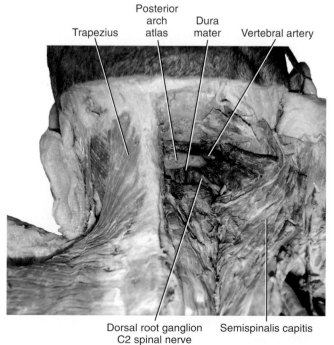

Trapezius   Posterior arch atlas   Dura mater   Vertebral artery

Dorsal root ganglion C2 spinal nerve   Semispinalis capitis

FIGURE 3-22. Dissection of suboccipital triangle exposing dura mater of spinal cord, dorsal root ganglion, vertebral artery, and posterior arch of atlas.

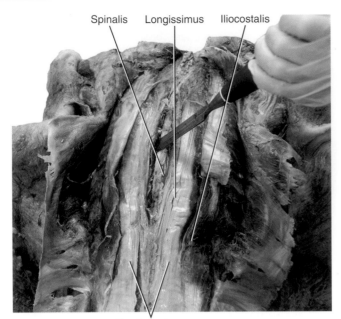

Spinalis Longissimus Iliocostalis

Erector spinae
muscle (group)

FIGURE 3-23. Superficial and intermediate muscles of back region reflected, revealing superficial layer of deep or native back muscles (erector spinae: spinalis, longissimus, iliocostalis).

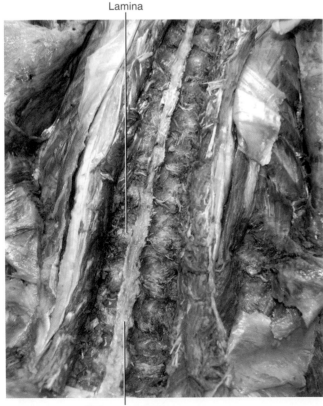

Lamina

Spinous process

FIGURE 3-24. The chisel or saw is angled laterally and short tapping blows of the mallet are used until the lamina is felt to fracture. Do not allow the chisel to be driven too deeply, or injury to the spinal cord or its rootlets will occur.

LAMINECTOMY

In preparation for the laminectomy, reflect or cut away the muscles of the back from the spines and transverse processes of the vertebrae as completely as possible using a scalpel, scissors, and chisel (Fig. 3-23). Clean away as much as possible all of the intrinsic muscles of the back from the laminae of the lower cervical, thoracic, and upper lumbar regions (Fig. 3-24).

With a bone saw or chisel and mallet, cut through the laminae longitudinally from the lower cervical to the lower lumbar regions (Fig. 3-25). Direct the blade of the saw or chisel anteromedially to avoid cutting the spinal nerves (Fig. 3-26).

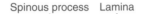

Spinous process Lamina

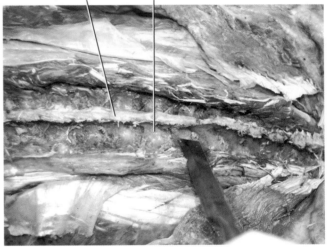

FIGURE 3-25. After removal of all muscles from the paraspinous region, the spinous processes and laminae are seen. The chisel is placed flat onto each lamina and angled away from the midline.

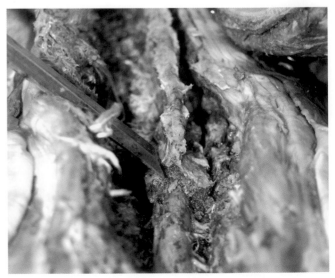

FIGURE 3-26. Direct blade of saw or chisel anteromedially to avoid cutting spinal nerves.

DISSECTION TIP: To facilitate the process, several laminae can be removed together as a block (Figs. 3-27 to 3-29). After excision of the vertebral laminae and spinous processes, the vertebral canal may not be exposed widely enough for clear visualization of its contents. If this is the case, remove additional bone as necessary with bone rongeurs or with a mallet and chisel. Exercise particular care in the regions of the intervertebral foramina to avoid cutting or tearing away the spinal nerve rootlets. Sharply pointed edges of bone may be present in the dissection field after the laminectomy is completed. Identify any sharp spicules and remove them to avoid injuries to your hands.

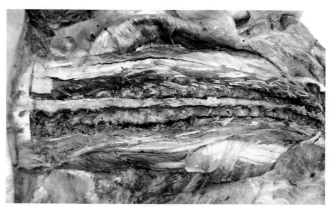

FIGURE 3-27. Bilateral dissection through laminae of vertebrae using chisel and mallet technique to reveal dura mater and spinal cord (Stryker-type electric saw can also be used).

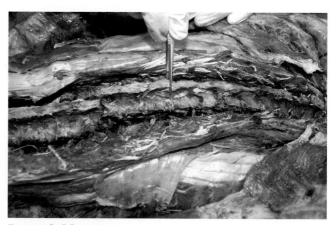

FIGURE 3-28. Using toothed forceps, gently lift spinous process–lamina unit away from spinal canal, revealing dura mater, dorsal root ganglia, and spinal cord.

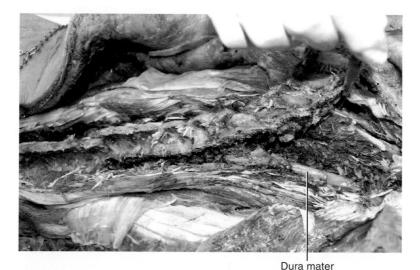

Dura mater

FIGURE 3-29. Removal of spinous process–lamina unit from lumbar region, exposing dura mater.

Remove the spinous processes and the laminae en bloc from the spinal canal (Fig. 3-30). Similarly, note the contents of the spinal canal: the epidural fat and the vertebral venous plexus of Batson (Fig. 3-31). Remove the fat and the venous plexus from the epidural space to expose the dura mater. Lift a part of the dura in the midline, and make a small, slitlike incision with scissors or a scalpel (Fig. 3-32). Continue the midline incision throughout the entire length of the dura mater (Fig. 3-33). If possible, avoid incising the underlying arachnoid layer by lifting and maintaining tension on the dura mater. Reflect the dura laterally to expose the contents of the dural sac. If the incision in the dura is made successfully, the arachnoid will appear as a thin, almost transparent layer (Fig. 3-33).

> ✋ *DISSECTION TIP:* Sometimes, arachnoid calcifications (plaques) may be present. These are usually incidental findings and have been attributed to trauma, myelography, subarachnoid hemorrhage, and spinal anesthesia (Fig 3-34).

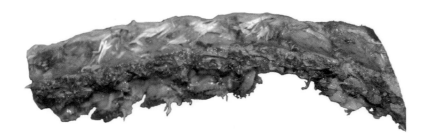

FIGURE 3-30. Section of spinous process–lamina unit removed from vertebral column.

Vertebral venous plexus

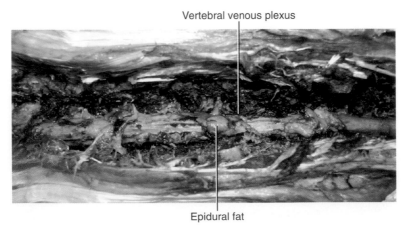

Epidural fat

FIGURE 3-31. Spinous process–lamina unit removed to expose epidural fat, dura mater, and vertebral venous plexus.

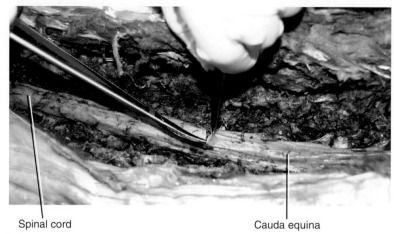

Spinal cord   Cauda equina

FIGURE 3-32. Spinous process–lamina unit removed from lumbar region, revealing dura mater covering spinal cord and cauda equina. Elevate dura mater during transverse cut.

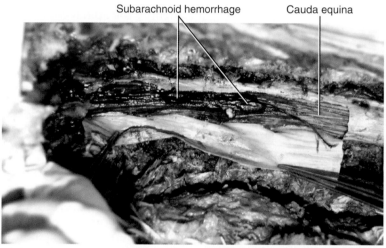

Subarachnoid hemorrhage   Cauda equina

FIGURE 3-33. Transverse and vertical incisions reflecting dura mater, revealing cauda equina and subarachnoid hemorrhage.

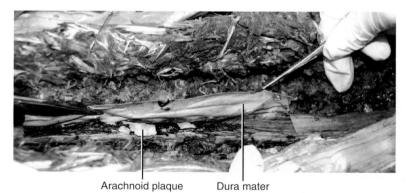

Arachnoid plaque   Dura mater

FIGURE 3-34. Transverse and vertical incisions reflecting dura mater, revealing arachnoid plaque among cauda equina.

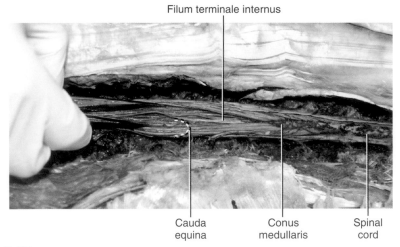

FIGURE 3-35. Dura mater reflected to reveal spinal cord, conus medullaris, and filum terminale among cauda equina.

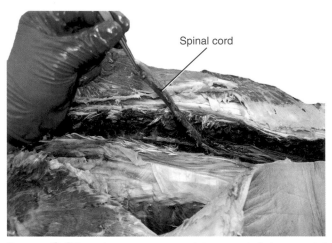

FIGURE 3-36. Reflecting spinal cord from cephalad to caudal reveals posterior longitudinal ligament.

Identify the spinal cord and its covering of pia mater. Observe the beginning of the filum terminale at its origin from the conus medullaris, the terminal part of the spinal cord. Note the cluster of large nerve rootlets on either side of the conus medullaris, the *cauda equina* (Fig 3-35; see also Figs. 3-32, 3-33, and 3-39). Transect and remove the spinal cord with its dural coverings. Identify the posterior longitudinal ligament on the vertebral bodies after the removal of the spinal cord and dura mater (Figs. 3-36 and 3-37). Look for the toothlike denticulate ligaments on each side of the spinal cord, lifting the cord carefully with forceps for inspection. These projections occur at the level of each vertebra, from the occipital bone to the last thoracic spinal nerve. The denticulate ligaments pierce the arachnoid mater to attach to the dura mater (Figs. 3-38 and 3-39).

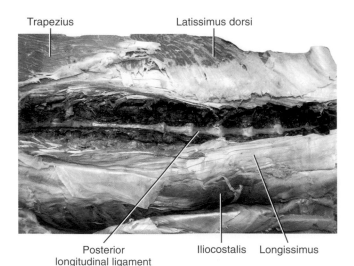

FIGURE 3-37. Spinal cord removed, revealing posterior longitudinal ligament.

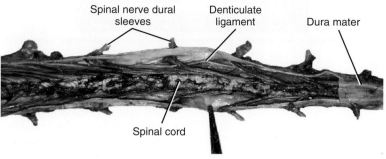

Spinal nerve dural sleeves Denticulate ligament Dura mater

Spinal cord

FIGURE 3-38. Transverse and vertical incisions reflecting dura mater, revealing spinal cord, denticulate ligament, and spinal nerve dural sleeves.

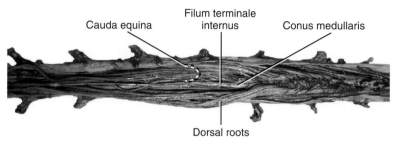

Cauda equina Filum terminale internus Conus medullaris

Dorsal roots

FIGURE 3-39. Transverse and vertical incisions reflecting dura mater, revealing conus medullaris, dorsal roots, and filum terminale.

LABORATORY IDENTIFICATION CHECKLIST

Nerves
- ❏ Greater occipital nerve (dorsal ramus C2)
- ❏ Lesser occipital nerve (ventral rami of C2 and C3)
- ❏ 3rd occipital nerve (dorsal ramus C3)
- ❏ Suboccipital nerve (dorsal ramus C1)
- ❏ Dorsal root ganglion
- ❏ Spinal nerve
- ❏ Spinal nerve dural sleeve

Arteries
- ❏ Occipital artery
- ❏ Vertebral artery

Vein
- ❏ Venous plexus (Batson's)

Muscles
- ❏ Trapezius
- ❏ Splenius capitis

Muscles—cont'd
- ❏ Semispinalis capitis
- ❏ Sternocleidomastoid
- ❏ Rectus capitis posterior major
- ❏ Rectus capitis posterior minor
- ❏ Superior capitis obliquus
- ❏ Inferior capitis obliquus
- ❏ Semispinalis capitis
- ❏ Erector spinae group
- ❏ Spinalis
- ❏ Longissimus
- ❏ Iliocostalis
- ❏ Multifidus

Bones
- ❏ Atlas
- ❏ Posterior arch
- ❏ Spinous processes
- ❏ Lamina
- ❏ Transverse processes
- ❏ Body
- ❏ Vertebral foramen

Ligaments
- ❏ Nuchal ligament (ligamentum nuchae)
- ❏ Ligamentum flavum (yellow/flaval ligaments)
- ❏ Posterior longitudinal ligament

Spinal Cord and Layers
- ❏ Dura mater
- ❏ Arachnoid mater
- ❏ Pia mater
- ❏ Denticulate ligaments
- ❏ Filum terminale
- ❏ Conus medullaris
- ❏ Cauda equina

LUMBAR PUNCTURE

Gray's Anatomy for Students: 108–116

Netter: 155–156, 163*

Clinical Application

A lumbar puncture uses a spinal needle to access the subarachnoid space between the 2nd and 4th lumbar vertebrae (L2 and L4) to withdraw cerebrospinal fluid for analysis (Fig. II-1).

*The Clinical Applications in each section are cross-referenced to the following sources: *Gray's Anatomy for Students*, 2e, and Netter: *Atlas of Human Anatomy*, 5e. Page references from each source are provided for procedures in the Clinical Applications.

Anatomic Landmarks

- Below the L2 vertebra. Feel spinous processes and space between processes (Fig. II-2).
- Supracristal plane crosses L4. Puncture is safe just superior or inferior to this point, which avoids the spinal cord.
- Superficial to deep:
  Skin
  Subcutaneous tissue
  Supraspinous ligament
  Interspinous ligament
  Ligamentum flavum (provides increased resistance to needle)
  Dura mater
  Subarachnoid space–cerebrospinal fluid

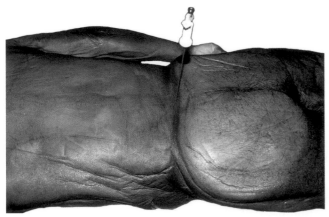

FIGURE II-1.

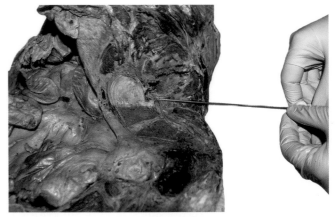

FIGURE II-2.

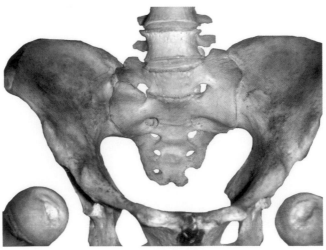

FIGURE II-3.

EXTRADURAL ANESTHESIA (CAUDAL OR SACRAL BLOCK)

Gray's Anatomy for Students: 116

Netter: 155, 158

Clinical Application

Introduce anesthetic solutions into the epidural space, which will anesthetize the spinal nerves exiting the dura mater.

Anatomic Landmarks (Figs. II-4 and II-5)

- Natal cleft
- Sacral cornu
- Superficial to deep:
  Skin
  Subcutaneous tissue
  Posterior sacrococcygeal ligament (increased resistance)
  Sacral canal

Sacralization is the anomalous fusion of the 5th lumbar vertebra (L5) to the 1st sacral vertebra (S1) (Fig. II-3).

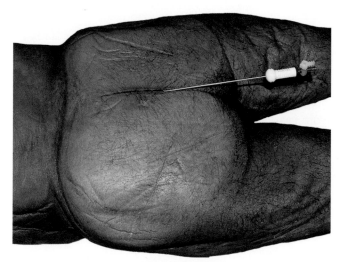

FIGURE II-4.

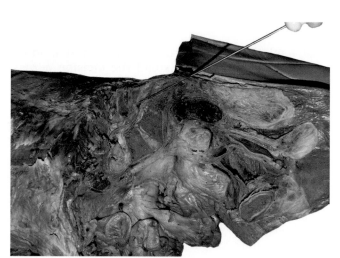

FIGURE II-5.

TRIANGLE OF AUSCULTATION

Gray's Anatomy for Students: 91

Netter: 171

Clinical Application

The triangle of auscultation defines an area that allows better auscultation with a stethoscope (due to less overlying muscle mass), to maximize listening to the lungs, 6th intercostal space, and the gastroesophageal junction on the left and assessing potential pathology.

Anatomic Landmarks

- Medial border of scapula
- Lateral border of trapezius
- Superior border of latissimus dorsi

Note: Area of triangle increases when arms are crossed and trunk is flexed.

CHAPTER 4

PECTORAL REGION AND BREAST

Netter: 175–187, 416

McMinn: 134–137, 144, 178–187

Gray's Atlas: 56–66, 359–363, 368

Make a midline incision from the suprasternal notch to the xiphoid process. Extend the incision across the border of the costal margin toward the midaxillary line. Make another incision from the suprasternal notch over the clavicle to the shoulder (Figs. 4-1 and 4-2). Continue the incision from the shoulder distally to a point approximately 2 inches (5 cm) above the elbow. An encircling incision around the midportion of the arm will permit removal of the skin from the upper arm. Reflect the skin from the thorax, shoulders, axillae, and proximal portions of the arms medially to the axillary space (Figs. 4-3 and 4-4). Remove the skin and the superficial fascia using blunt and sharp dissection.

> **✋ DISSECTION TIP:** Start the dissection at the junction of the suprasternal notch and the clavicle (see Fig. 4-2). As the superficial fascia and skin are retracted, you will encounter anterior cutaneous branches of ventral primary rami and vessels emerging near the sternum. The vessels are the perforating branches of the internal thoracic artery and the perforating tributaries to the internal thoracic vein. Cut through these cutaneous nerves and vessels.

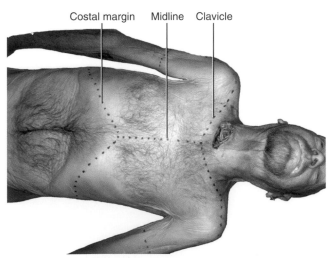

FIGURE 4-1. Skin markings of anterior thoracic wall for superficial dissection incisions.

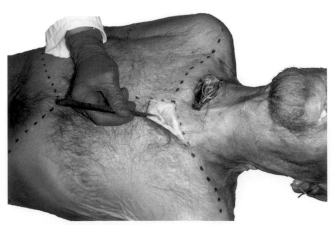

FIGURE 4-2. Skin reflection of anterior thoracic wall, medial to lateral.

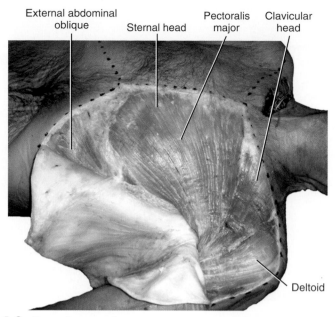

External abdominal oblique

Sternal head

Pectoralis major

Clavicular head

Deltoid

FIGURE 4-3. Skin reflection of anterior thoracic wall exposing deltopectoral region.

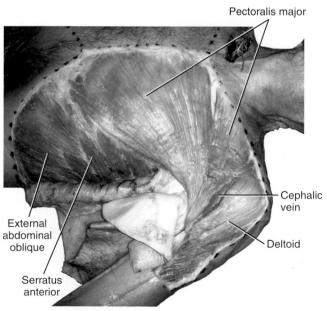

Pectoralis major

Cephalic vein

Deltoid

External abdominal oblique

Serratus anterior

FIGURE 4-4. Skin reflection of anterior thoracic wall exposing deltopectoral triangle, serratus anterior muscle, and external abdominal oblique muscle.

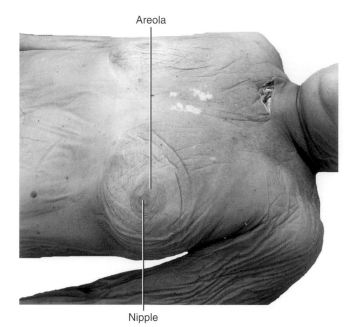

FIGURE 4-5. Skin of female breast with nipple-areolar complex.

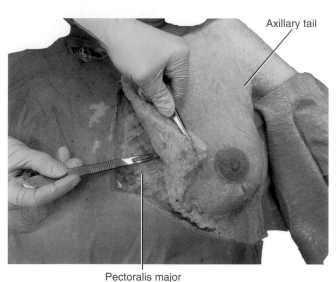

FIGURE 4-7. Reflecting left breast, deep to superficial fascia.

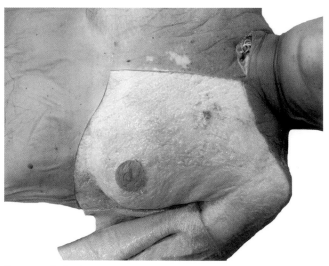

FIGURE 4-6. Skin reflection from anterior thoracic wall (same technique as Fig. 4-3) revealing superficial fascia and nipple-areolar complex.

In female cadavers, in addition to the incisions described in the removal of the skin, make an oblique incision through the skin of the breast from the midpoint of the clavicle toward the anterior axillary line, encircling the areola (Fig. 4-5). Lift the skin at the edge of the incision with a forceps, and start reflecting the adipose tissue from the pectoralis major with a scalpel (Figs. 4-6 and 4-7) Note the retinacula cutis, which begins at the dermis and extends deeply into the breast, forming fibrous septae and irregular bands of dense connective tissue. Cut through the middle of the areola (Figs. 4-8 and 4-9). Try to identify one or more lactiferous ducts (Fig. 4-10); the ducts may possess an expanded part (lactiferous sinus or ampulla) deep to the nipple. The lactiferous ducts narrow as they pass through the nipple tissue, each terminating separately on its surface. In most older cadavers, little will remain of the duct system or glandular tissue, which is replaced with fibrous tissue infiltrated with fat.

> ✋ *DISSECTION TIP:* In some cadavers an injection reservoir may be identified under the skin (Fig. 4-11). These reservoirs are connected to a catheter implanted in a deeper vein to allow direct access to a large vein without having to "stick" the vein each time and are used for long-term injections (e.g., chemotherapy).

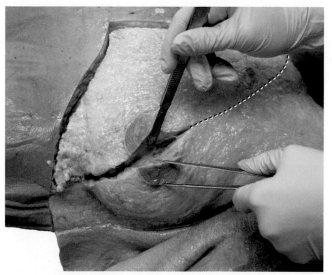

FIGURE 4-8. Sagittal incision through nipple-areolar complex revealing glandular tissue, ducts, connective tissue, and fat of breast.

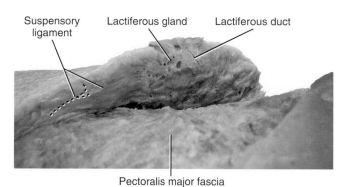

FIGURE 4-10. Sagittal incision through nipple-areolar complex revealing lactiferous gland and duct and suspensory ligament of breast.

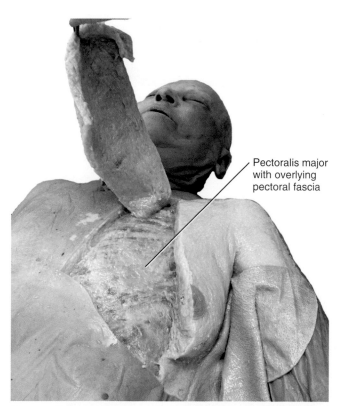

FIGURE 4-9. Partial removal of left breast revealing pectoralis major and fascia lying deep to breast and superficial fascia.

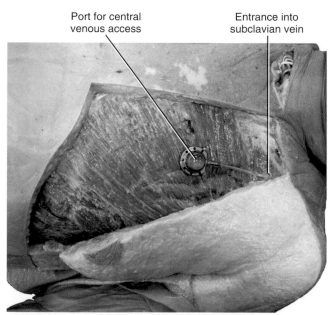

FIGURE 4-11. Left pectoralis major fascia removed, revealing its muscle with central venous port in situ.

Identify the pectoralis major muscle invested in a thin, tough fascia, the pectoral fascia (part of the deep fascia system) (see Figs. 4-3 and 4-10). After cleaning the fascia from the pectoralis major, note the separation of the pectoralis major from the deltoid muscle by the deltopectoral groove (see Fig. 4-4). Detach the clavicular, sternal, and abdominal attachments of the pectoralis major with a scalpel, and reflect the muscle laterally to its insertion onto the humerus (Figs. 4-12 and 4-13). Transect the clavicular portion of the pectoralis major muscle from the suprasternal notch to the midclavicular line in order to avoid cutting important vessels and nerves, including the lateral pectoral nerve.

> ✋ *DISSECTION TIP:* When the pectoralis major is reflected, pay special attention so as not to transect the medial pectoral nerve as it passes through, or lies lateral or inferior to, the pectoralis minor muscle to enter the pectoralis major.

After the pectoralis major has been reflected, identify the upper border of the pectoralis minor muscle, and dissect out the clavipectoral fascia to expose the subclavian vein (Fig. 4-14). This fascia attaches proximally to the clavicle and invests the subclavius muscle. The clavipectoral fascia then passes as a sheet toward the pectoralis minor muscle, invests it, and then blends distally with axillary fascia, forming the so-called suspensory ligament of the axilla.

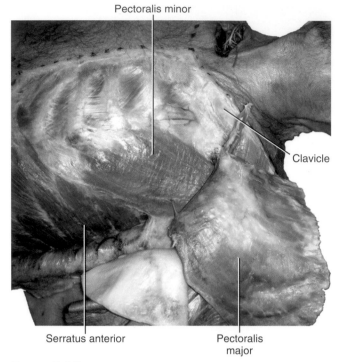

FIGURE 4-13. Reflection of pectoralis major muscle highlighting pectoralis minor attachment to ribs 3 to 5.

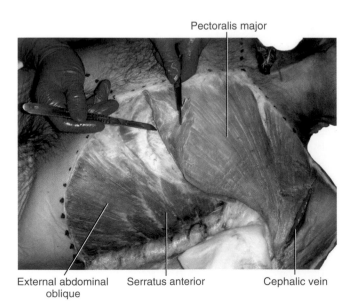

FIGURE 4-12. Left pectoralis major muscle reflected from anterior chest wall.

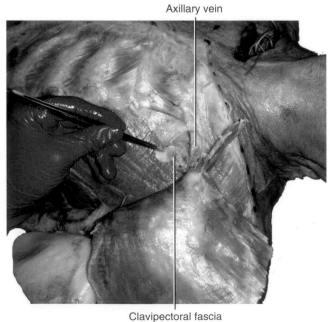

FIGURE 4-14. Reflection of pectoralis major muscle and its fascia revealing clavipectoral fascia.

Next, observe the subclavian vein, the lateral pectoral nerves, and the pectoral branches of the thoracoacromial artery as they emerge to reach the pectoralis major muscle (Figs. 4-15 and 4-16). Trace the pectoral arteries to their origin from the thoracoacromial artery, and preserve these as the dissection proceeds.

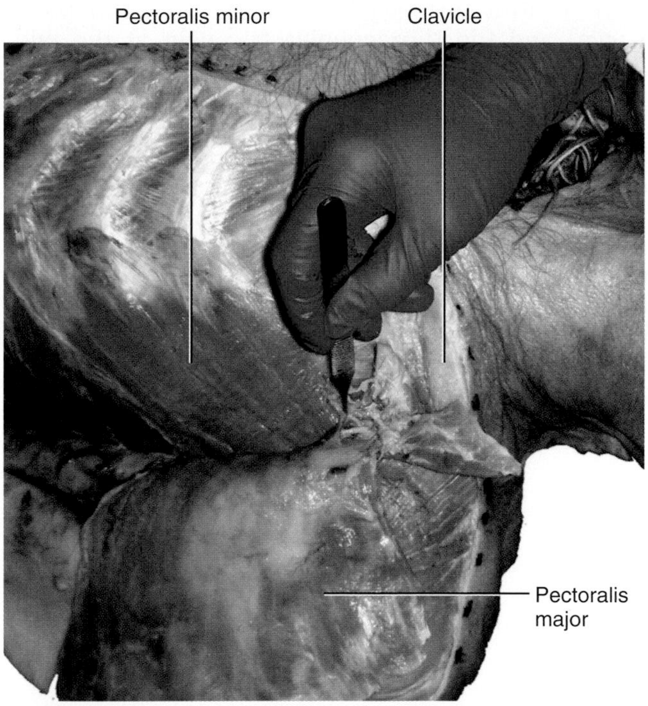

Insert the scissors at the inferior border of the pectoralis minor muscle, and split the connective tissue underneath (Fig. 4-17). With a scalpel, reflect the pectoralis minor from ribs 3, 4, and 5 (Fig 4-18).

> ✋ *DISSECTION TIP:* Often in older cadavers, large lymph nodes located deep to the pectoralis minor (retropectoral nodes) may be evident.

FIGURE 4-15. Removal of clavipectoral fascia and identification of axillary vein (see Fig. 4-16).

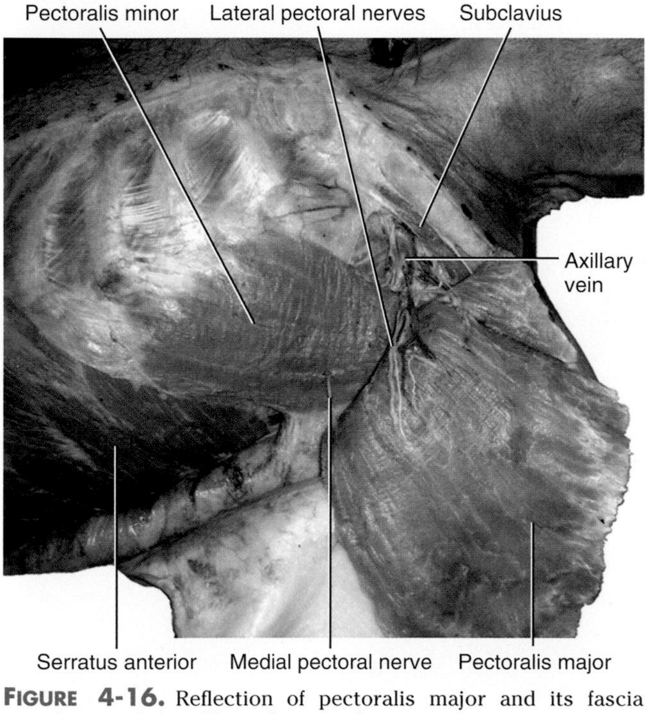

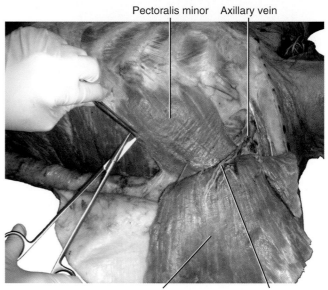

FIGURE 4-17. Reflection of pectoralis major and its fascia revealing pectoralis minor muscle. Scissor blades are positioned along lateral inferior border of pectoralis minor.

FIGURE 4-16. Reflection of pectoralis major and its fascia revealing medial and lateral pectoral nerves.

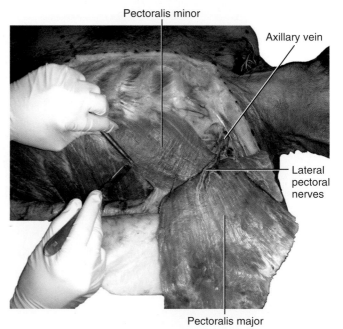

FIGURE 4-18. Reflection of pectoralis major and its fascia revealing pectoralis minor muscle. Place scalpel tip at lateral inferior border of pectoralis minor.

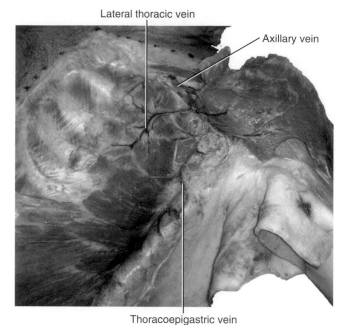

Lateral thoracic vein

Axillary vein

Thoracoepigastric vein

FIGURE 4-19. Reflection of pectoralis major and minor muscles revealing venous network, including axillary, lateral thoracic, and thoracoepigastric veins.

As the superficial fascia is reflected from the anterolateral aspect of the thoracic wall, look for the thoracoepigastric vein. The thoracoepigastric vein is a tributary to the axillary vein by direct or indirect connections. During the reflection of the fascia near the midaxillary line, lateral cutaneous branches of ventral primary rami may be exposed where they enter the superficial fascia (Figs. 4-19 and 4-20). Try to preserve as many of these as possible. A few centimeters inferior to the junction of the 2nd thoracic (T2) ventral primary ramus (intercostobrachial nerve) and the thoracoepigastric vein at the midaxillary line over the serratus anterior muscle, identify and trace the long thoracic nerve, which innervates the serratus anterior muscle (Figs. 4-21 to 4-23). Clean the intercostobrachial nerve (T2), which emerges from the 2nd intercostal space. This nerve supplies the skin of the axilla and the upper medial aspect of the arm. In some specimens, the 3rd intercostal nerve may communicate with the intercostobrachial nerve. Clean this nerve toward the skin of the axilla (Fig. 4-24).

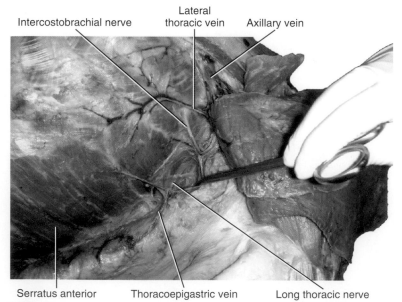

Intercostobrachial nerve

Lateral thoracic vein

Axillary vein

Serratus anterior

Thoracoepigastric vein

Long thoracic nerve

FIGURE 4-20. The thoracoepigastric vein is retracted laterally with scissors to reveal the long thoracic nerve.

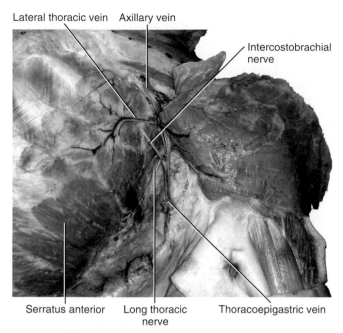

Lateral thoracic vein   Axillary vein

Intercostobrachial nerve

Serratus anterior   Long thoracic nerve   Thoracoepigastric vein

FIGURE 4-21. Reflection of pectoralis major and minor muscles and deep fascia revealing venous network, intercostobrachial nerve, and long thoracic nerve.

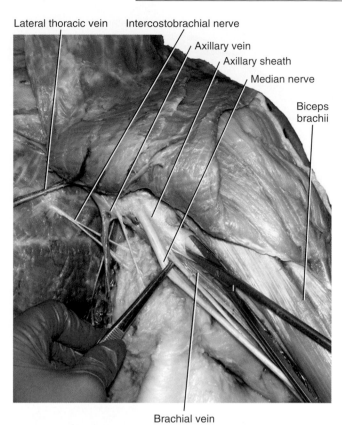

Lateral thoracic vein   Intercostobrachial nerve

Axillary vein

Axillary sheath

Median nerve

Biceps brachii

Brachial vein

FIGURE 4-22. Reflection of pectoralis major and minor muscles and deep fascia revealing axillary sheath, axillary and brachial veins, and median nerve.

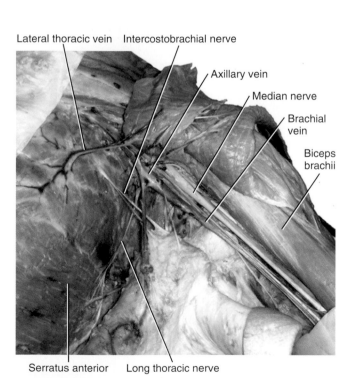

Lateral thoracic vein   Intercostobrachial nerve

Axillary vein

Median nerve

Brachial vein

Biceps brachii

Serratus anterior   Long thoracic nerve

FIGURE 4-23. Reflection of pectoralis major and minor muscles and deep fascia revealing neurovenous structures of the axillary region.

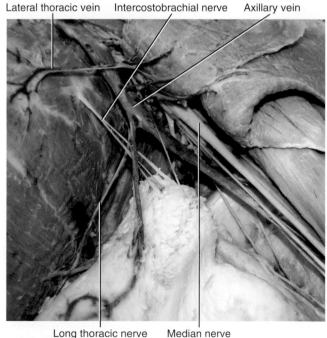

Lateral thoracic vein   Intercostobrachial nerve   Axillary vein

Long thoracic nerve   Median nerve

FIGURE 4-24. Reflection of pectoralis major muscle and fascia revealing pectoralis minor and relationship to axillary vein and long thoracic artery.

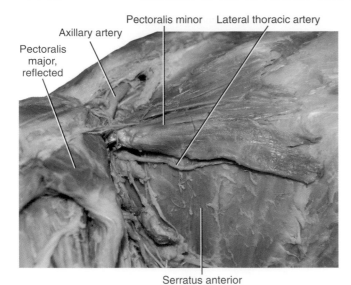

FIGURE 4-25. Reflection of pectoralis major muscle exposing lateral thoracic artery, seen traveling along the lateral border of the pectoralis minor muscle.

At the lateral border of the pectoralis minor on the surface of the serratus anterior muscle, expose the lateral thoracic artery (Fig. 4-25). Its origin is typically from the 2nd portion of the axillary artery (see Chapter 7); however, this may vary. Look carefully for a small artery penetrating the musculature of the 1st or 2nd intercostal spaces. This is the supreme (superior, highest) thoracic artery, which arises from the 1st part of the axillary artery (Fig. 4-26).

The cephalic vein is found within the deltopectoral groove. This vein can be exposed by dividing the fascia that lies superficial to it. The cephalic vein is an important landmark for identifying the first part of the axillary artery (Fig. 4-27).

Remove part of the axillary sheath and the axillary fascia deep to the pectoralis major muscle. This tube-like fascia covers the axillary artery, axillary vein, and the brachial plexus and derives from the prevertebral fascia. With scissors, separate the fascia and remove most of it (see Figs. 4-22 and 4-23). Once the fascia is removed, replace the pectoralis minor muscle over the axillary artery. This muscle divides the axillary artery into three parts.

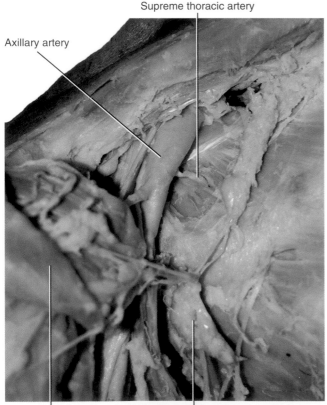

FIGURE 4-26. Dissection of axillary region revealing reflected pectoralis minor muscle, axillary and supreme thoracic artery, and axillary lymph nodes.

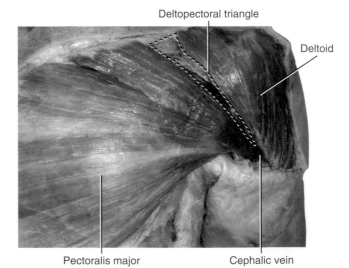

FIGURE 4-27. Skin reflected from anterolateral thoracic wall revealing deltopectoral muscles, deltopectoral triangle, and cephalic vein.

Place a probe or the scissors between the external intercostal membrane and the internal intercostal muscle (Fig. 4-28). The external intercostal membrane travels between the lateral border of the sternum and the midclavicular line. Cut this membrane and expose the internal intercostal muscle (Fig. 4-29). This muscle layer runs in a direction opposite to the external intercostals, like "hands in your back pockets." The external intercostal muscles are oriented in a direction medially and downward, like "hands in your front pockets" (Fig. 4-30).

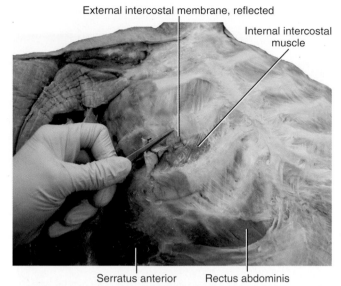

FIGURE 4-29. External intercostal membrane is cut and reflected laterally to reveal internal intercostal muscle.

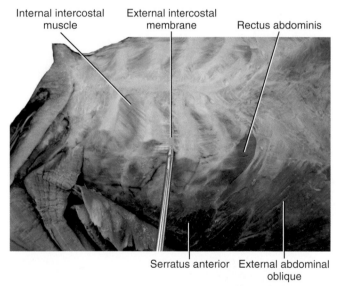

FIGURE 4-28. Anterior thoracic wall musculature revealing external intercostal membrane (over scissors) and internal intercostal, external abdominal oblique, rectus abdominis, and serratus anterior muscles.

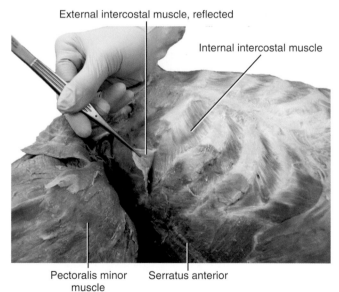

FIGURE 4-30. Anterolateral chest wall with reflected pectoralis muscle and fascia revealing external intercostal, internal intercostal, and serratus anterior muscles.

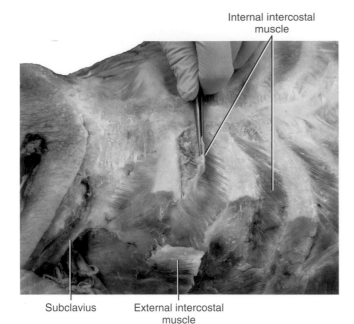

FIGURE 4-31. Anterolateral chest wall revealing subclavius, external intercostal, and internal intercostal muscles. The internal intercostal muscle is cut superiorly and reflected inferiorly to expose the endothoracic fascia.

Near the sternum, the external intercostal layer is continued medially by the external intercostal membrane. Reflect the internal intercostal muscle adjacent to the sternum, and expose the contents of the intercostal space (Figs. 4-31 and 4-32). Identify the endothoracic fascia and carefully reflect it (Fig. 4-33). Identify the internal thoracic artery and vein (Figs. 4-34 and 4-35).

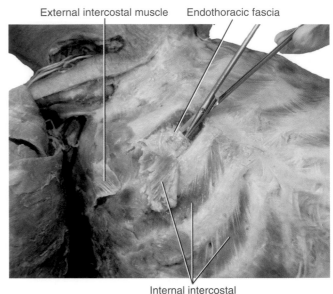

FIGURE 4-33. Anterolateral chest wall with reflected internal intercostal muscle revealing endothoracic fascia with external and internal intercostal muscles (note that between T1 and T4, intercostal segments do not have innermost muscle fibers).

FIGURE 4-32. Anterolateral chest wall with reflected internal intercostal muscle revealing endothoracic fascia and external and internal intercostal muscles (note that between T1 and T4, intercostal segments do not have innermost muscle fibers).

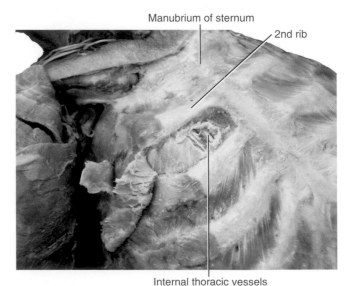

FIGURE 4-34. Anterior chest wall with reflected internal intercostal muscle and endothoracic fascia revealing internal thoracic artery and vein.

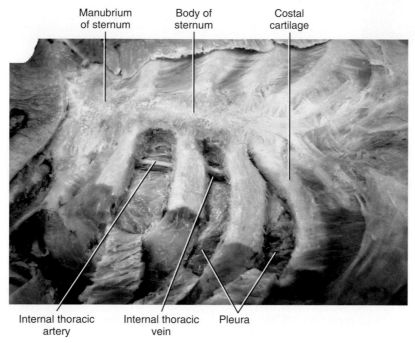

Manubrium of sternum   Body of sternum   Costal cartilage

Internal thoracic artery   Internal thoracic vein   Pleura

Figure 4-35. Anterolateral chest wall with manubrium, body of sternum, and costal cartilage. Endothoracic fascia removed to highlight internal thoracic artery and vein.

LABORATORY IDENTIFICATION CHECKLIST

Some of the nerves and arteries listed here will have been dissected during the laboratory for the superficial back (and upper limb) but are also seen when dissecting the breast.

Nerves
- ❑ Anterior intercostal
- ❑ Intercostobrachial (T2)
- ❑ Lateral intercostal (T3-T7)
- ❑ Lateral pectoral
- ❑ Medial pectoral
- ❑ Axillary
- ❑ Long thoracic
- ❑ Thoracodorsal
- ❑ Subscapular

Arteries
- ❑ Thoracoacromial trunk
- ❑ Pectoral branches
- ❑ Deltoid branches
- ❑ Clavicular branches
- ❑ Acromial branches
- ❑ Internal (mammary) thoracic
- ❑ Lateral thoracic
- ❑ Anterior intercostal
- ❑ Posterior intercostal

Veins
- ❑ Axillary
- ❑ Internal thoracic
- ❑ Intercostal veins

Muscles
- ❑ Pectoralis major
  - ❑ Clavicular head
  - ❑ Sternal head
  - ❑ Abdominal head (not always present)
- ❑ Pectoralis minor
- ❑ Subclavius
  Serratus anterior
- ❑ External/internal intercostals

Bones
- ❑ Sternum
  - ❑ Manubrium
  - ❑ Body
  - ❑ Xiphoid process
  - ❑ Manubriosternal joint (angle of Louis, T4-T5)
- ❑ Clavicle
- ❑ 1st rib
- ❑ Ribs 2-12

Lymphatics
- ❑ Axillary node drainage (generally 6 recognized nodal groups with total of 35-40 nodes)
- ❑ Internal thoracic node drainage (~5 per side)
- ❑ Thoracic duct

Ligaments
- ❑ Suspensory ligaments of Cooper

Breast
- ❑ Areolar-nipple complex
- ❑ Superficial fascia (from anterior chest wall)
- ❑ Lobes (15-20)
- ❑ Tail of breast (Spence) into axilla
- ❑ Deep fascia

CHAPTER 5

LUNGS, REMOVAL OF HEART, AND POSTERIOR MEDIASTINUM

Netter: 184–206

McMinn: 187–188, 196–217

Gray's Atlas: 66–87, 102–113

OPENING THE THORACIC CAVITY

With a scalpel, transect the intercostal muscles, serratus anterior muscle, and a portion of the external abdominal oblique muscle (Figs. 5-1 to 5-3). Make sure that you start your dissection above the emergence of the intercostobrachial nerve and then descend toward the midaxillary line. With a saw or bone cutter, carefully cut the intercostal musculature

in the first intercostal space lateral to the manubrium, then extend these incisions downward, just anterior to the emergence of the anterior cutaneous branches of the intercostal nerves, cutting the ribs

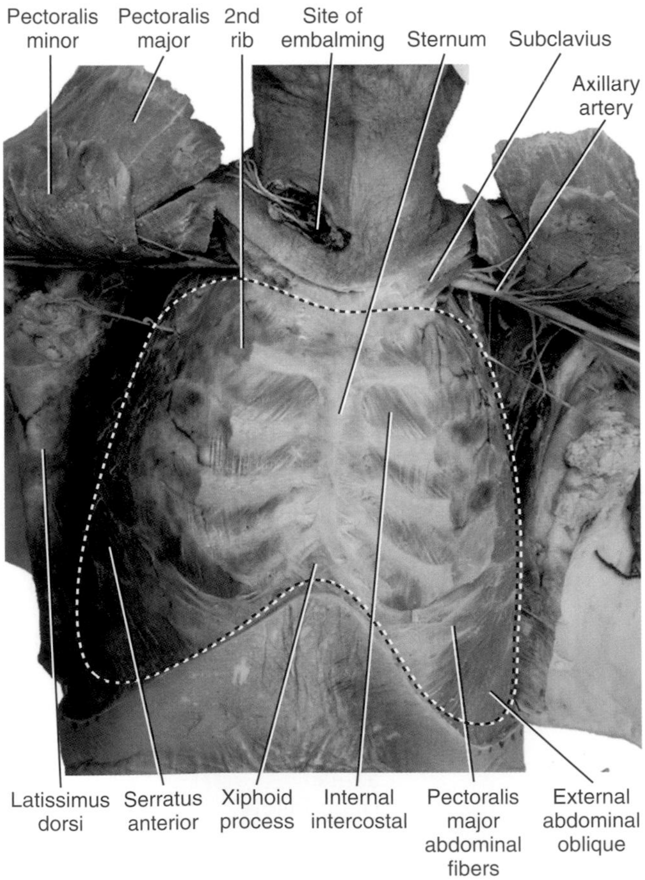

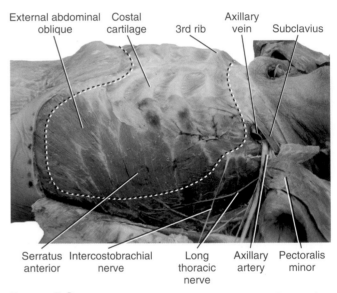

FIGURE 5-2. Anterolateral view of chest with tracing for incision to reveal deep chest structures.

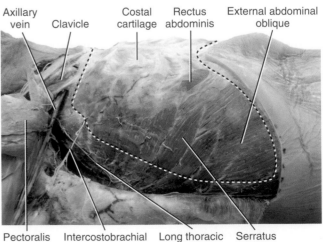

FIGURE 5-3. Anterolateral view of chest with tracing for incision to reveal deep chest structures.

FIGURE 5-1. Anterior chest wall with skin, fascia, and pectoralis major and minor reflected, revealing tracing of rib cage for deep dissection of chest contents.

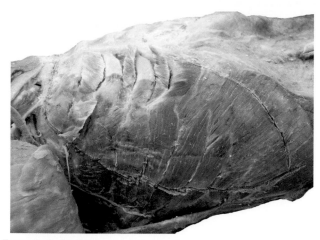

FIGURE 5-4. Anterolateral view of chest with incision to allow for thoracotomy.

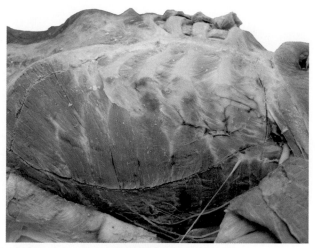

FIGURE 5-5. Anterolateral view of chest with incision to allow for thoracotomy.

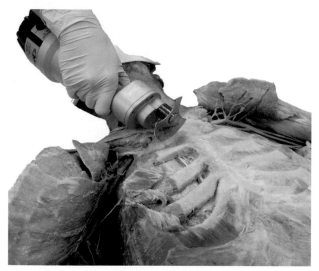

FIGURE 5-6. Skin, fascia, and pectoralis muscles reflected from anterior chest wall to reveal intercostal dissection of external intercostal muscles, as well as internal thoracic (mammary) artery and vein. Bone saw, cutters, or scalpel is used to make the bone incisions.

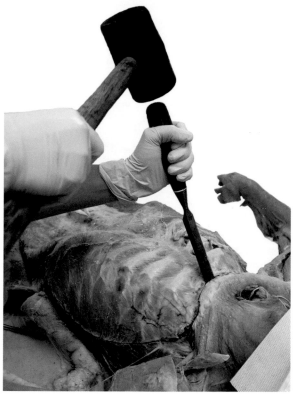

FIGURE 5-7. Anterolateral view of chest with incision to reveal deep chest structures. Use mallet and chisel to release bone and connective tissue to allow removal of anterior chest wall plate.

and intercostal musculature to the level of the 10th rib (Figs. 5-4 and 5-5). Divide the manubrium transversely above the sternal angle (Fig. 5-6). After making the saw cuts, use a scalpel and bone cutters to free the anterior thoracic wall completely. Try to avoid damage to the underlying lungs (Figs. 5-7 and 5-8).

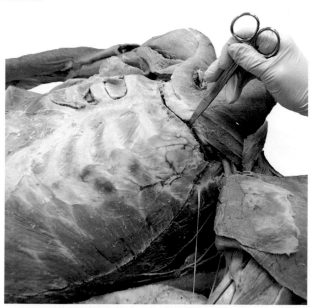

FIGURE 5-8. Anterolateral view of chest with incision to reveal deep chest structures. Once bone and connective tissue have been transected, use blunt scissors to lift chest plate.

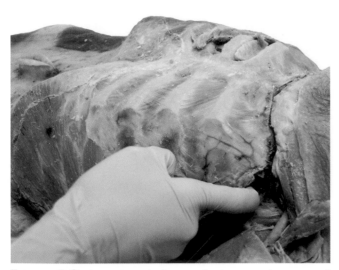

FIGURE 5-9. Anterolateral chest wall plate can be removed manually.

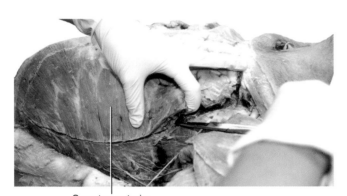

Serratus anterior

FIGURE 5-10. Anterolateral view of chest with incision to reveal deep chest structures. Use blunt dissection with scissors to remove the chest plate.

> ☝ *DISSECTION TIP:* Often, in the first and second intercostal spaces, you will be able to place your fingertips underneath the internal surface of the anterior thoracic wall and lift it up (Fig. 5-9). If some parts are still connected to the wall, use a scalpel and bone cutters to free the anterior thoracic wall (Figs. 5-10 and 5-11). Be careful when you place your fingertips under the exposed ribs; sharp spicules are often present and may cause injury. Use a bone cutter or rongeur to remove these.

Place you fingertips underneath the openings of the thoracic wall and pull up (Fig. 5-12). If the internal thoracic vessels are still intact, cut them and then pull the chest wall inferiorly, exposing the thoracic contents (Fig. 5-13). As you reflect the wall inferiorly, incise the parietal pleura from the internal surface of the anterior thoracic wall with a scalpel, leaving it intact over the lungs (Fig. 5-14). Cut the sternopericardial ligaments that connect the pericardial sac to the posterior surface of the sternum. Continue the reflection of the anterior thoracic wall downward, until the thoracic viscera can be clearly seen (Fig. 5-15). Keep the wall turned downward as the dissection proceeds (Fig. 5-16). Forcing the wall down will usually result in sufficient stretching or tearing of tissues so that the anterior wall remains reflected inferiorly. If this is not the case, you can remove the anterior thoracic wall (Fig. 5-17).

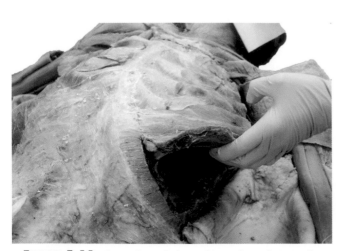

FIGURE 5-11. Anterolateral chest plate reflected manually.

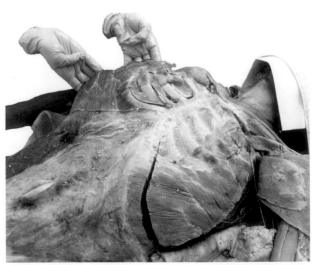

FIGURE 5-12. Anterolateral chest plate reflected manually. Release connective tissue deep to anterior chest wall plate bilaterally.

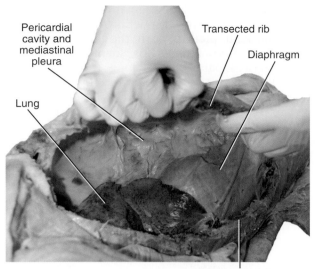

FIGURE 5-13. Partial reflection of anterior chest wall plate revealing deeper structures.

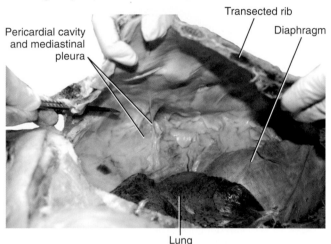

FIGURE 5-14. Partial reflection of anterior chest wall plate revealing deep structures.

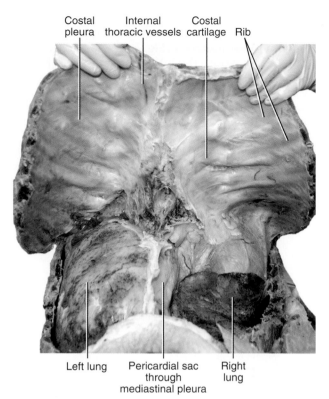

FIGURE 5-16. Bilateral reflection of anterior chest wall plate revealing deep internal structures.

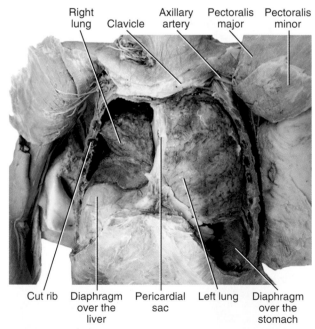

FIGURE 5-17. Anterior chest wall plate removed, revealing internal chest structures. Note that the right lung is collapsed. This is probably due to a pneumothorax that occurred during life.

FIGURE 5-15. Bilateral reflection of anterior chest wall plate revealing deep internal structures.

> ✋ *DISSECTION TIP:* The pleura is attached to the thoracic wall by a continuous layer of connective tissue, the endothoracic fascia. In some cadavers with previous pathology of the thorax, such as infections, the pleura may be thickened and adherent to the thoracic walls, making efforts to preserve it difficult.

Observe the internal surface of the anterior thoracic wall, and identify the internal thoracic arteries and veins and their branches (Fig. 5-18). Reflect the parietal pleura to expose the intercostal muscles. Reflecting the parietal pleura in the 1st and 2nd intercostal spaces exposes the internal thoracic artery. To expose the internal thoracic artery and vein further, reflect the transverse thoracis muscles. Identify the branches of the internal thoracic artery, such as the perforating and anterior intercostal branches (Fig. 5-19). Typically, the terminal branches of the internal thoracic artery—the superior epigastric and musculophrenic branches—are located close to the xiphoid process.

Identify the costodiaphragmatic and costomediastinal recesses. After inspecting the subdivisions of the parietal pleura, push the lung away from the heart with your fingertips. Identify the mediastinal pleura separating the lung from the heart. Insert the scissors and separate the mediastinal pleura from the pericardium (Figs. 5-20 and 5-21). Identify the phrenic nerve traveling anterior to the hilum of the lung and preserve it (Fig. 5-22). Use the separation technique to expose the pulmonary arteries and veins (Figs. 5-23 and 5-24). Use the

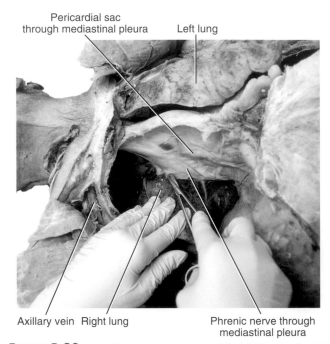

FIGURE 5-20. Anterior chest structures with right lung reflected to expose mediastinum to dissect for lung evacuation.

FIGURE 5-18. Undersurface of removed chest plate, revealing structures intimate with the chest plate.

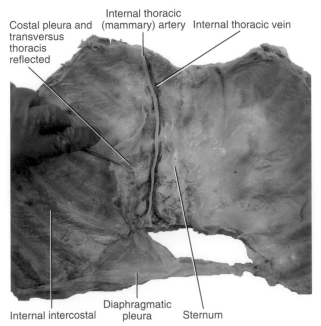

FIGURE 5-19. Undersurface of removed chest plate highlighting internal thoracic (mammary) artery.

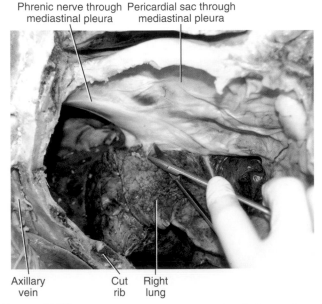

FIGURE 5-21. Anterior chest structures with right lung reflected to expose mediastinum.

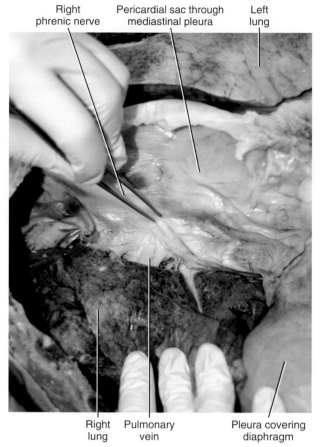

FIGURE 5-22. Anterior chest structures with right lung reflected to reveal mediastinum highlighting phrenic nerve intimate with pericardial sac.

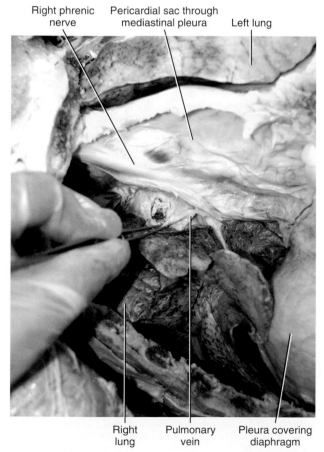

FIGURE 5-23. Anterior chest structures with right lung reflected to reveal the mediastinum and highlighting the phrenic nerve, which is in intimate contact with pericardial sac.

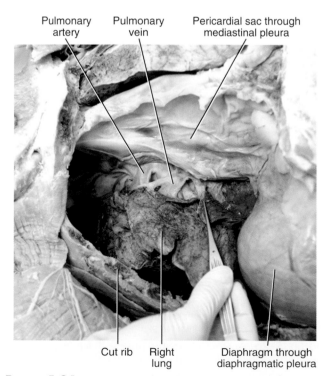

FIGURE 5-24. In the right pleural cavity, the pulmonary artery and vein are seen.

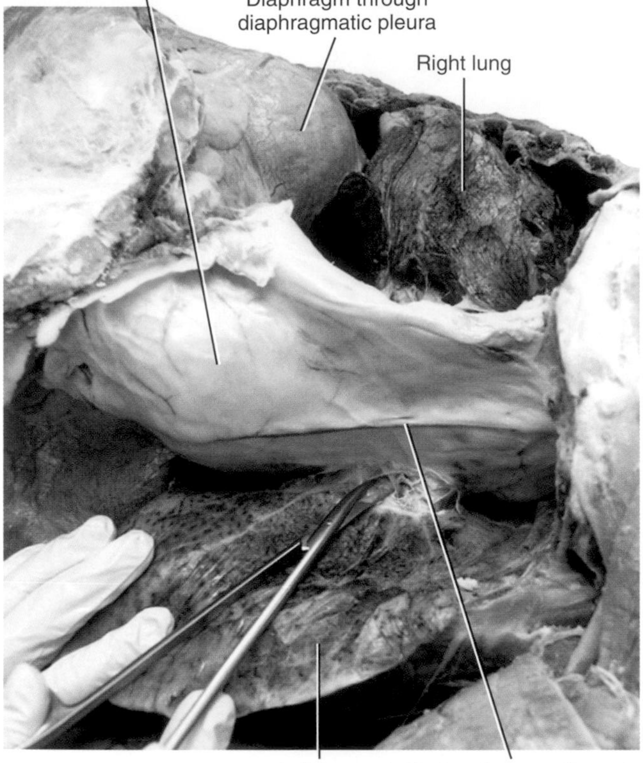

Pericardial sac through
mediastinal pleura

Diaphragm through
diaphragmatic pleura

Right lung

Left lung   Left phrenic nerve through
mediastinal pleura

FIGURE 5-25. Anterior chest structures with left lung reflected for hilar dissection.

Pericardial sac through
mediastinal pleura   Right lung

Left lung   Left phrenic nerve
and vessels through
mediastinal pleura

Left
pulmonary
artery

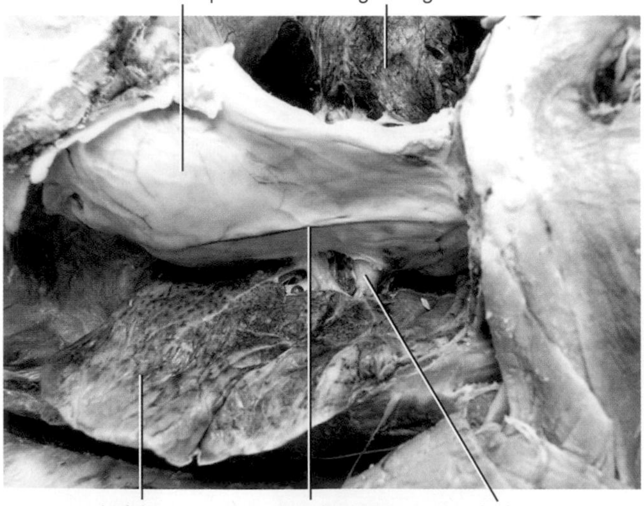

FIGURE 5-26. Anterior chest structures with left lung reflected for hilar dissection revealing pulmonary vessels.

same technique for the contralateral lung (Figs. 5-25 and 5-26).

> ✋ *DISSECTION TIP:* The costodiaphragmatic recess is usually the location where excess embalming fluids accumulate during dissection. Drain the fluid using a syringe, and place paper towels into the recess (Figs. 5-27 and 5-28). Also, once the lungs are removed, holes can be made in the posterior intercostal spaces so that fluid exits onto the dissection table. This method may necessitate placing a wedge or block under the thorax to lift the body slightly off of the dissecting table.

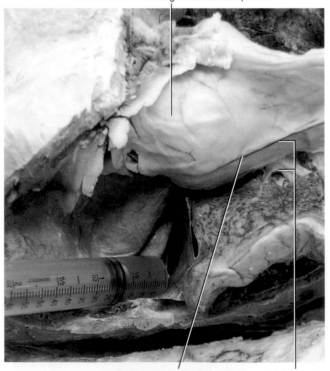

Pericardial sac through mediastinal pleura

Left phrenic nerve and vessels
through mediastinal pleura   Pulmonary
vessels

FIGURE 5-27. Anterolateral view of deep chest dissection. Syringe is placed into the costodiaphragmatic recess, and excess fluid is aspirated.

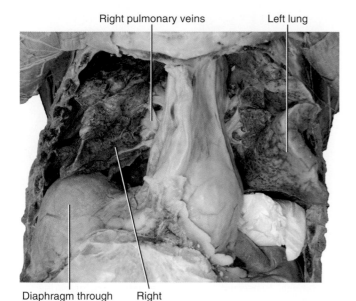

Right pulmonary veins — Left lung

Diaphragm through diaphragmatic pleura — Right lung

FIGURE 5-28. Breast plate removed, revealing deep chest structures. Right and left pulmonary veins are exposed.

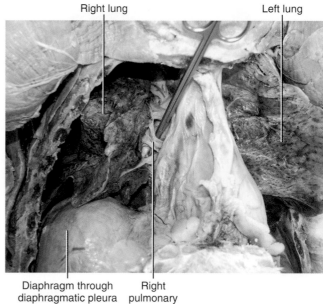

Right lung — Left lung

Diaphragm through diaphragmatic pleura — Right pulmonary veins

FIGURE 5-29. Right pulmonary vein exposed and lifted upward for transection.

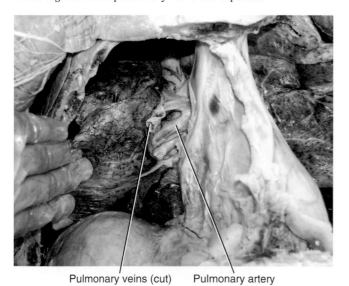

Pulmonary veins (cut) — Pulmonary artery

FIGURE 5-30. Right lung retraction revealing pulmonary artery after pulmonary veins have been removed.

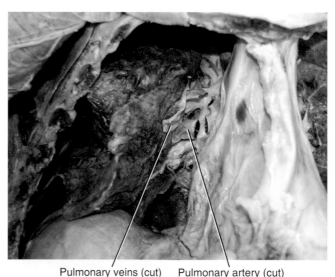

Pulmonary veins (cut) — Pulmonary artery (cut)

FIGURE 5-31. Right lung pulmonary vasculature transected.

After exposing the pulmonary arteries, pulmonary veins, and primary bronchi at the hila of the left and right lungs, transect them with scissors or a scalpel (Figs. 5-29 to 5-32). Remove the lungs from the thoracic cavity, and observe the posterior mediastinum covered with parietal pleura (Figs. 5-33 to 5-36).

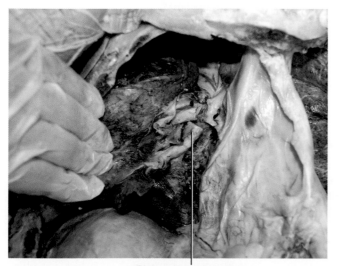

Right primary bronchus

FIGURE 5-32. Right lung pulmonary vasculature and airway (primary bronchus) transected.

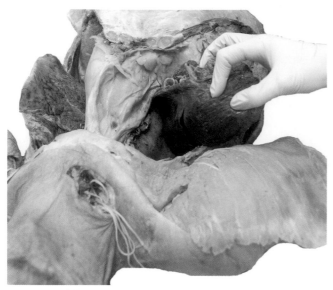

FIGURE 5-33. Removal of right lung from superior to inferior with medial retraction.

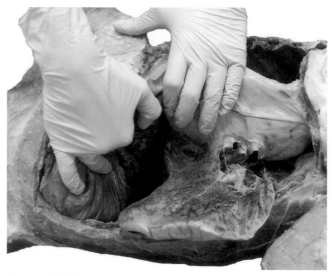

FIGURE 5-34. Removal of left lung with pulmonary vasculature and bronchi transected, using medial retraction, preparing for lung removal.

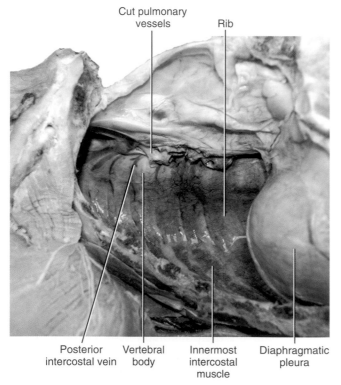

Cut pulmonary vessels   Rib

Posterior intercostal vein   Vertebral body   Innermost intercostal muscle   Diaphragmatic pleura

FIGURE 5-35. Right hemithorax with lung removed, revealing vertebral column and posterior chest wall.

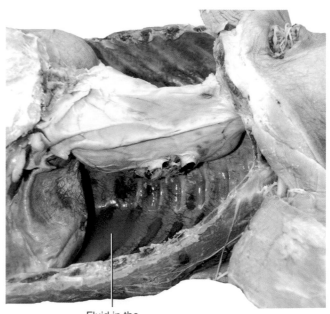

Fluid in the costodiaphragmatic recess

FIGURE 5-36. Bilateral lung removal with intact pericardial sac and contents.

> **DISSECTION TIP:** Often the lungs have adhesions far inferior and posterior to the hilum of the lung. To remove the lung completely, you will need to push the diaphragm inferiorly and explore with your fingertips the area posterior and inferior to the hilum so that such adhesions can be dissected free (Fig. 5-34).

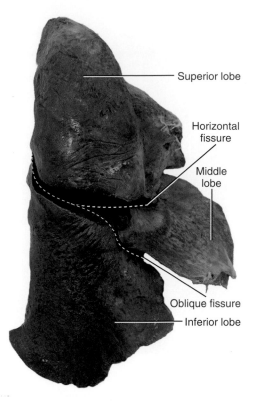

FIGURE 5-37. Right lung removed, revealing anterolateral external surfaces.

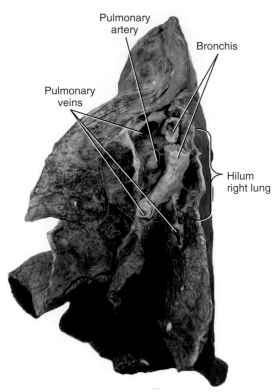

FIGURE 5-38. Isolated right lung with medial view highlighting structures of the hilum.

Place the lungs onto a tray, and examine the internal surface of each lung separately. For the right lung, identify the oblique and horizontal fissures and their corresponding upper, middle, and lower lobes (Fig. 5-37). Inspect the hilum of the lung, and identify the pulmonary arteries, pulmonary veins, and primary bronchi (Fig. 5-38).

> *DISSECTION TIP:* Note that the horizontal fissure will often appear to be incomplete in right lungs. To identify the pulmonary arteries and pulmonary veins at the hilum of the right lung, note that the pulmonary veins are located in the anterior aspect of the hilum, where the pulmonary arteries are usually located superior and anterior to the bronchi (Fig. 5-38).

Similar to the right lung, identify the oblique fissure in the left lung and the corresponding upper and lower lobes (Fig. 5-39). Inspect the hilum of the lung, and identify the pulmonary arteries, pulmonary veins, and primary bronchi (Fig. 5-40). Inferior to the hilum, trace the two layers of visceral pleura fusing together to form the pulmonary ligament (Fig. 5-41). Identify the cardiac notch on the superior lobe of the left lung and lingula at its inferior medial portion.

> ☝ *DISSECTION TIP:* To identify the pulmonary arteries and pulmonary veins at the hilum of the left lung, note that the pulmonary veins are located along the anterior aspect of the hilum, whereas the pulmonary arteries are usually found superior to the bronchi (Fig. 5-38).

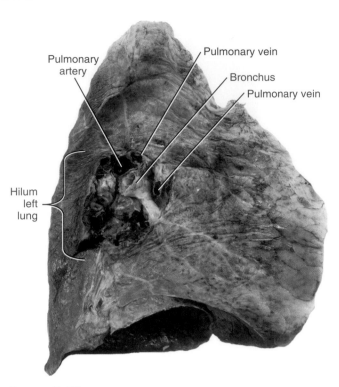

FIGURE 5-40. Removal of left lung with medial view highlighting hilum structures.

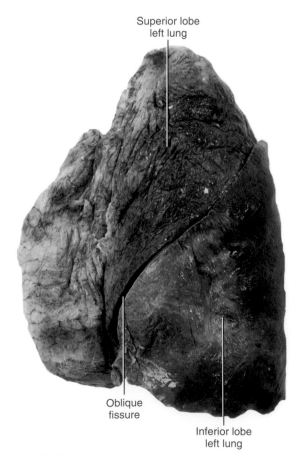

FIGURE 5-39. Removal of left lung revealing external surfaces.

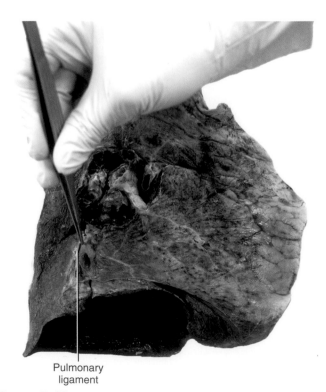

FIGURE 5-41. Removal of left lung with medial view highlighting pulmonary ligament.

Optional Lung Dissection

The lung contents can be dissected to expose a single segmental bronchus, segmental artery, and segmental vein. The portion of lung supplied by the segmental bronchus, artery, and vein is defined as a *bronchopulmonary segment*. With your forceps, lift the bronchus, and using blunt dissection, separate it from the lung parenchyma. Remove most of the internal lung parenchyma with your forceps and scissors, leaving its borders and lateral walls intact (Fig. 5-42). In the right lung, you will be able to dissect the superior, middle, and inferior lobar bronchi. Each lobar bronchus branches off into several segmental bronchi, and each of these supply one bronchopulmonary segment. The right lung contains 10 to 12 bronchopulmonary segments, and the left lung contains 10. When you reach a bronchopulmonary segment, note the relationships among the artery, vein, and bronchus. The segmental arteries are located posterior to the segmental bronchi, and the segmental veins are between two adjacent bronchopulmonary segments.

> ✋ *DISSECTION TIP:* As it passes superior to the right pulmonary artery, the right superior lobar bronchus is named the *eparterial bronchus.*

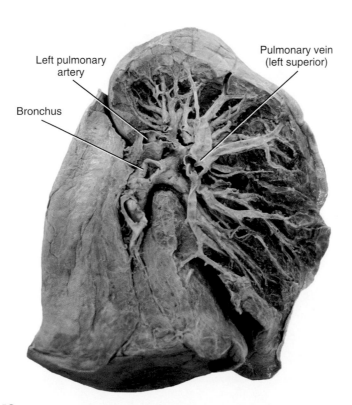

Left pulmonary artery

Pulmonary vein (left superior)

Bronchus

FIGURE 5-42. Removal of left lung with medial view revealing bronchopulmonary segments.

REMOVAL OF HEART

Before removing the heart from the pericardial cavity, the phrenic nerves need to be identified and preserved. Observe the pericardiacophrenic vein at the lateral border of the pericardial sac bilaterally. Dissect out the pericardium next to the pericardiacophrenic vein, and identify the phrenic nerve (Figs. 5-43 and 5-44). The phrenic nerve is accompanied by the pericardiacophrenic artery, a branch of the internal thoracic artery. Dissect the phrenic nerve along its entire length, from the top of the thoracic cavity to its penetration into the diaphragm (Figs. 5-45 and 5-46).

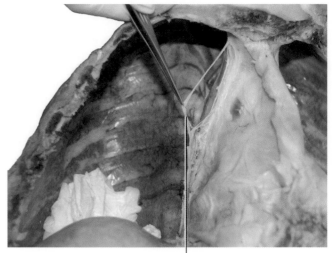

Right phrenic nerve

FIGURE 5-45. Bilateral lung removal with intact pericardial sac and contents revealing right phrenic nerve.

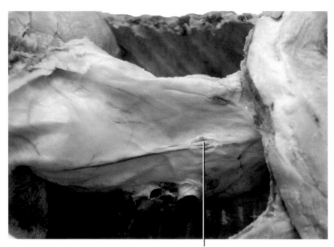

Left phrenic nerve and
pericardiacophrenic vein

FIGURE 5-43. Bilateral lung removal with intact pericardial sac and contents.

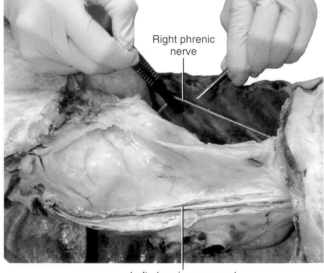

Right phrenic nerve

Left phrenic nerve and
pericardiacophrenic vessels

FIGURE 5-46. Intact pericardial sac and contents with dissected phrenic nerve and pericardiacophrenic vessels.

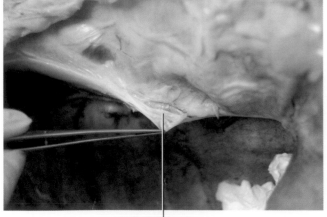

Left phrenic nerve

FIGURE 5-44. Left hemithorax with intact pericardial sac revealing left phrenic nerve.

With toothed forceps, lift the right inferolateral edge of the pericardium near the diaphragm, and make a small incision (Fig. 5-47). Note the attachment of the pericardium to the central tendon of the diaphragm. Make a transverse incision in the pericardium parallel to the diaphragmatic surface (Fig. 5-48). Make a second, connecting vertical incision through the pericardium along the side of the right atrium (Fig. 5-49) and along the side of the left ventricle (Fig. 5-50). Note that the parietal pericardium and the visceral pericardium (epicardium) are continuous with the great vessels as they pierce the fibrous pericardium.

> **✦ DISSECTION TIP:** When the pericardial sac is first opened, a small amount of serous fluid is often seen.

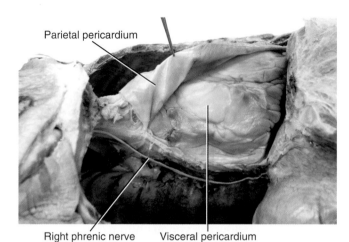

FIGURE 5-49. Reflected pericardial sac revealing visceral pericardium of heart.

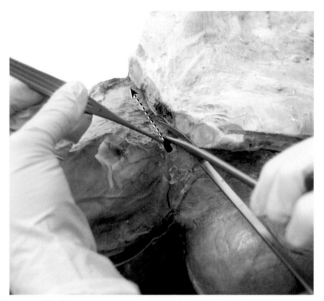

FIGURE 5-47. Anterior view of pericardial sac with tracing for transverse incision *(dotted arrow)* of pericardial sac.

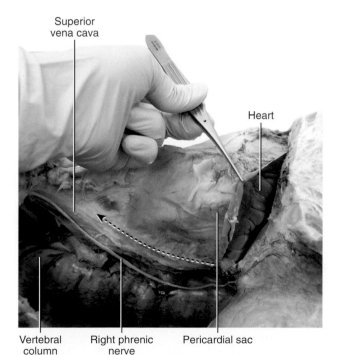

FIGURE 5-48. Anterolateral view of pericardial sac with base reflected and tracing for lateral vertical incision *(dotted arrow)*.

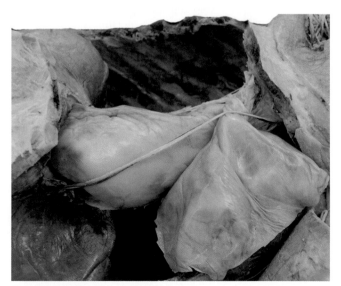

FIGURE 5-50. Anterolateral reflection of pericardial sac while maintaining an intact left phrenic nerve.

External Inspection

For orientation of the heart within the pericardial cavity, observe the position of the right atrium, right auricle, right ventricle and its outflow tract, and pulmonary trunk. Note the left atrium, left ventricle and apex of the heart, and anterior and posterior interventricular grooves. The right ventricle forms the sternocostal surface and part of the diaphragmatic surface of the heart. The left or pulmonary surface is composed mainly of the left ventricle. The right ventricle forms the sternocostal surface and part of the diaphragmatic surface of the heart. Note that the right ventricle is the most anterior part of the heart and is almost in contact with the sternum.

Sinuses

Note the position of the inferior vena cava, which is located inferior and to the right between the heart and the diaphragm. The reflections of the pericardium lead to the formation of two so-called sinuses within the pericardial cavity, the transverse and oblique pericardial sinuses. To identify the oblique pericardial sinus, lift the apex of the heart laterally and to the right with your fingertips, and expose the blindly ending space in the pericardial cavity behind the heart and below the venous hilum (Fig. 5-51). The venous hilum contains the four pulmonary veins and the superior and inferior venae cavae. The sleevelike investment of visceral pericardium around these vessels and the roof of the left atrium reflects to show the parietal pericardial sac, forming the inverted, U-shaped oblique sinus. If you place your fingers in front of the atria and directly behind the aorta and pulmonary artery, you will occupy the space known as the *transverse pericardial sinus* (Fig. 5-52).

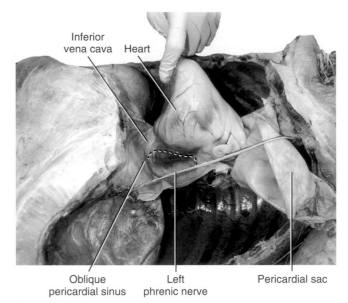

FIGURE 5-51. Reflected pericardial sac with apex of heart reflected anteriorly to reveal the oblique sinus *(dotted line)*.

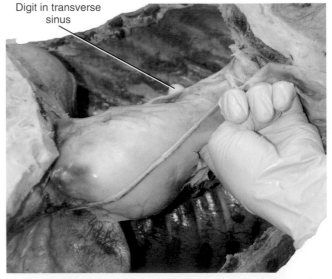

FIGURE 5-52. Reflected pericardial sac with placement of digit through transverse sinus.

Technique

To remove the heart, first lift its apex upward and expose the inferior vena cava, then transect it (Figs. 5-53 and 5-54). With scissors, separate the adhesions between the heart (posteriorly) and pericardium, and lift the heart upward to expose the left atrium (Figs. 5-55 and 5-56).

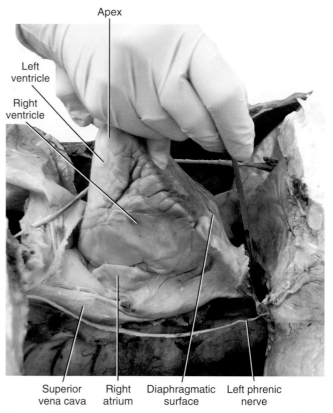

FIGURE 5-54. Apex of heart reflected anteriorly to allow transection of inferior vena cava.

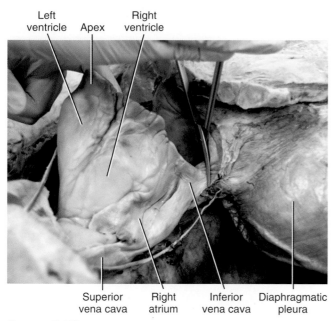

FIGURE 5-53. Apex of heart reflected anteriorly to allow transection of inferior vena cava.

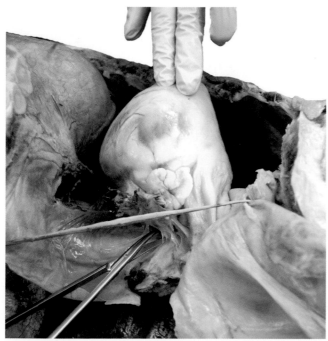

FIGURE 5-55. With the apex of the heart lifted, scissors are used to separate the pericardium from the posterior surface of heart.

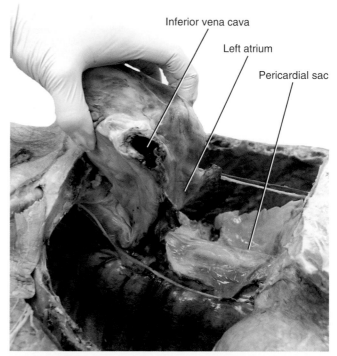

FIGURE 5-56. Apex of heart reflected anterosuperiorly, revealing cut inferior vena cava, left atrium, and posterior pericardial structures.

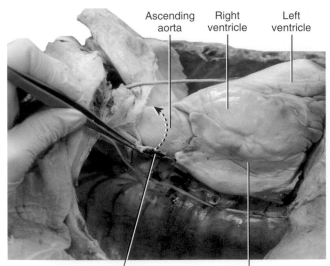

FIGURE 5-57. With the pericardial sac displaced laterally and the superior vena cava cut, the ascending aorta is identified. The dotted arrow notes the region of the aorta to be transected.

Cut the superior vena cava (Fig. 5-57). Next, cut the ascending aorta and the pulmonary trunk (Figs. 5-58 and 5-59). Remove the heart from the pericardial cavity.

> ☞ *DISSECTION TIP:* In some hearts, the pulmonary veins are adherent to the pericardium. Place some tension on the heart and lift it upward. If necessary, place the scissors between the pulmonary veins and the pericardium and separate the two.

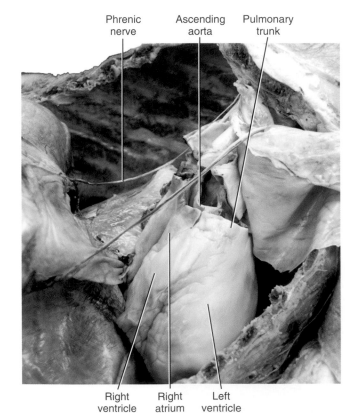

FIGURE 5-58. External view of heart with transected great vessels.

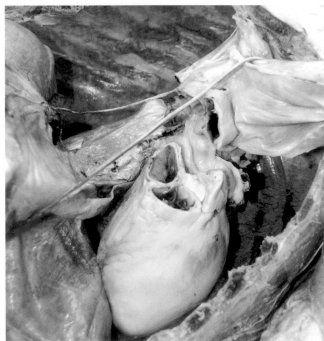

FIGURE 5-59. External view of heart with transected great vessels.

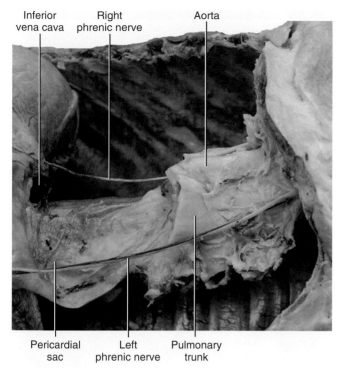

Inferior vena cava   Right phrenic nerve   Aorta

Pericardial sac   Left phrenic nerve   Pulmonary trunk

FIGURE 5-60. Bilateral lung removal, with the anterior part of the pericardial sac and heart removed.

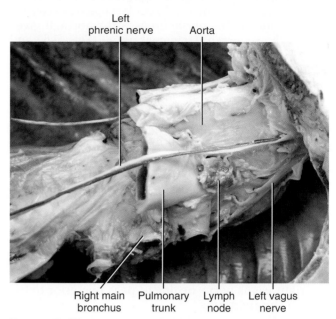

Left phrenic nerve   Aorta

Right main bronchus   Pulmonary trunk   Lymph node   Left vagus nerve

FIGURE 5-61. A closer view of Fig. 5-60 shows the left vagus nerve and a regional lymph node.

Observe the left side of the thoracic cavity, specifically the lateral side of the aortic arch and the pulmonary trunk (Figs. 5-60 and 5-61). Identify and trace the left vagus nerve over the arch of the aorta (Fig. 5-60). Note the relationship between the vagus and phrenic nerves. With forceps, pull the pulmonary trunk downward, and dissect the space (aortopulmonary window) between the aorta and the pulmonary trunk (Fig. 5-62). Identify the ligamentum arteriosum,

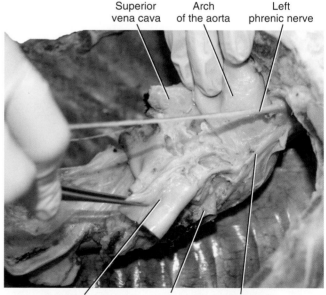

Superior vena cava   Arch of the aorta   Left phrenic nerve

Pulmonary trunk pulled inferiorly   Left pulmonary artery   Left vagus nerve

FIGURE 5-62. With the pulmonary trunk displaced inferiorly, note the relationship of the phrenic and vagus nerves to the hilum of the lung. The phrenic nerve travels anterior and the vagus nerve posterior to the hilum of the lung.

the connection between the left pulmonary artery and the arch of the aorta. Identify the trachea and its bifurcation into the left and right bronchi. The vagus nerves give rise to the recurrent laryngeal nerves. On the left side, as the nerve crosses the aorta, it gives rise to the recurrent laryngeal nerve (Figs. 5-63 and 5-64). Clean the left vagus nerve, and where the left vagus crosses the aortic arch, locate the left recurrent laryngeal nerve.

The left recurrent laryngeal nerve passes under the ligamentum arteriosum and courses upward between the trachea/esophagus and the ascending aorta in the tracheoesophageal groove. The right recurrent laryngeal nerve arises from the right vagus nerve at the level of the right subclavian artery and turns back superiorly behind this vessel, to pass upward and medially toward the larynx and enter the tracheoesophageal groove.

Along the right side of the trachea (or esophagus) identify and clean the right vagus nerve. This nerve can be found by probing between the azygos vein and the lateral aspect of the trachea, at which point the right vagus nerve begins to pass posterior to the root of the right lung.

Expose the tracheal bifurcation, and identify the carinal (inferior tracheobronchial) lymph nodes. A nerve plexus anterior to the carina can be seen by cutting into the trachea at its bifurcation. The nerves represent the deep cardiac plexus formed by sympathetic and vagal fibers.

> ✋ *DISSECTION TIP:* Dissect the tracheobronchial lymph nodes; these nodes often are enlarged from malignant disease (Fig. 5-65).

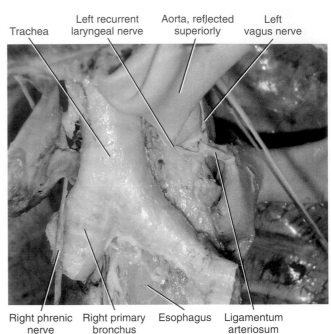

FIGURE 5-64. Deep mediastinal structures include right and left bronchus and vagus, phrenic, and recurrent laryngeal nerves.

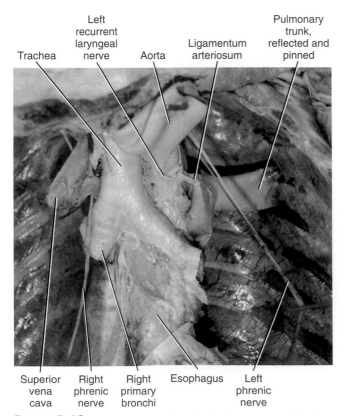

FIGURE 5-63. Anterior view of mediastinal structures, including the aorta, trachea, and esophagus.

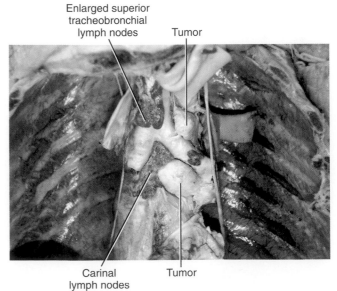

FIGURE 5-65. Anterior view of mediastinal structures revealing lymph nodes, right and left bronchus, reflected ascending aorta, and tumor intimate with left bronchus.

Remove the pericardium over the esophagus. With forceps, lift the esophagus and remove the pleura from the esophagus and the vertebral column (Figs. 5-66 and 5-67). After removal of the pleura, dissect the fatty layer present over the vertebral bodies. Dissect between the esophagus and the vertebral bodies to identify the thoracic duct (Fig. 5-68), which often looks similar to adipose tissue. Clean and preserve the thoracic duct (Fig. 5-69). With forceps, lift the pleura, and with the aid of scissors, separate the pleura from the underlying tissues over the ribs (Figs. 5-70 and 5-71).

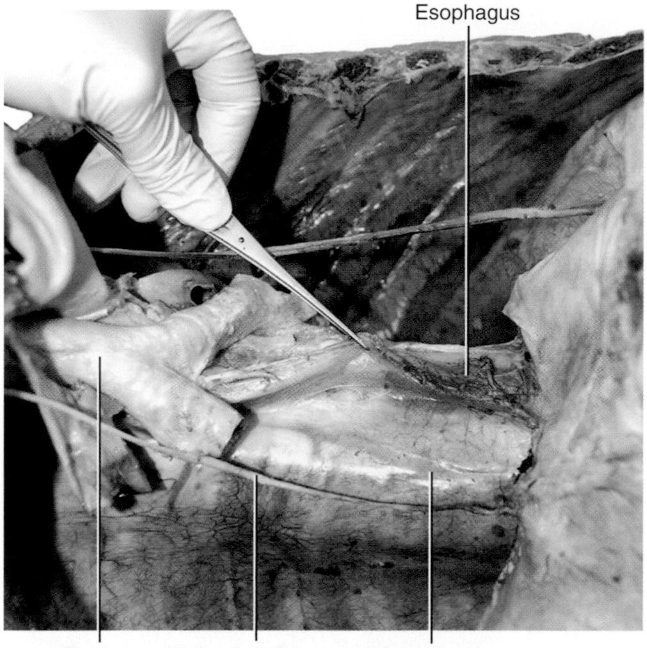

Esophagus

Trachea   Right phrenic nerve   Azygos vein

FIGURE 5-66. Anterolateral view of the posterior mediastinum. Note that the esophagus is being retracted laterally.

Esophagus

Azygos vein

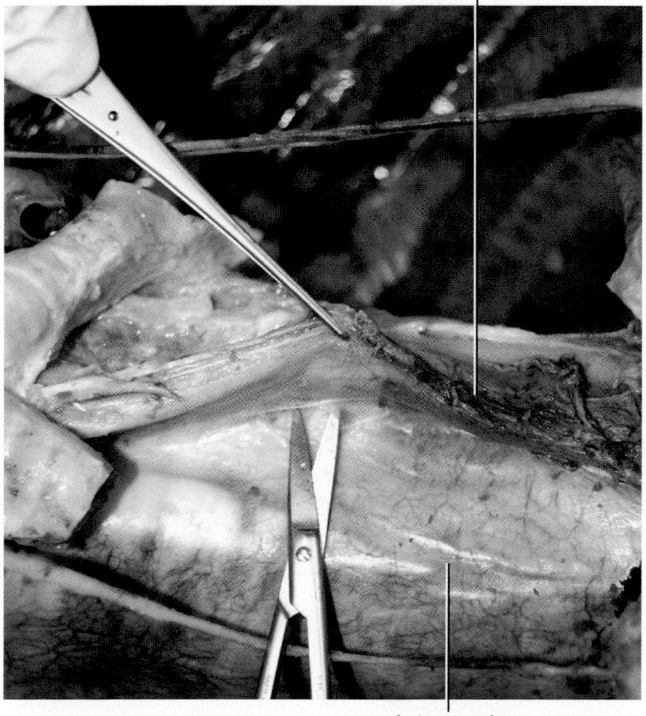

FIGURE 5-67. Anterolateral view of deep posterior mediastinal structures with tension on mediastinal pleura.

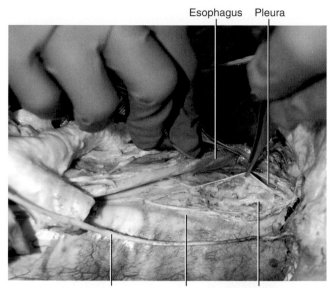

Esophagus   Pleura

Phrenic nerve   Azygos vein   Thoracic duct

FIGURE 5-68. Anterolateral view of deep posterior mediastinal structures highlighting the thoracic duct, esophagus, and azygos vein.

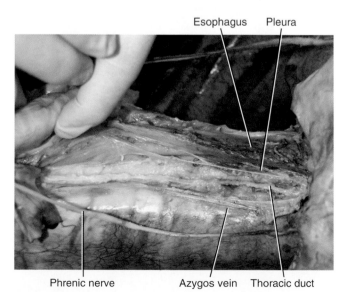

Esophagus   Pleura

Phrenic nerve   Azygos vein   Thoracic duct

FIGURE 5-69. Anterolateral view of deep posterior mediastinal structures demonstrating the thoracic duct, esophagus, and azygos vein.

> ☝ *DISSECTION TIP:* To reflect the pleura, use the tip of the scissors or a probe, and scrape the tissue between the pleura and the ribs. Do not cut any tissue with the forceps; use it as a probe (Figs. 5-70 and 5-71).

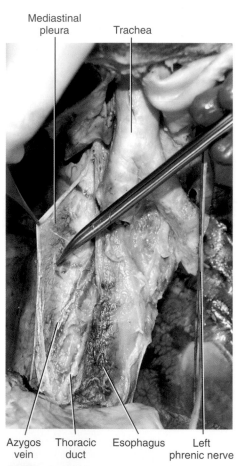

FIGURE 5-70. Anterior view of deep mediastinal structures revealing azygos vein, thoracic duct, and esophagus.

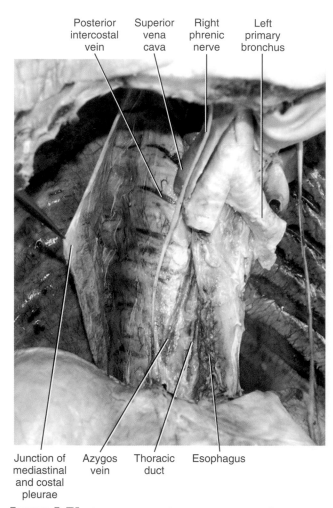

FIGURE 5-71. Anterior view of posterior chest wall structures revealing posterior intercostal vein, azygos vein, superior vena cava, and interface between mediastinal and costal pleurae.

Remove the majority of pleura from the thoracic cavity (Fig. 5-72). Trace the intercostal vein, artery, and nerve traveling in one of the posterior intercostal spaces.

> ☝ *DISSECTION TIP:* Use the handle of your scissors to remove fat over the intercostal space (Fig. 5-73).

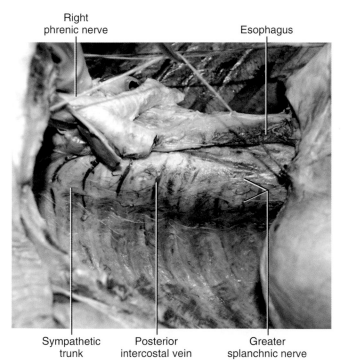

FIGURE 5-72. Right lateral view of posterior chest wall revealing sympathetic trunk, greater splanchnic nerves, and posterior intercostal vein.

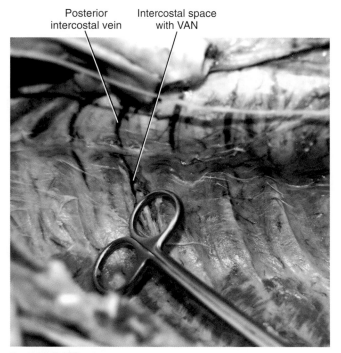

FIGURE 5-73. Right lateral view of posterior chest wall revealing neurovascular structures of the intercostal space at T4. *VAN,* Vein, artery, nerve.

Trace and identify the sympathetic trunk that runs along the junction between the vertebral bodies and ribs and appears as a white line. Near the midportion of the thoracic vertebral column, identify a bundle of nerve fibers originating from the sympathetic chain and running obliquely toward the midline (Fig. 5-74). This is the *greater splanchnic nerve,* formed primarily from fibers derived from the 5th to 9th thoracic (T5-T9) nerves. Clean the sympathetic chain and identify the greater (T5-T9), lesser (T10-11), and least (T12) splanchnic nerves (Fig. 5-75). After cleaning out the sympathetic chain and thoracic splanchnic nerves, dissect and clean the communicating rami connecting the sympathetic chain with the intercostal nerves. Identify the white and gray rami communicantes (Fig. 5-76). Trace the left and right vagus nerves as they descend behind the right and left primary bronchi to form the esophageal plexus on the anterior surface of the esophagus (Fig. 5-77).

> **DISSECTION TIP:** The origin of the greater, lesser, and least splanchnic nerves is subject to variation. Also, the lesser and least splanchnic nerves are often difficult to see in the thorax before removal of the liver on the right, and because of an immobile descending thoracic aorta on the left.

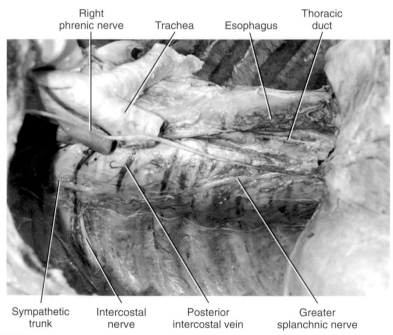

Right phrenic nerve   Trachea   Esophagus   Thoracic duct

Sympathetic trunk   Intercostal nerve   Posterior intercostal vein   Greater splanchnic nerve

FIGURE 5-74. Right lateral view of posterior chest wall demonstrating the sympathetic trunk, greater splanchnic nerve, and intercostal nerve.

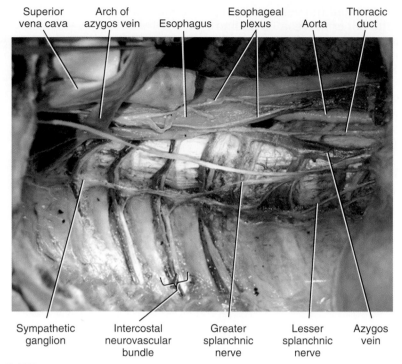

FIGURE 5-75. Right lateral view of posterior chest wall highlighting sympathetic trunk, sympathetic ganglion, and greater and lesser splanchnic nerves.

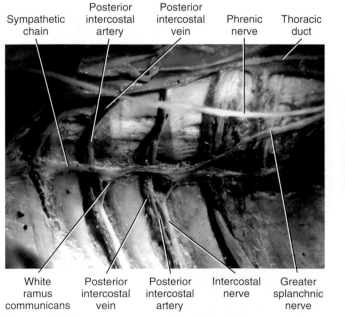

FIGURE 5-76. Right lateral view of posterior chest wall with sympathetic trunk, white ramus communicans, and intercostal nerve.

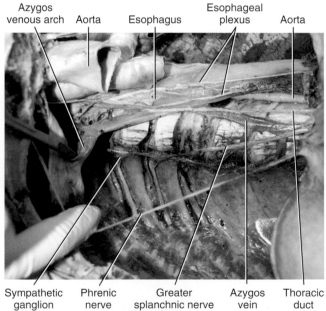

FIGURE 5-77. Right lateral view of posterior chest wall revealing azygos vein, sympathetic trunk, ganglion, and splanchnic nerve.

Trace the superior vena cava and the veins draining into it. To the right of the superior vena cava, find the azygos vein draining into it (Fig. 5-77). Identify the right posterior intercostal veins anterior and superior to the vertebral bodies. On the left side of the thorax, identify the hemiazygos vein with the lowest three or four left posterior intercostal venous tributaries. Lift the esophagus at the midline, and note the accessory hemiazygos vein crossing the midline to join the azygos vein (Fig. 5-78).

✍ *DISSECTION TIP:* The arch of the aorta and the descending thoracic aorta can be displaced or atherosclerotic, making the dissection of the left posterior thorax difficult. Often the greater, lesser, and least splanchnic nerves, as well as the hemiazygos and accessory hemiazygos veins, are hidden behind the aorta.

Lift the midportion the thoracic aorta, and note the origin of the posterior intercostal arteries. Identify the esophageal and bronchial arteries arising from the anterior aspect of the aorta (Figs. 5-79 and 5-80).

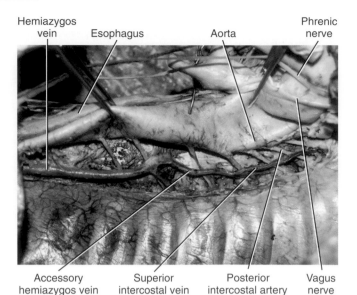

FIGURE 5-78. Left lateral view of posterior thoracic wall revealing accessory azygos and accessory hemiazygos veins.

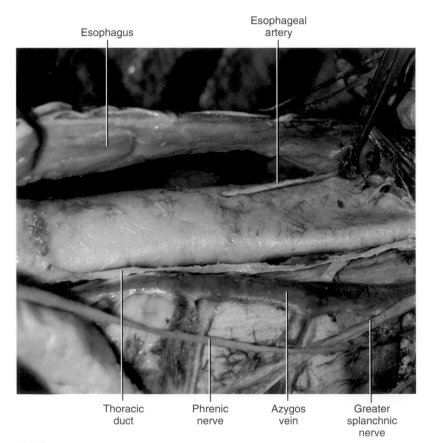

FIGURE 5-79. Right lateral view of posterior chest wall demonstrating the esophagus, esophageal artery, aorta, thoracic duct, and azygos vein.

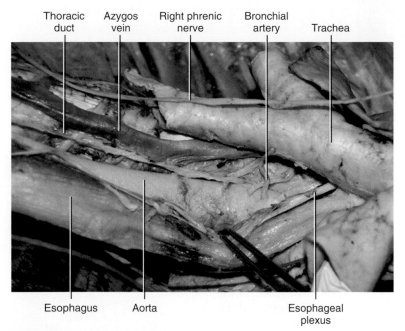

FIGURE 5-80. Left lateral view of posterior mediastinum with the esophagus and esophageal plexus reflected demonstrating the aorta, thoracic duct, and azygos vein.

LABORATORY IDENTIFICATION CHECKLIST

Nerves
- ❐ Anterior intercostal
- ❐ Intercostobrachial T2
- ❐ Lateral intercostal T3-T7
- ❐ Intercostal
- ❐ Sympathetic trunk
- ❐ Sympathetic ganglia
- ❐ Gray and white rami communicantes
- ❐ Stellate ganglion
- ❐ Phrenic
- ❐ Vagus
- ❐ Right recurrent laryngeal
- ❐ Left recurrent laryngeal
- ❐ Esophageal plexus
- ❐ Cardiac plexus

Arteries
- ❐ Aorta
- ❐ Subclavian
- ❐ Internal thoracic
- ❐ Superior epigastric
- ❐ Musculophrenic
- ❐ Pericardiacophrenic
- ❐ Pulmonary
- ❐ Bronchial
- ❐ Esophageal
- ❐ Anterior intercostal
- ❐ Posterior intercostal

Veins
- ❐ Superior vena cava
- ❐ Inferior vena cava
- ❐ Subclavian
- ❐ Internal thoracic
- ❐ Superior epigastric
- ❐ Brachiocephalic
- ❐ Anterior intercostal
- ❐ Posterior intercostal
- ❐ Azygos
- ❐ Accessory hemiazygos
- ❐ Hemiazygos

Muscles
- ❐ External intercostal
- ❐ Internal intercostal
- ❐ Innermost intercostal
- ❐ Transverse thoracis (sternocostalis) muscle
- ❐ Subcostals
- ❐ Diaphragm

Lymphatics
- ❐ Thoracic duct

Ligament
- ❐ Ligamentum arteriosum

Gland
- ❐ Thymus

Organ Tissues
- ❐ Lung
- ❐ Parietal pleura
- ❐ Visceral pleura
- ❐ Pulmonary ligament
- ❐ Lobes of right and left lungs
- ❐ Hilum
- ❐ Primary bronchi
- ❐ Secondary bronchi
- ❐ Tertiary bronchi
- ❐ Lingula
- ❐ Apex of heart
- ❐ Base of heart
- ❐ Oblique fissure
- ❐ Esophagus

Bones
- ❐ Sternum
- ❐ Ribs
- ❐ Bodies of thoracic vertebrae with intervertebral discs

CHAPTER 6

HEART

Netter: 208–220, 462, 465

McMinn: 189–195

Gray's Atlas: 88–100

INSPECTION

Inspect the heart externally and identify the right atrium, right auricle, superior vena cava (SVC), inferior vena cava (IVC), conus or infundibulum, pulmonary artery, ascending aorta, left atrium, pulmonary veins, and left auricle (Figs. 6-1 to 6-4). Identify the *sulcus terminalis,* a shallow groove in the roof of the right atrium, which extends between the right side of the orifice of the SVC and that of the IVC.

The dissection typically begins with the exposure and identification of the coronary arteries. Note the apex of the left ventricle and the *acute* (right) and *obtuse* (left) margins of the heart.

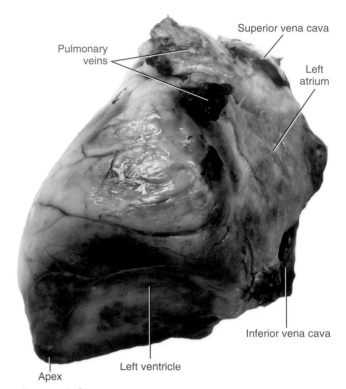

FIGURE 6-2. Topographic view of left atrium and ventricle.

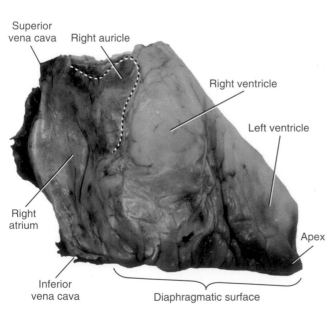

FIGURE 6-1. Anterior view of external surfaces of the heart; *dotted outline*, right auricle.

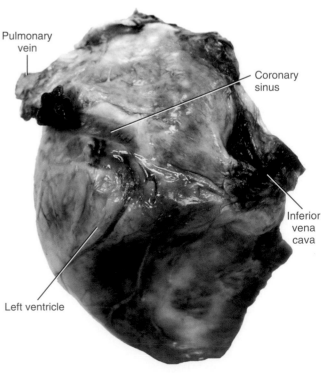

FIGURE 6-3. Topographic view of the posterior heart.

82

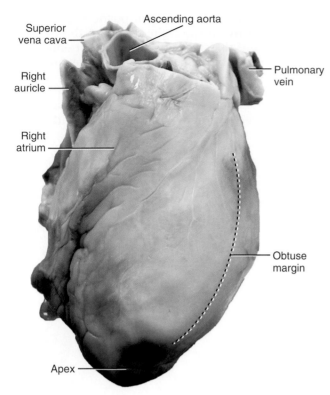

Superior
vena cava

Ascending aorta

Pulmonary
vein

Right
auricle

Right
atrium

Obtuse
margin

Apex

FIGURE 6-4. Base, margin, and apex of topographic heart; *dotted line,* obtuse margin.

Coronary Arteries

To remove the epicardium (visceral pericardium) and the fat covering the right coronary artery, identify the right auricle and retract it laterally. Palpate the space between the right auricle and the atrioventricular (AV, coronary) groove or sulcus, and expose the proximal part of the right coronary artery (Fig. 6-5).

> ✋ *DISSECTION TIP:* Most of the coronary arteries in adults can be felt with palpation because of their increased hardening from atherosclerotic changes of aging. The terms *atrium* and *auricle* are not synonymous. The auricles are appendages of the atria.

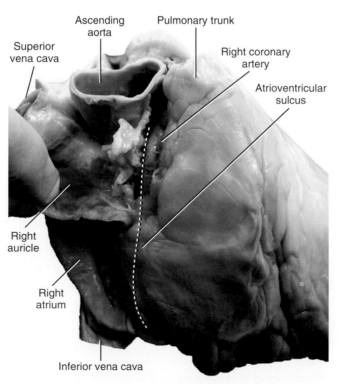

Ascending
aorta

Pulmonary trunk

Superior
vena cava

Right coronary
artery

Atrioventricular
sulcus

Right
auricle

Right
atrium

Inferior vena cava

FIGURE 6-5. Topographic view of base of heart structures; *dotted line,* tracing of right coronary artery.

Expose the superficial portion of the *right coronary artery* (RCA) by cleaning away the epicardium and fat covering the vessel (Figs. 6-6 to 6-8). Trace the RCA toward the right side of the diaphragmatic surface of the heart, taking care to protect its branches. As the artery passes near the edge of the right auricle, it usually gives off the artery of the sinu-atrial node (Fig. 6-9). The sinu-atrial (SA) nodal artery arises in 65% of cases from the proximal portion of the RCA, traveling upward to the right atrium at the junction of the SVC and the right auricle, where it enters the sinus node. In the remaining cases, the SA nodal artery arises from the proximal portion of the left coronary artery. The second branch of the RCA is the artery of the conus, or *conal artery.* The conal artery arises from the proximal part of the RCA and passes

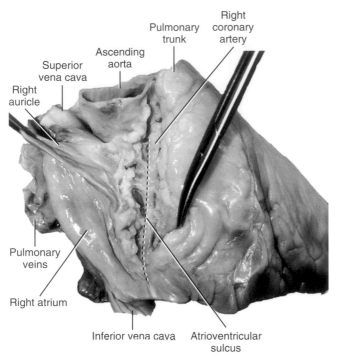

FIGURE 6-6. Early dissection between right atrium and ventricle revealing right coronary artery.

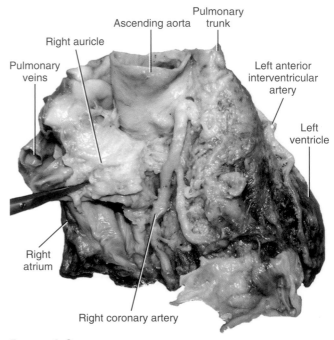

FIGURE 6-8. Dissection of right coronary artery from its origin.

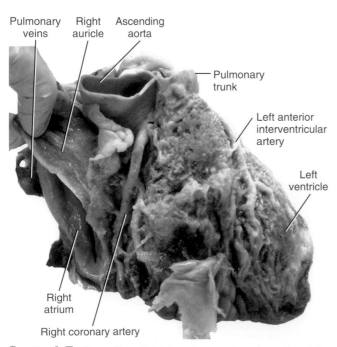

FIGURE 6-7. Dissection of right coronary artery from its origin.

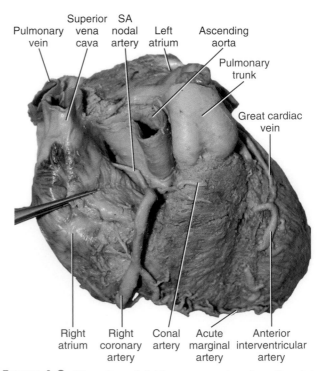

FIGURE 6-9. Dissection of right coronary artery from its origin. *SA,* Sinu-atrial.

to the left, around the right ventricle, at the level of the subpulmonary infundibulum (Fig. 6-9). Close to the diaphragmatic surface of the heart, the RCA typically gives rise to the right marginal artery, which supplies the inferior border of the right ventricle.

The RCA continues posteriorly in the AV groove and in most cases will descend and terminate in the posterior interventricular groove as the posterior interventricular (descending) artery (Fig. 6-10). This artery supplies the inferior third of the interventricular septum and a portion of the inferior wall of the left ventricle. Lastly, before it becomes the posterior interventricular artery, the RCA will give off the artery of the atrioventricular (AV) node. In 80% of specimens, the AV nodal artery arises from the RCA near the posterior interventricular groove as it crosses the "crux" of the heart (Fig. 6-11).

> ✍ *DISSECTION TIP:* To identify the artery to the AV node, carefully lift the left atrium at the posterior AV groove, and clean away the fat (Fig. 6-11, *B*). The crux of the heart is the center point of the anatomic base where the atria and ventricles are most closely approximated posteriorly.

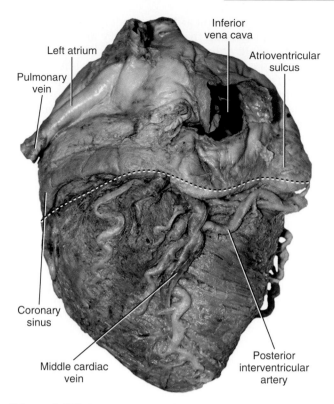

FIGURE 6-10. Posterior view of heart with the posterior interventricular artery and middle cardiac vein exposed.

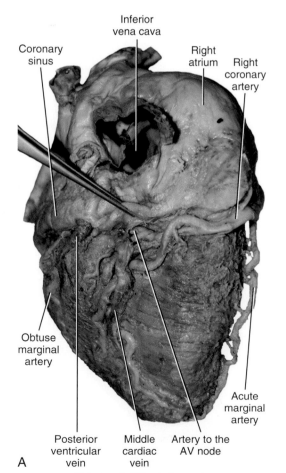

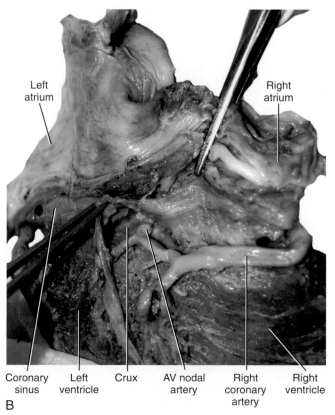

FIGURE 6-11. A, Posterior view of heart with posterior interventricular artery and artery to the atrioventricular (AV) node exposed. **B,** Left atrium pulled back to reveal AV nodal artery within crux of heart.

To remove the epicardium (visceral pericardium) and the fat covering the left coronary artery, identify the left auricle and retract it laterally (Figs. 6-12 and 6-13). Palpate the space between the left auricle, the AV (coronary) sulcus, and expose the proximal part of the left coronary artery (Figs. 6-14 and 6-15). The left coronary artery is typically very small (a few centimeters in length) and divides into the anterior interventricular coronary artery (left anterior descending) and left circumflex artery.

Palpate the anterior interventricular groove, and feel for the anterior interventricular artery. Use the separation technique to expose the anterior interventricular artery. This vessel gives off relatively large diagonal branches to the anterior surface of the left ventricle (Fig. 6-16). Deeply penetrating septal branches arise from the deep surface of the anterior interventricular artery and enter the muscular interventricular septum (Figs. 6-17 and 6-18) at the level of the subpulmonary infundibulum, to supply the proximal parts of the left and right bundle branches.

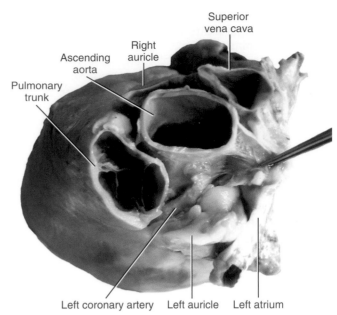

FIGURE 6-13. Superior view of the great vessels. To the left of the great vessels, fat is reflected and the origin of the left coronary artery is exposed.

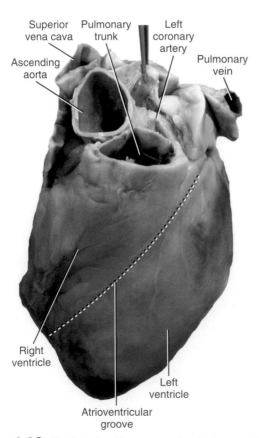

FIGURE 6-12. Vertical tilt of heart revealing its base and apex.

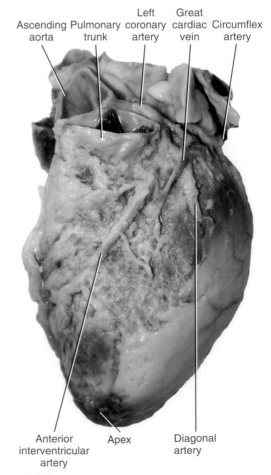

FIGURE 6-14. Epicardial fat is removed from the surface of the left ventricle and the anterior interventricular artery is exposed.

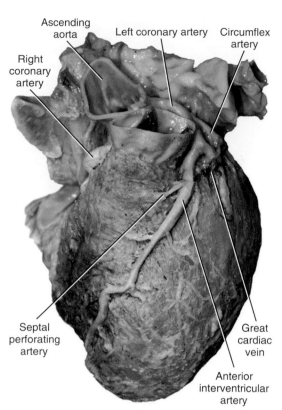

FIGURE 6-15. Epicardial fat removed from left ventricle with the anterior interventricular artery exposed.

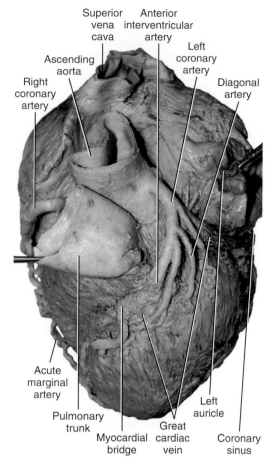

FIGURE 6-16. Removing epicardial fat from the left ventricle and exposing the anterior interventricular artery to reveal diagonal branches and a myocardial bridge.

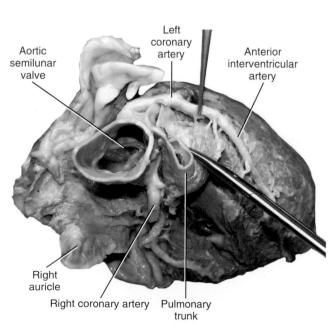

FIGURE 6-17. Anterior interventricular artery is retracted, and septal perforating branches are exposed.

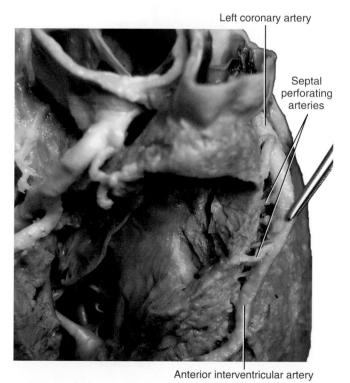

FIGURE 6-18. Left coronary artery with septal and anterior interventricular branches.

The circumflex coronary artery runs in the left AV groove toward the left border and around to the base of the heart. This vessel typically gives off the left marginal artery crossing the left border of the heart, supplying the left ventricular free wall (Fig. 6-19).

☞ *DISSECTION TIP:* Numerous variations exist in the pattern of distribution of the right and left coronary arteries. Among the most common of the variations is the source of the posterior interventricular coronary artery. In the majority of cases, the RCA provides the source for this artery. In about 15% of cases, however, the left circumflex artery gives off this branch. Many times during this dissection, it is possible to identify hearts that have undergone coronary artery bypass graft (CABG) procedures (Figs. 6-20 and 6-21). Try to expose the graft vessel and identify to which vessel it is connected. Another often encountered variation is the presence of myocardial bridges covering the left anterior interventricular artery, which penetrates the myocardium for a few centimeters and emerges distally as an epicardial artery (see Fig 6-16).

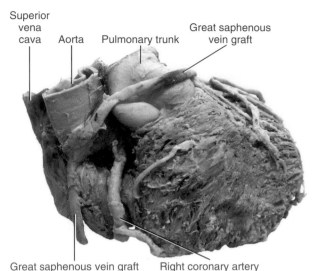

FIGURE 6-20. Anterior view of the heart demonstrating a great saphenous vein graft.

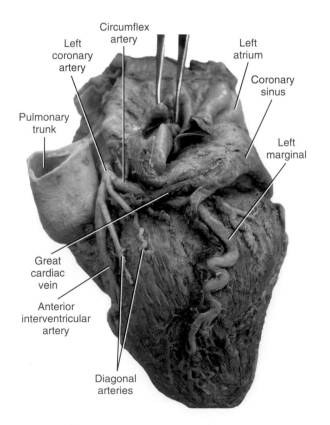

FIGURE 6-19. Lateral view with vertical tilt revealing left coronary artery, circumflex and marginal branches.

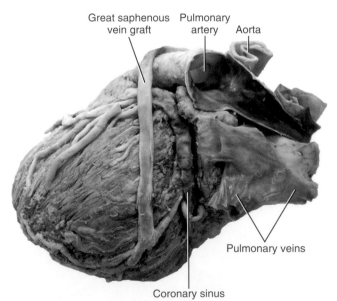

FIGURE 6-21. Posterior view revealing the great saphenous vein graft.

On the posterior surface of the heart at the AV sulcus between the IVC and the left atrium, identify the *coronary sinus,* a small confluence of veins approximately 2 cm long. It receives the great cardiac vein, the middle cardiac vein, and occasionally, the small cardiac vein and the oblique vein of the left atrium. Identify the great cardiac vein, which lies in the anterior interventricular groove, accompanying the left anterior interventricular artery. The middle cardiac vein lies in the posterior interventricular groove and accompanies the posterior interventricular artery. The small cardiac vein lies in the AV groove next to the opening of the coronary sinus. This vein usually joins the right marginal vein or separately opens into the right atrium.

> ☝ *DISSECTION TIP:* The cardiac veins have very thin walls and are often damaged during dissection.

DISSECTION OF HEART

Incise the right atrium laterally, making a vertical incision from the inferior vena cava to the superior vena cava (Fig 6-22) and avoid cutting the IVC valve. With forceps, reflect the flap made by the lateral incision in the right atrium, and observe the muscular ridge within the chamber, the *crista terminalis* (Fig. 6-23). Note the pectinate muscles arising from the crista terminalis and fanning out through the wall of the right auricle.

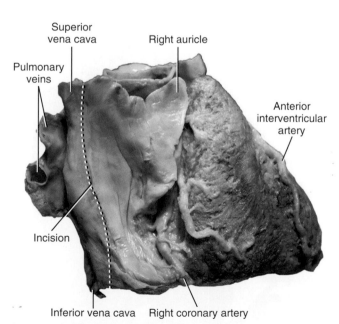

FIGURE 6-22. Anterior view of the right atrium with incision landmark between the inferior and superior venae cavae.

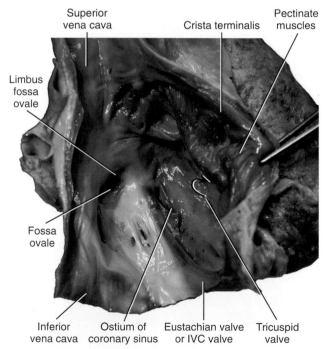

FIGURE 6-23. Superior and inferior venae cavae opened with a vertical incision, revealing internal structures of the right atrium; *IVC,* inferior vena cava.

Observe the smooth roof of the right atrium between the orifices of the two venae cavae, the *sinus venarum*. Within the right atrium, note the valve of the IVC (eustachian valve), and medial to the opening of the IVC, note the valve (thebesian valve) and ostium of the coronary sinus (coronary os). Note also the venae cordis minimi (thebesian veins), which are small openings in the internal surface of the right atrium. The interatrial septum forms the medial wall of the right atrium. Within the septum is a depressed region, the *fossa ovalis* (fossa ovale), bordered by a thicker rim of muscle, the superior limbus fossa ovalis (Fig. 6-24). The fossa ovalis marks the line of fusion between the original embryonic septum secundum with the septum primum, closing the ostium secundum. In 20% of cases, the area of fusion in the interatrial septum is incomplete, and an oblique fissure of communication between the two atria is retained. This is known as a "probe-patent foramen ovale" (Fig. 6-25).

Turn the right atrium upward, and note the *tricuspid valve* and its three leaflets: septal, anterior, and posterior. The separation of the three leaflets may not be well delineated. Identify the membranous septum between the septal and anterior leaflets of the tricuspid valve. Place one finger deeply within the aorta (below the level of its valve) while palpating the base of the interatrial septum with the thumb of the same hand. The small area where the thumb and the finger are separated by the thinnest amount of tissue marks the site of the membranous septum (Figs. 6-26 and 6-27).

Incise the left atrium laterally, making a horizontal incision from the right to the left pulmonary veins (Fig. 6-28). With forceps, reflect the flap made by the lateral incision in the left atrium, and observe within the chamber a smooth surface and limited number of pectinate muscles in the left auricle (Fig. 6-29).

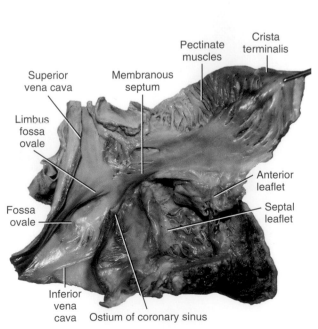

FIGURE 6-24. Internal aspect of the heart and superior vena cava.

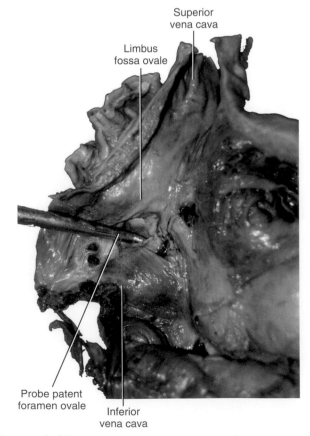

FIGURE 6-25. Right atrium reflected to reveal patent foramen ovale.

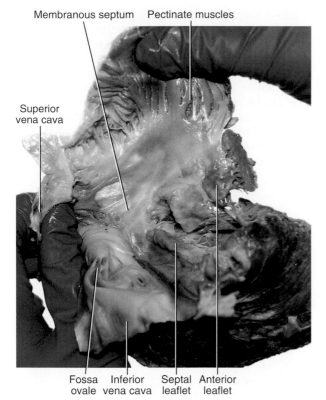

Membranous septum   Pectinate muscles

Superior
vena cava

Fossa   Inferior   Septal   Anterior
ovale   vena cava   leaflet   leaflet

FIGURE 6-26. Anterior atrial wall is lifted upward, and with a light behind it (transillumination), the membranous septum is seen.

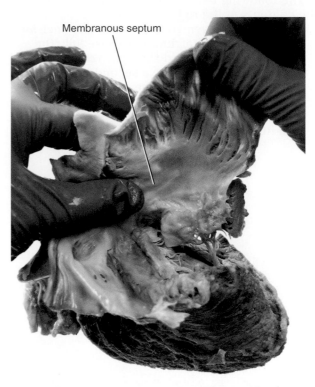

Membranous septum

FIGURE 6-27. Right atrium reflected with dissector's left thumb palpating the membranous septum.

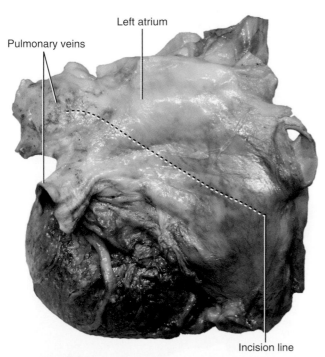

Left atrium

Pulmonary veins

Incision line

FIGURE 6-28. Base of heart with outline used for making incision in order to see contents of the left atrium.

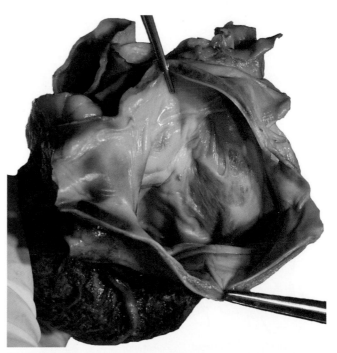

FIGURE 6-29. Left atrium incised superiorly, revealing internal structures.

The following two techniques are used to expose the contents of the right ventricle:

1. Open the right ventricle by making an incision through the right atrium to expose fully the tricuspid valve toward the right ventricle (ventricular inlet). Make a second incision from the pulmonary valve to the apex of the right ventricle (ventricular outlet). The major problem with this technique is that the moderator band and RCA are often cut (Figs. 6-30 and 6-31).

2. Make a small, circular incision a few centimeters below the subpulmonary infundibulum. This area is typically occupied by the right ventricular free wall (Figs. 6-32 and 6-33). Carefully, start cutting larger pieces of the right ventricular free wall, keeping in mind not to cut the moderator band (Fig. 6-34). Once you identify the moderator band, cut around the papillary muscle toward the tricuspid valve, and expose as much of the right ventricle as possible (Fig. 6-35).

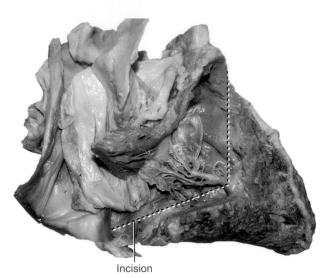

FIGURE 6-30. Deep dissection of right ventricle using V-shaped incisions revealing internal structures.

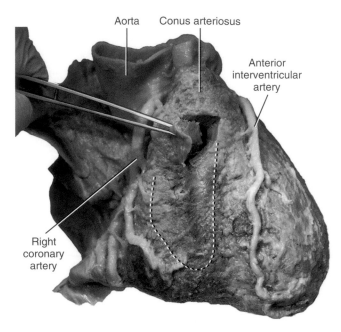

FIGURE 6-32. Transverse and vertical incision into right ventricle, creating window into conus arteriosus; dotted lines show continuation of incision.

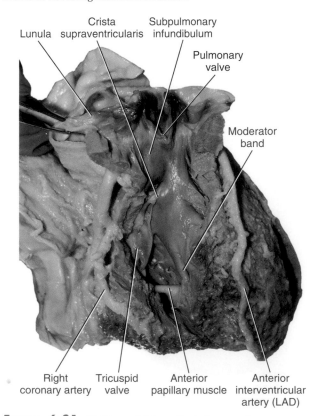

FIGURE 6-31. Right ventricle reflected away from apex and in line with pulmonary valve; *LAD,* left anterior descending artery.

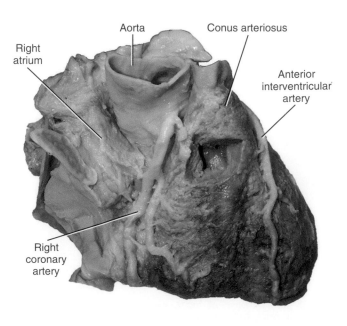

FIGURE 6-33. Window revealing internal conus arteriosus.

DISSECTION TIP: The majority of hearts will have a significant amount of coagulated blood around the cordae tendineae and the papillary muscles (Fig. 6-36). With forceps, carefully clean out the coagulated blood (Fig. 6-37). Water may also be run through the heart to aid in this cleaning process.

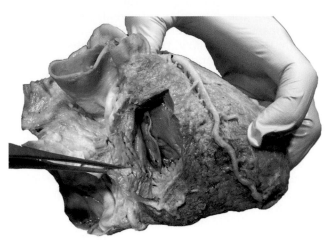

FIGURE 6-34. Reflected anterior wall of right ventricle revealing internal structures.

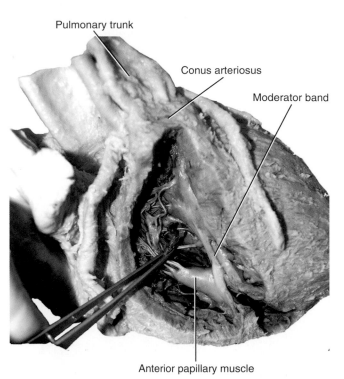

FIGURE 6-36. Reflected anterior wall of the right ventricle revealing internal structures.

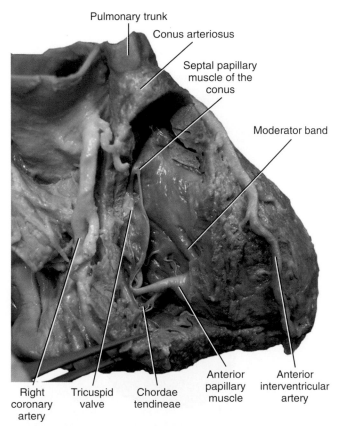

FIGURE 6-35. Reflected anterior wall of right ventricle revealing internal structures.

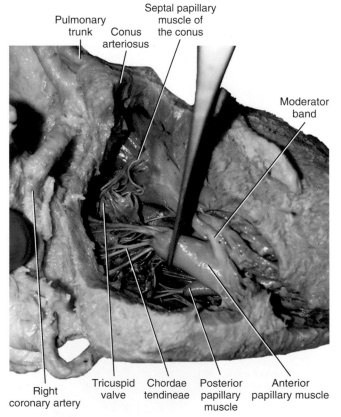

FIGURE 6-37. Reflected anterior wall of right ventricle revealing internal structures.

Identify the anterior, posterior, and septal cusps of the tricuspid valve. Observe that the cusps are anchored to papillary muscles within the ventricle by slender, tough, chordae tendineae (see Figs. 6-36 and 6-37). Identify the large anterior papillary

muscle. Posterior and inferior to this muscle is the posterior papillary muscle. The septal papillary muscle may consist of several small, septal papillary muscles arising from the interventricular septum, with short chordae tendineae passing to the septal leaflet of the valve. The highest and largest is called the septal papillary muscle of the conus, or of Luschka or Lancisi (see Fig. 6-31).

Note the thick, irregular-shaped bundles of muscle within the right ventricle, the *trabeculae carneae*. The *moderator band* (or septomarginal trabeculation) passes from the muscular interventricular septum to the base of the anterior papillary muscle. Cut through the pulmonary trunk, and note that the three semilunar-shaped cusps join together at the commissures. Note the *lunula* (free margin) and nodule of each cusp. Observe the horizontal muscle tissue in which the pulmonary (pulmonic) valve sits; this is the subpulmonary muscular infundibulum. The area between the septal papillary muscle of the conus and subpulmonary infundibulum is demarcated by the crista supraventricularis (see Fig. 6-31).

Identify the right coronary cusp, the noncoronary cusp, and the left coronary cusp of the aortic valve (Fig. 6-38).

Make a parallel incision from the anterior interventricular artery to the bifurcation of the left coronary artery into left anterior interventricular and coronary circumflex arteries (Figs. 6-39 and 6-40). With

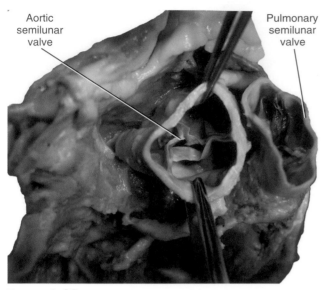

FIGURE 6-38. Aorta and pulmonary vessels transected superior to base of heart revealing their valves, respectively.

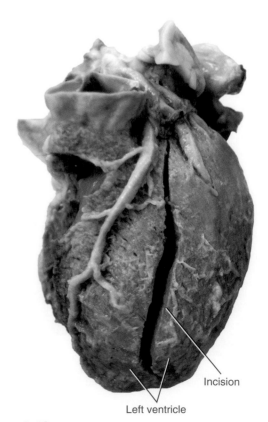

FIGURE 6-39. Lateral view with vertical tilt revealing the left coronary artery and dominant branches, with tracing *(dotted line)* for incision into the left ventricle.

FIGURE 6-40. Lateral view with vertical tilt revealing the left coronary artery and dominant branches, with incision into the left ventricle.

your fingers or a retractor, open the left ventricle and observe the muscular ridges, the trabeculae carneae (Fig. 6-41). Identify the mitral valve (left AV valve) with its two leaflets, an anterior and a posterior leaflet attaching by chordae tendineae to two papillary muscles, the posteromedial papillary muscle (closer to intraventricular septum, *septophilic*) and the anterolateral papillary muscle (farther away from the intraventricular septum, *septophobic*).

Make a vertical incision toward the aorta and cut through the aortic valve (Fig. 6-42). Identify the cusps of the aortic valve and the lunula (free margin) and nodule of each cusp. Identify the ostia of the coronary arteries and the depressions in the wall of the aorta, the "aortic sinuses of Valsalva." Beneath the noncoronary cusp of the aorta, identify the membranous portion of the interventricular septum (Fig. 6-43).

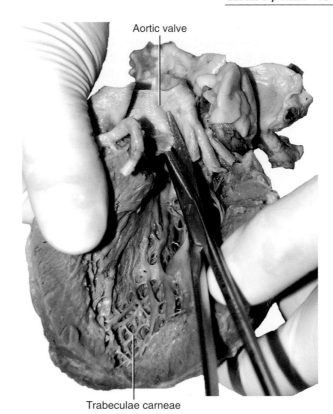

FIGURE 6-42. Opened left ventricle demonstrating internal structures and the scissors incising aortic valve.

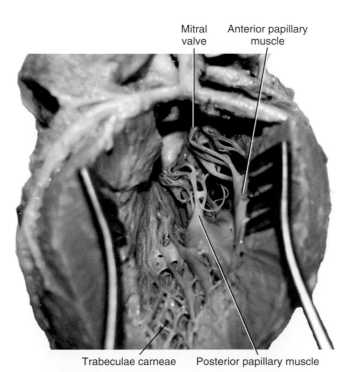

FIGURE 6-41. Lateral view with vertical tilt revealing internal structures of the left ventricle.

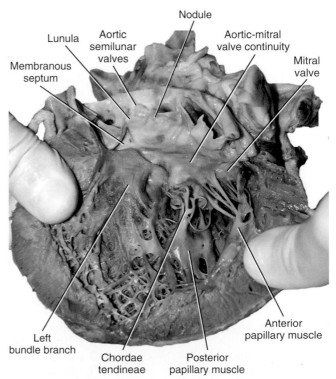

FIGURE 6-43. Left ventricle reflected revealing internal structures, and highlighting the aortic and mitral valves.

Make an incision from the lateral border of the left ventricle behind the anterolateral papillary muscle (Fig. 6-44). Observe the leaflets of the mitral valve and the aortic-mitral valve continuity. Notice the layer of lighter-colored tissue, which appears to travel inferiorly down the interventricular septum, between the coronary cusp and the noncoronary cusp of the aorta. This tissue forms the left bundle branch of the cardiac conduction system. Some of its fibers may be seen crossing the ventricular lumen freely as so-called false tendons (see Fig. 6-43).

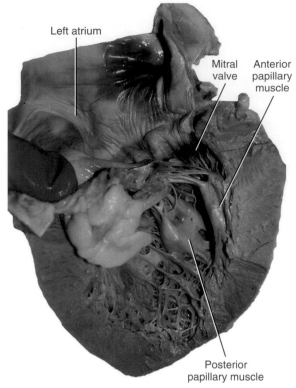

FIGURE 6-44. Left ventricle reflected open, revealing left atrioventricular valve and papillary muscles.

LABORATORY IDENTIFICATION CHECKLIST

Arteries
- ❏ Aorta
- ❏ Common carotid
- ❏ Brachiocephalic trunk
- ❏ Pulmonary
- ❏ Left coronary
- ❏ Anterior interventricular
- ❏ Circumflex
- ❏ Interventricular septal branches
- ❏ Right coronary
- ❏ Marginal
- ❏ Sinu-atrial (SA) nodal
- ❏ Atrioventricular (AV) nodal
- ❏ Posterior interventricular

Veins
- ❏ Superior vena cava
- ❏ Inferior vena cava and eustachian valve
- ❏ Right and left pulmonary veins
- ❏ Coronary sinus and thebesian valve
- ❏ Great cardiac
- ❏ Middle cardiac
- ❏ Small cardiac
- ❏ Anterior interventricular
- ❏ Posterior interventricular

Heart
- ❏ Right auricle
- ❏ Right atrium
- ❏ Superior vena cava
- ❏ Inferior vena cava
- ❏ Fossa ovalis
- ❏ Opening of coronary sinus
- ❏ Crista terminalis
- ❏ Pectinate muscle
- ❏ Sinus venosus region (smooth aspcct)
- ❏ Right ventricle
- ❏ Right atrioventricular (AV) valve, or tricuspid valve
- ❏ Chordae tendineae
- ❏ Anterior papillary muscle
- ❏ Posterior papillary muscle
- ❏ Septal papillary muscle
- ❏ Septomarginal trabeculation (moderator band)
- ❏ Interventricular septum
- ❏ Trabeculae carneae
- ❏ Conus arteriosus
- ❏ Pulmonary (pulmonic) valve
- ❏ Aortic valve
- ❏ Left auricle
- ❏ Left atrium
- ❏ Right and left pulmonary veins

Heart—cont'd
- ❏ Left atrioventricular (AV) valve, or bicuspid/mitral valve
- ❏ Left ventricle
- ❏ Chordae tendineae
- ❏ Anterior papillary muscle
- ❏ Posterior papillary muscle
- ❏ Chordae tendineae
- ❏ Anterior papillary muscle
- ❏ Posterior papillary muscle
- ❏ Trabeculae carneae

THORACENTESIS

Gray's Anatomy for Students: 235

Netter: 224, 225

Clinical Application

Introduce a needle or trocar into the intrathoracic cavity, creating a conduit to allow air (pneumothorax) to escape or to help remove fluid.

Anatomic Landmarks

- *Needle:* 2nd intercostal space at midclavicular line
  Skin
  Subcutaneous
  External intercostal fascia/muscle
  Internal intercostal fascia/muscle
  Parietal pleura
- *Tube:* 5th intercostal space at midaxillary line
  Skin
  Subcutaneous tissue
  Inferior angle of scapula
  Lateral pectoralis major border
  Lateral breast tissue
  Intercostal muscles
  Parietal pleura

Note: Needle placement for pneumothorax is 2nd intercostal space at midclavicular line; tube placement is at midaxillary line (Fig. III-1).

CENTRAL VENOUS LINE (CATHETERIZATION OF SUBCLAVIAN VEIN OR INTERNAL JUGULAR VEINS)

Gray's Anatomy for Students: 972, 979

Netter: 192

Clinical Application

Introduce a line (catheter) into the subclavian vein above and behind the clavicle and lateral to the sternocleidomastoid muscle for long-term infusion of fluids or medicines (Fig. III-2).

Anatomic Landmarks

- Skin
- Subcutaneous tissue
- Sternocleidomastoid muscle
- Clavicle
- Costoclavicular ligament
- Subclavian vein
- Anterior scalene, phenic nerve, lymphatic ducts
- Pleura

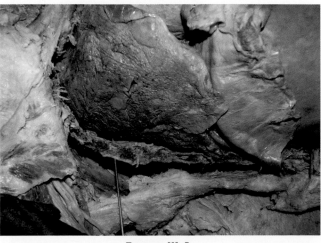

FIGURE III-1.

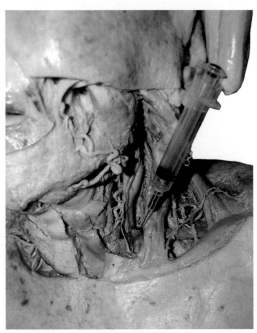

FIGURE III-2.

PERICARDIOCENTESIS

Gray's Anatomy for Students: 177–179

Netter: 206, 209

Clinical Application

Withdraw fluid from the pericardial space (Fig. III-3).

Anatomic Landmarks

Subxiphoid Approach

- Xiphoid process of sternum
- Skin
- Subcutaneous tissue
- Rectus abdominis
- Diaphragmatic pericardium
- Pericardial space

Parasternal approach

- Left 5th intercostal space
- Left sternal border
- Skin
- Subcutaneous tissue
- External intercostal
- Internal intercostal
- Innermost intercostal
- Sternal space/pleura
- Pericardial space

Note: Liver, stomach, and internal thoracic artery may be in danger of injury (Fig. III-4).

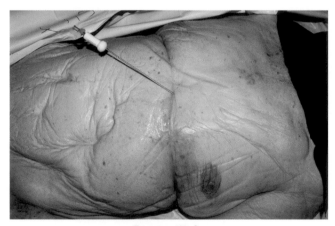

FIGURE III-3.

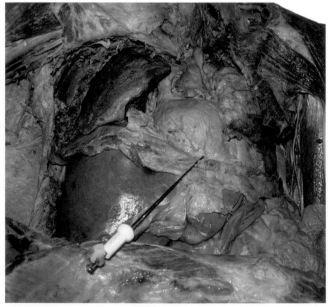

FIGURE III-4.

OTHER LANDMARKS AND OBSERVATIONS

- Figure III-5 shows an example of enlarged malignant lymph nodes in the axilla.
- The sternalis muscle is one of the most common variations found in the musculature of the anterior thoracic wall (Fig. III-6).
- Figure III-7 shows a cadaver with a pacemaker.

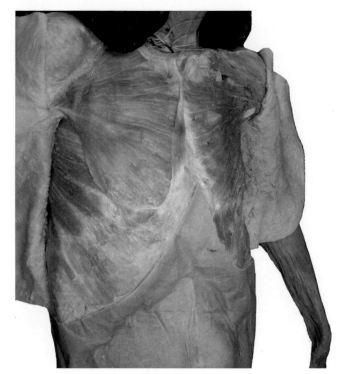

FIGURE III-6.

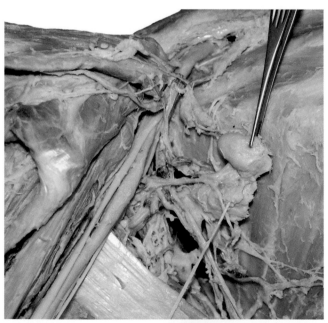

FIGURE III-5.

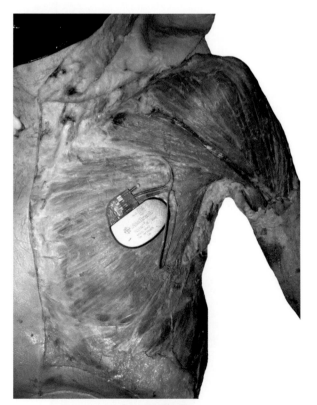

FIGURE III-7.

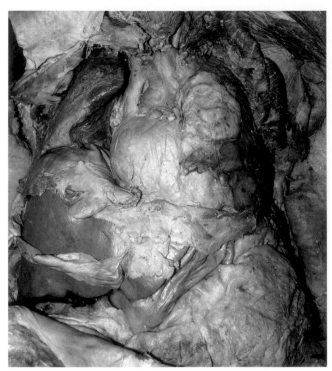

FIGURE III-8.

- See Figures III-8 to III-11 for examples of lungs with malignant lesions.
- The *myocardial bridge* is a muscular bridge that covers the anterior interventricular artery for a short distance within the myocardium. It is a common finding during dissection (Fig. III-12).
- Figures III-13 and III-14 show the effects of myocardial infarction on the heart.

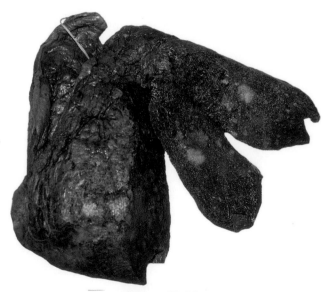

FIGURE III-10.

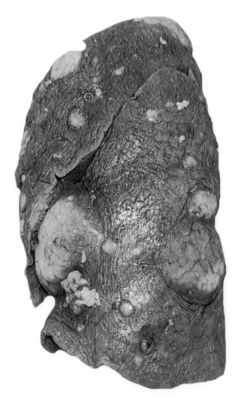

FIGURE III-9.

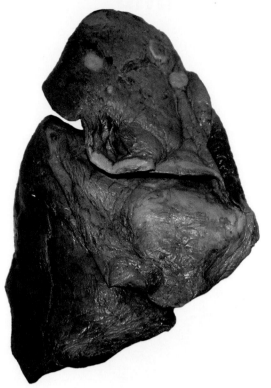

FIGURE III-11.

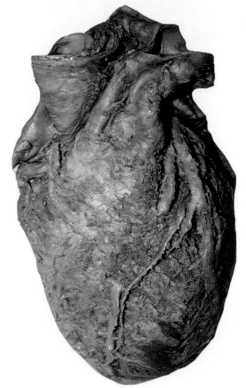

FIGURE III-12.

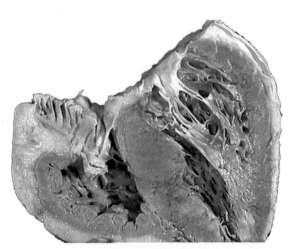

FIGURE III-13.

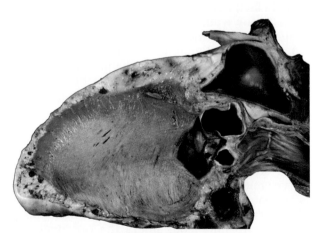

FIGURE III-14.

CHAPTER 7

AXILLA AND ARM

Netter: 403, 412, 417–426

McMinn: 144–149

Gray's Atlas: 368–389

Make a skin incision from the shoulder distally to a point 2 to 3 inches (5-7.5 cm) above the elbow. An encircling incision around the midportion of the arm allows for medial retraction of the skin from the upper arm. Reflect the skin from the thorax, shoulders, axillae, and proximal portions of the arms medially to the axillary space (as shown previously in Fig. 4-4). See Chapter 8 for the incisions used in the forearm.

Axillary Borders

The pectoral region should have been dissected before the study of the axilla is begun. Refer to Chapter 4 for the regional anatomy of the pectoral region and breast. Review the following borders of the axilla:

- **Anterior wall:** Pectoralis major and minor muscles and clavipectoral fascia
- **Posterior wall:** Latissimus dorsi, teres major, and subscapularis muscles
- **Lateral wall:** Humerus, short head of biceps brachii muscle, and coracobrachialis muscle
- **Medial wall:** Upper five ribs, their intercostal muscles, and adjacent serratus anterior muscle
- **Base:** Axillary fascia
- **Apex** *(cervicoaxillary canal):* Superior border of scapula, 1st rib, and clavicle

Identify the long thoracic nerve running over the serratus anterior muscle. Note the intercostobrachial nerve emerging from the 2nd intercostal space, which is the lateral cutaneous branch of the 2nd thoracic (T2) nerve crossing over the long thoracic nerve, to supply with cutaneous fibers the proximal, medial aspect of the brachium and axilla (Fig. 7-1). Preserve these two nerves. Keep the pectoralis major and minor muscles reflected laterally.

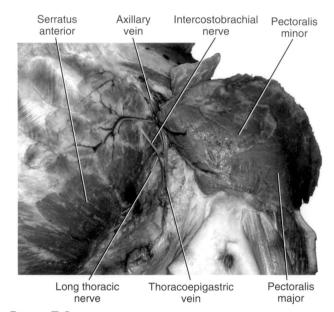

Serratus anterior   Axillary vein   Intercostobrachial nerve   Pectoralis minor

Long thoracic nerve   Thoracoepigastric vein   Pectoralis major

FIGURE 7-1. Anterior axillary region with skin removed and pectoralis muscles reflected, exposing intercostobrachial and long thoracic nerves.

☝ *DISSECTION TIP:* Adipose tissue and lymphatics occupy most of the space in the axilla. Do not attempt to remove them at this stage. Push them away from the structures you identify, and remove them at a later stage.

Identify the fascia that invests the axillary artery, axillary vein, and the brachial plexus, called the *axillary sheath.* Excise the axillary sheath between the axillary artery and the brachial plexus by gently pulling away the nerves (Fig. 7-2). Remove the axillary sheath, and push the adipose tissue away from the brachial plexus (Fig. 7-3) Identify and clean the axillary artery and vein (Fig. 7-4).

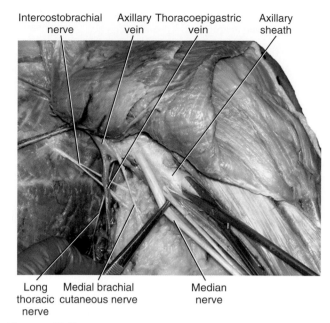

FIGURE 7-2. Anterior axillary region with pectoralis muscles reflected, revealing excision of axillary sheath to expose terminal branches of brachial plexus.

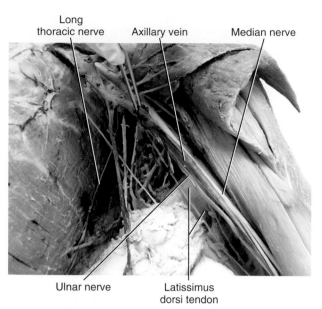

FIGURE 7-4. Anterior axillary view of deep dissection, revealing axillary vein and terminal branches of brachial plexus.

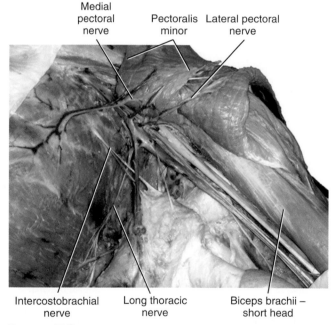

FIGURE 7-3. Anterior axillary region with pectoralis muscles reflected and most of axillary sheath removed, revealing terminal branches of brachial plexus.

The axillary vein is formed at the base of the axilla by the confluence of the venae comitantes of the brachial artery with the basilic vein. (Large arteries, such as the axillary or femoral, are accompanied by a single vein. Smaller arteries, such as the brachial, have two or more accompanying veins, which are found on either side of the artery and are called "venae comites" or *venae comitantes*). The axillary

☝ *DISSECTION TIP:* The arteries are typically named based on the structures they supply, not according to their origin.

artery extends from the lateral border of the 1st rib to the lower border of the teres major muscle. Just before it crosses the 1st rib, the artery is named the *subclavian artery.* Distal to the teres major, the name of the vessel changes to the *brachial artery.*

Clean the adipose tissue between the pectoralis minor muscle and brachial plexus (Fig. 7-4). Identify the axillary artery and its three divisions, demarcated with its relationship to the pectoralis minor muscle (Fig. 7-5). Identify the superior thoracic artery arising from the 1st part of the axillary artery. To identify this vessel, look for an artery penetrating the

☝ *DISSECTION TIP:* Do not attempt to identify any lymph nodes associated with the axillary vein and its tributaries. Nodes are evident and easily dissected only in cadavers with cancer. Similarly, do not attempt to identify the central axillary nodes within the fat of the central portion of the axilla. Smaller tributaries to the axillary vein that obscure the dissecting field can be excised and removed.

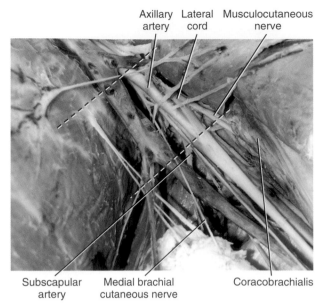

FIGURE 7-5. Anterior axillary view revealing the second part of the axillary artery, thoracoacromial artery, and lateral cord. Red dashed lines represent the borders on the pectoralis minor muscle over the axillary artery, dividing its three portions.

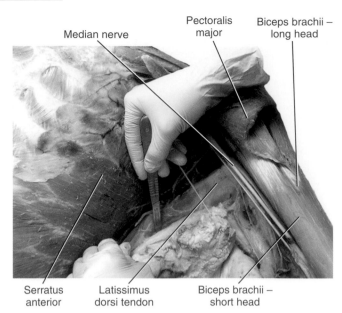

FIGURE 7-6. Anterior axillary view revealing removal of the fat from the latissimus dorsi muscle.

musculature of the 1st or 2nd intercostal space. From the 2nd part of the axillary artery (deep to pectoralis minor muscle), identify the thoracoacromial trunk and the lateral thoracic artery (Fig. 7-5). Look for the pectoral branches of the thoracoacromial trunk supplying the pectoralis major and minor muscles. Do not look for the remaining branches of the thoracoacromial trunk (deltoid, acromial, and clavicular).

Anatomic Landmarks

- **Supreme thoracic artery:** 1st or 2nd intercostal spaces
- **Lateral thoracic artery:** Lateral border of pectoralis minor muscle. Often, the lateral thoracic artery will arise as a branch of the thoracoacromial trunk.
- **Thoracoacromial trunk:** 2nd part of axillary artery
- **Pectoral branches:** Look for these on the internal surface of the pectoralis major and minor muscles, and trace them backward to the axillary artery and thoracoacromial trunk. The pectoral branches often originate directly from the 2nd part of the axillary artery.

Separate the axillary artery from the branches of the brachial plexus, and remove fat from the latissimus dorsi muscle (Figs. 7-5 and 7-6). Do not remove fat deep to the axilla. Continue removing the axillary sheath from the brachial artery and vein, and expose the median nerve distally to the midportion of the arm (Fig. 7-7). Cut the axillary vein at the point where the 1st part of the axillary artery originates, and reflect the vein and its tributaries toward the forearm. Do not completely remove the vein from the cadaver.

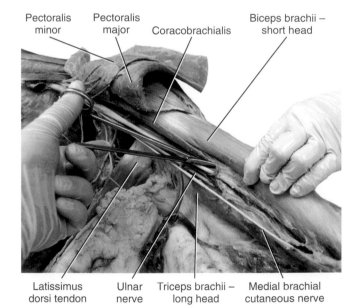

FIGURE 7-7. Removing the axillary sheath and soft tissue, exposing median and ulnar nerves and medial antebrachial cutaneous nerve.

> ✎ *DISSECTION TIP:* Exposing the branches of the brachial plexus to the midportion of the humerus allows greater mobility and facilitates the identification of structures deep in the axilla.

Distal to the pectoralis minor muscle, from the 3rd portion of the axillary artery, identify the anterior circumflex humeral, posterior circumflex humeral,

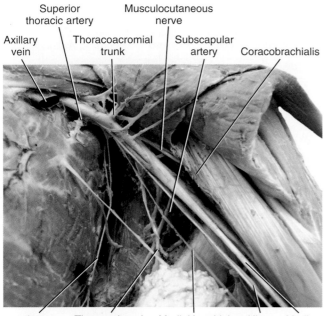

Superior thoracic artery Musculocutaneous nerve

Axillary vein Thoracoacromial trunk Subscapular artery Coracobrachialis

Long thoracic nerve Thoracodorsal nerve Medial brachial cutaneous nerve Ulnar nerve Median nerve

FIGURE 7-8. Anterior axillary view with reflected pectoralis muscles, removed axillary vein, revealing the axillary artery and associated nerves.

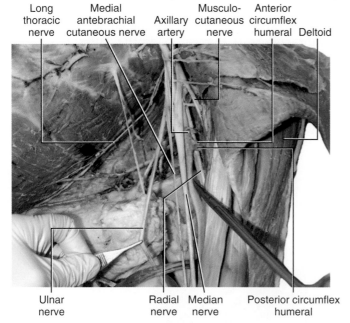

Long thoracic nerve Medial antebrachial cutaneous nerve Axillary artery Musculo-cutaneous nerve Anterior circumflex humeral Deltoid

Ulnar nerve Radial nerve Median nerve Posterior circumflex humeral

FIGURE 7-9. Axillary artery and ulnar and median nerves are pulled laterally to expose radial nerve and anterior and posterior circumflex humeral arteries.

and subscapular arteries. The subscapular artery runs vertically toward the latissimus dorsi and branches into the thoracodorsal artery, supplying the latissimus dorsi muscle, and the circumflex scapular artery, traveling posteriorly to the muscles of the posterior scapula (Figs. 7-8 and 7-9).

The brachial plexus is divided into roots, trunks, divisions, cords, and terminal branches. The roots,

trunks, and divisions are indentified later in the root of the neck dissection. In this dissection, you will be able to identify the cords and terminal branches of the brachial plexus. The cords are named with respect to their positions in relationship to the axillary artery. As a result, the *lateral cord* is situated lateral to the axillary artery, the *medial cord* medial to the axillary artery, and the *posterior cord* posterior (deep) to the axillary artery. The lateral cord gives off two branches: the lateral pectoral nerve supplies the pectoralis major muscle, and the musculocutaneous nerve supplies the biceps brachii, coracobrachialis, and brachialis muscles (Fig. 7-8).

> ✋ *DISSECTION TIP:* A landmark for identifying the musculocutaneous nerve is that the nerve pierces the proximal portion of the coracobrachialis muscle.

Identify and clean the branches of the medial cord: the medial pectoral nerve, ulnar nerve, medial root of median nerve, medial brachial cutaneous nerve, and medial antebrachial cutaneous nerve. Alongside the medial antebrachial cutaneous nerve, identify the basilic vein (formed at the medial aspect of the dorsal venous arch of the hand; see Chapters 8 and 9). Trace and expose the median nerve to the elbow (Fig. 7-9).

> ✋ *DISSECTION TIP:* The medial brachial cutaneous nerve (medial cutaneous nerve to the arm) is often severed during the removal of the skin over the brachium. The medial antebrachial cutaneous nerve (medial cutaneous nerve to the forearm) runs parallel to the ulnar nerve. The landmark for identifying the ulnar nerve is to trace it as it crosses posterior to the medial epicondyle of the humerus. In contrast, the medial antebrachial cutaneous nerve runs more superficially and terminates in the skin of the forearm (see Fig. 7-16).

The posterior cord gives rise to the following branches: upper, middle, and lower subscapular nerves; axillary nerve; and radial nerve. To identify the posterior cord, pull the medial cord and the axillary artery away from the coracobrachialis muscle (Figs. 7-8 to 7-10). Deep to the axillary artery, identify the posterior cord. Trace the radial nerve as it penetrates the triceps brachii. At the level of the surgical neck of the humerus, dissect and expose the anterior and posterior circumflex humeral arteries. Identify the axillary nerve running alongside the posterior circumflex humeral artery passing posterior to the surgical neck of the humerus to reach the quadrangular space.

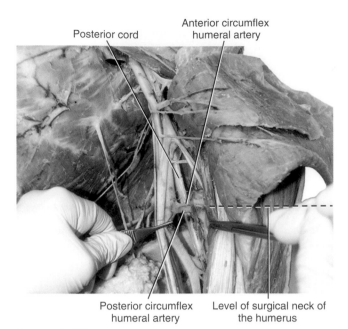

Posterior cord

Anterior circumflex humeral artery

Posterior circumflex humeral artery

Level of surgical neck of the humerus

FIGURE 7-10. Anterior axillary view with reflected pectoralis muscles, traction from axillary artery, revealing lateral cord, posterior cord, and musculocutaneous nerve. Red dashed line shows level of the surgical neck of the humerus.

DISSECTION TIP: The posterior circumflex humeral artery is typically much larger than the anterior circumflex humeral artery. In some specimens, the posterior humeral artery may arise from the subscapular artery.

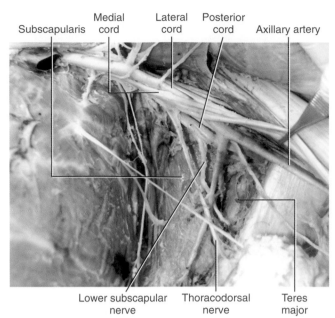

Subscapularis

Medial cord

Lateral cord

Posterior cord

Axillary artery

Lower subscapular nerve

Thoracodorsal nerve

Teres major

FIGURE 7-12. Deep anterior axillary view with reflected pectoralis muscles, removed axillary vein, revealing neurovascular structures.

Pull the medial cord upward, and observe the subscapular artery and the posterior cord of the brachial plexus. Identify the middle subscapular nerve (thoracodorsal) that supplies the latissimus dorsi muscle and runs alongside the thoracodorsal artery, which also supplies the latissimus dorsi (Figs. 7-11 to 7-13). Distal to the origin of the middle subscapular

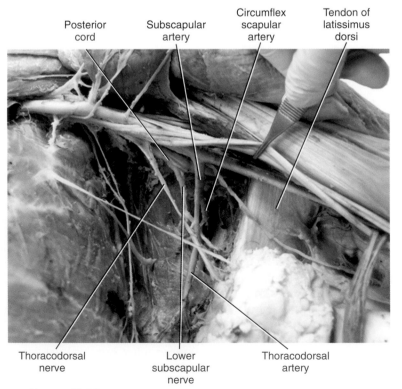

Posterior cord

Subscapular artery

Circumflex scapular artery

Tendon of latissimus dorsi

Thoracodorsal nerve

Lower subscapular nerve

Thoracodorsal artery

FIGURE 7-11. Anterior axillary view revealing posterior structures.

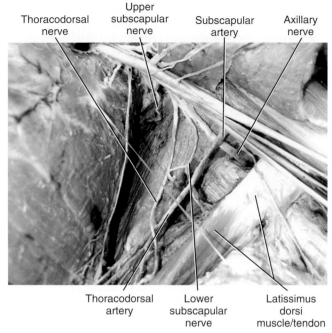

Thoracodorsal nerve · Upper subscapular nerve · Subscapular artery · Axillary nerve

Thoracodorsal artery · Lower subscapular nerve · Latissimus dorsi muscle/tendon

FIGURE 7-13. Deep anterior axillary view revealing upper, middle, and lower subscapular nerves.

nerve, identify the lower subscapular nerve running at the lateral border of subscapularis with the scapular circumflex artery. The lower subscapular nerve supplies part of the subscapularis and the entire teres major muscle. Clean out the subscapularis muscle and at its deeper portion, identify the upper subscapular nerve supplying the subscapularis muscle (Figs. 7-12 to 7-14).

Anatomic Landmarks

- **Subscapular artery:** Arises from the 3rd part of the axillary artery (pull the medial cord upward to expose it) and runs vertically down between the latissimus dorsi and subscapularis muscles.
- **Thoracodorsal artery:** Arises from the subscapular artery and continues to run downward to supply the latissimus dorsi muscle. This artery is found on the surface of the latissimus dorsi accompanied by the middle subscapular nerve (trace the artery backward to its origin).
- **Scapular circumflex artery:** Arises from the subscapular artery and turns around to enter the gap between the lateral border of the subscapularis and latissimus dorsi muscles alongside the lower subscapular nerve (trace the nerve backward to its origin from the posterior cord).
- **Posterior circumflex humeral artery:** Pull the axillary artery away from the coracobrachialis at the level of the surgical neck of the humerus, and identify the artery. It runs alongside the axillary nerve.
- **Posterior cord:** Pull the axillary artery laterally. Look posteriorly and deep to it for the posterior cord.
- **Radial nerve:** Look at the medial surface of the arm for the nerve penetrating the triceps brachii muscle (see Fig. 7-18). Trace the nerve backward to the axilla and posterior cord.
- **Axillary nerve:** Identify the posterior circumflex humeral artery. The axillary nerve runs next to it. Trace the nerve backward to the posterior cord.

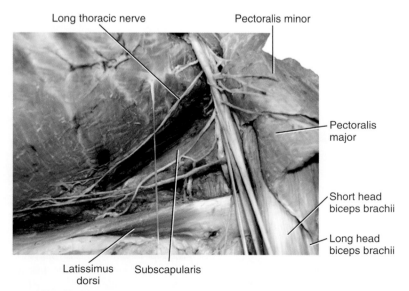

Long thoracic nerve · Pectoralis minor · Pectoralis major · Short head biceps brachii · Long head biceps brachii

Latissimus dorsi · Subscapularis

FIGURE 7-14. Deep anterior axillary view revealing posterior nerve structures.

- **Ulnar nerve**: Look for the nerve traveling along the medial aspect of the arm, not providing any branches to the arm, and crossing posterior to the medial epicondyle.
- **Median nerve**: Look for the nerve traveling along the medial aspect of the arm without giving off any branches to the arm. It is easily found as it dives underneath the bicipital aponeurosis.
- **Medial antebrachial cutaneous nerve**: Runs parallel and superficial to the ulnar nerve, and is distributed to the skin of the forearm. The basilic vein runs together with this nerve.
- **Medial brachial cutaneous nerve**: Runs parallel for a short distance in the arm with the medial antebrachial cutaneous nerve, and is distributed to the skin of the arm. This nerve is often cut when the skin of the arm is reflected.
- **Upper subscapular nerve**: Look deep in the axilla for the nerve that penetrates the subscapularis muscle. It is located deep and medial to the subscapularis muscle.
- **Middle subscapular nerve (thoracodorsal)**: Found on the surface of the latissimus dorsi muscle running alongside the thoracodorsal artery.
- **Lower subscapular nerve**: It runs with the scapular circumflex artery in the gap between the lateral border of the subscapularis and latissimus dorsi muscles.

Continue the dissection by exposing the terminal branches of the brachial plexus in the arm (Fig. 7-15). The *axillary* artery changes its name to *brachial* artery as it crosses the lower border of the teres major tendon. Identify the first branch of the brachial artery, the *deep* brachial artery (profunda brachii

artery) running deep to the triceps brachii muscle with the radial nerve (Figs. 7-16 and 7-17).

Continue the dissection, reflecting the skin over the medial portion of the triceps brachii muscle, and expose all the branches of the radial nerve (Fig. 7-18). Reflect the skin medially over the biceps brachii

---

✋ *DISSECTION TIP:* If time permits, expose the short head of the biceps brachii from its origin at the coracoid process of the scapula. The tendon of the long head of the biceps brachii lies lateral to the short head. You may expose the tendon of the long head of the biceps brachii muscle from the supraglenoid tubercle, just above the glenoid fossa of the scapula.

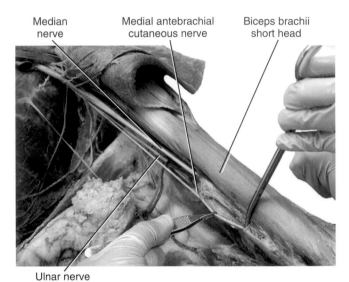

FIGURE 7-16. Complete exposure of median, ulnar, and medial antebrachial cutaneous nerves in the arm.

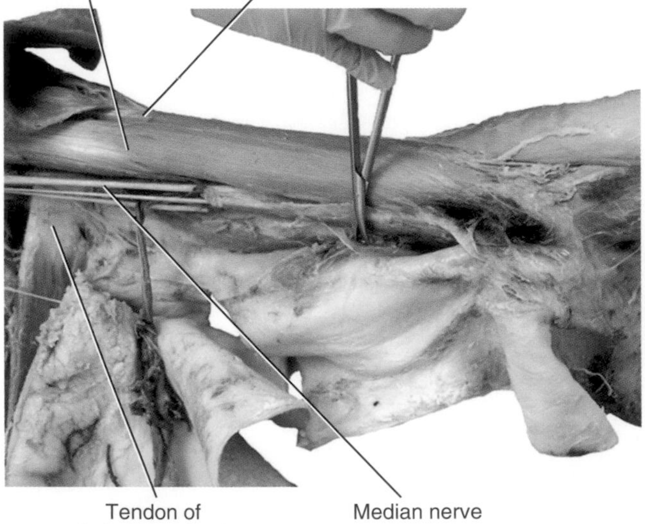

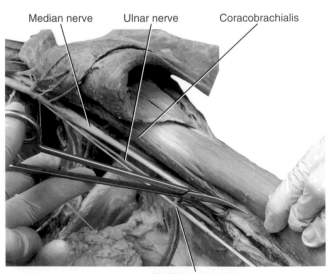

FIGURE 7-17. Complete exposure of median and ulnar nerves and medial antebrachial cutaneous nerve in the arm.

FIGURE 7-15. Lower axillary and upper arm view with skin reflected, revealing muscular and nerve structures.

DISSECTION TIP: The brachialis muscle is innervated primarily by the musculocutaneous nerve; however, the radial nerve may also contribute to its innervation.

muscle (Figs. 7-19 and 7-20). Identify the long and short heads of the biceps brachii.

Just inferior to the biceps brachii, identify the brachialis muscle (Fig. 7-20). Identify the coracobrachialis muscle, noting the musculocutaneous nerve passing through the muscle.

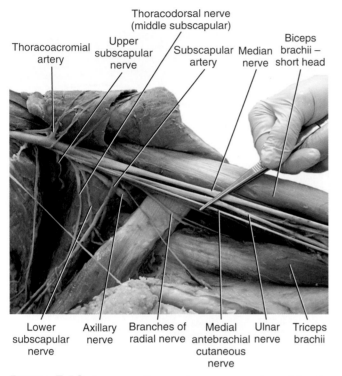

FIGURE 7-18. Lower axillary and upper arm view with skin reflected, revealing muscles and nerves.

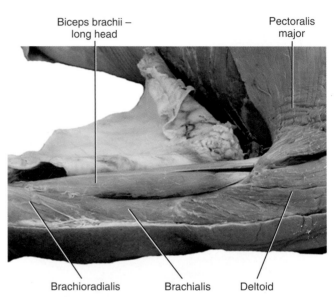

FIGURE 7-20. Upper arm view with skin reflected, revealing biceps brachii, brachialis, and deltoid muscles.

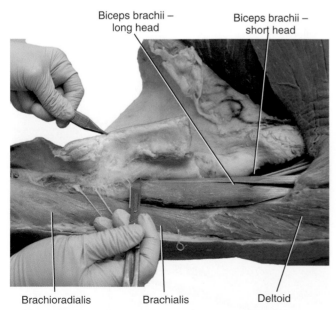

FIGURE 7-19. Upper arm view with skin reflected, revealing biceps brachii, brachialis, and deltoid muscles.

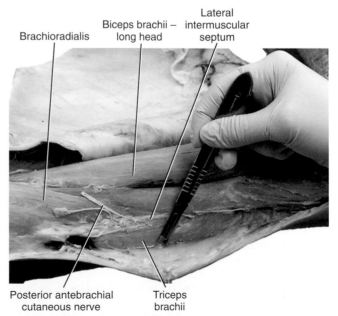

FIGURE 7-21. Dissection and reflection of skin over lateral head of triceps brachii, with exposure of posterior cutaneous nerve to the forearm.

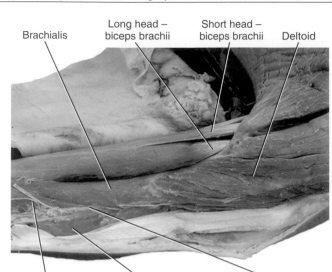

FIGURE 7-22. Upper arm view with skin reflected, revealing superficial musculature.

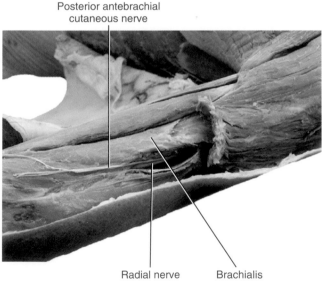

FIGURE 7-23. Reflection of deltoid muscle and exposure of the origin of the posterior cutaneous nerve to the forearm.

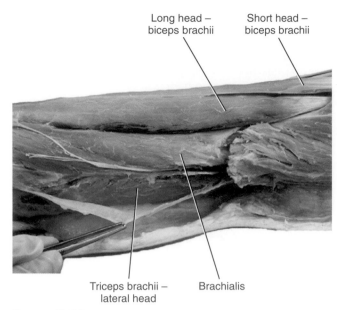

FIGURE 7-24. Reflection of deltoid and lateral head of triceps brachii, with exposure of posterior cutaneous nerve to the forearm.

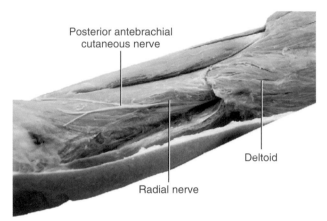

FIGURE 7-25. Reflection of deltoid and lateral head of triceps, with exposure of posterior cutaneous nerve to the forearm and radial nerve.

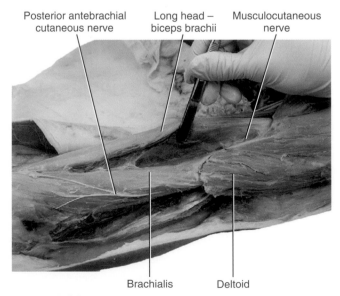

FIGURE 7-26. Anterior arm view, with traction to biceps brachii revealing musculature and nerve.

Reflect the skin over the lateral aspect of the arm inferiorly (Fig. 7-21).

Identify the posterior cutaneous nerve to the forearm (branch of radial nerve) emerging between the brachialis and triceps brachii muscles (Fig. 7-22). Trace the origin of the posterior cutaneous nerve to the forearm by separating the brachialis from the triceps brachii (Fig. 7-23). Lift the inferior portion of the deltoid muscle from the humeral surface. Reflect the fascia covering the triceps, and expose the lateral head of the triceps brachii muscle (Fig. 7-24).

Trace the radial nerve to the spiral groove of the humerus between the medial and long heads of the triceps brachii muscle (Fig. 7-25).

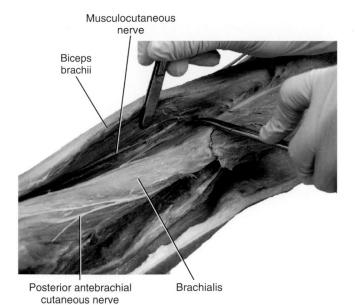

Musculocutaneous nerve

Biceps brachii

Posterior antebrachial cutaneous nerve

Brachialis

FIGURE 7-27. Anterior view of the arm with elevation of the biceps brachii demonstrating the underlying musculotaneous nerve.

Trace the musculocutaneous nerve as it penetrates the coracobrachialis muscle, then lift the biceps brachii and observe the course of the musculocutaneous nerve (Fig. 7-26). Clean all soft tissues between the biceps brachii and brachialis muscles, and dissect the musculocutaneous nerve to the lateral aspect of the brachium as it emerges to become the lateral antebrachial cutaneous nerve (Fig. 7-27). Identify the three heads of the triceps brachii muscle.

> **DISSECTION TIP:** The *lateral* head is the most inferior part of the triceps brachii muscle and is recognizable on the lateral surface of this muscle. The *medial* head arises from the posterior and medial surfaces of the humerus distal to the spiral groove. The *long* head arises from the infraglenoid tubercle of the scapula and is located medial and proximal to the spiral groove.

If time permits, trace the ascending branch of the deep brachial artery, and look for its anastomoses with the posterior circumflex humeral artery.

LABORATORY IDENTIFICATION CHECKLIST

Nerves

Lateral cords
- ❏ Musculocutaneous
- ❏ Lateral pectoral

Medial cords
- ❏ Medial pectoral
- ❏ Medial brachial cutaneous
- ❏ Medial antebrachial cutaneous
- ❏ Ulnar nerve

Posterior cords
- ❏ Axillary
- ❏ Upper subscapular
- ❏ Lower subscapular
- ❏ Thoracodorsal
- ❏ Radial

Arteries
- ❏ Axillary
- ❏ Superior thoracic
- ❏ Thoracoacromial
- ❏ Pectoral

Arteries—cont'd
- ❏ Lateral thoracic
- ❏ Subscapular
- ❏ Thoracodorsal
- ❏ Circumflex scapular
- ❏ Anterior circumflex humeral
- ❏ Posterior circumflex humeral

Veins
- ❏ Axillary
- ❏ Thoracoepigastric
- ❏ Cephalic
- ❏ Brachial
- ❏ Venae comitantes

Lymph Nodes
- ❏ Infraclavicular
- ❏ Apical
- ❏ Lateral
- ❏ Central
- ❏ Subscapular
- ❏ Pectoral

Muscles
- ❏ Short head of biceps brachii
- ❏ Long head of biceps brachii
- ❏ Long head of triceps brachii
- ❏ Lateral head of triceps brachii
- ❏ Latissimus dorsi
- ❏ Pectoralis major
- ❏ Pectoralis minor
- ❏ Serratus anterior
- ❏ Subclavius
- ❏ Deltoid
- ❏ Subscapularis
- ❏ Teres major
- ❏ Teres minor

Fascia
- ❏ Clavipectoral fascia

Bones
- ❏ Clavicle
- ❏ Humerus
- ❏ Scapula

CHAPTER 8

FOREARM (ANTEBRACHIUM)

Netter: 427–439, 463–464, 466

McMinn: 152–157

Gray's Atlas: 390–391, 396–405

BEFORE DISSECTION

Palpate the following bony landmarks on the cadaver or on yourself:

- Lateral and medial epicondyles of the humerus
- Styloid process of the radius
- Head, styloid process, olecranon process, and shaft of the ulna
- Carpal bones

Continue the incision from the lateral side of the shoulder with a vertical incision across the length of the forearm toward the wrist. Make an encircling incision around the wrist (Fig 8-1). Reflect the skin medially from the anterior compartment of the forearm, and expose the antebrachial fascia and the extensor retinaculum (Fig. 8-2). Identify the posterior cutaneous nerve of the forearm (posterior antebrachial nerve) (Fig. 8-2), lateral cutaneous nerve to the forearm (lateral antebrachial cutaneous nerve), and medial cutaneous nerve to the forearm (medial antebrachial cutaneous nerve) (Fig. 8-3).

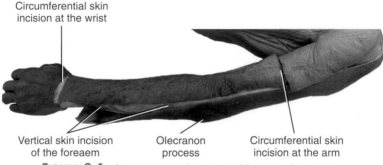

FIGURE 8-1. Skin incisions for arm and forearm dissections.

Circumferential skin incision at the wrist

Vertical skin incision of the foreaem Olecranon process Circumferential skin incision at the arm

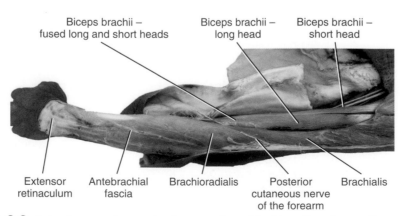

Biceps brachii – fused long and short heads   Biceps brachii – long head   Biceps brachii – short head

Extensor retinaculum   Antebrachial fascia   Brachioradialis   Posterior cutaneous nerve of the forearm   Brachialis

FIGURE 8-2. Lateral arm and posterior forearm view with skin reflected, revealing superficial structures.

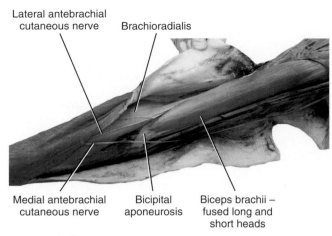

Lateral antebrachial
cutaneous nerve   Brachioradialis

Medial antebrachial   Bicipital   Biceps brachii –
cutaneous nerve   aponeurosis   fused long and
short heads

FIGURE 8-3. Lateral arm view with skin reflected, revealing superficial structures.

> ✎ *DISSECTION TIP:* Preserve as many of the cutaneous nerve branches as possible. Typically, the posterior cutaneous nerve to the forearm will emerge between the triceps brachii and brachialis muscles; the lateral cutaneous nerve to the forearm will emerge lateral to the bicipital aponeurosis between the biceps brachii and brachioradialis muscles; and the medial cutaneous nerve to the forearm can be traced proximally to the medial cord of the brachial plexus.

Biceps brachii –
fused long and
short heads

Brachioradialis

Lateral antebrachial
cutaneous nerve

Medial antebrachial   Bicipital   Medial antebrachial
cutaneous nerve   aponeurosis   cutaneous nerve

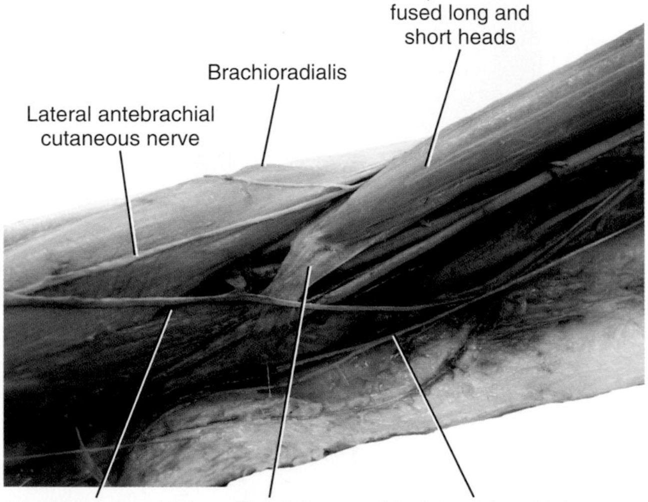

FIGURE 8-4. Cubital region with skin reflected, showing superficial structures.

Reflect the skin over the bicipital aponeurosis, and expose the cubital fossa. The biceps brachii tendon enters the cubital fossa as an aponeurotic expansion. Remove the deep fascia and the fat on the anterior surface of the cubital fossa, preserving the bicipital aponeurosis. Identify the lateral and medial cutaneous nerves to the forearm as they relate to the bicipital aponeurosis (Fig. 8-4). Lateral to the tendon of the biceps brachii, separate the brachioradialis muscle from the brachialis muscle, and identify the radial nerve as it enters the forearm. Reflect the bicipital aponeurosis laterally, and identify the brachial artery, just deep to the veins of the cubital fossa. Retract the brachial artery laterally, and on its medial side, identify the median nerve.

Continue the dissection by reflecting the skin over the extensor compartment of the forearm, and identify the distribution of the medial and lateral cutaneous nerves to the forearm (Fig. 8-5). Identify the

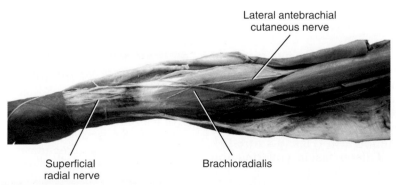

Lateral antebrachial
cutaneous nerve

Superficial   Brachioradialis
radial nerve

FIGURE 8-5. Anterior arm and forearm view with skin reflected, revealing superficial structures.

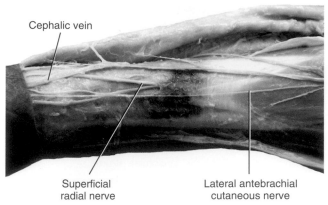

Cephalic vein

Superficial radial nerve

Lateral antebrachial cutaneous nerve

FIGURE 8-6. Cubital fossa view with skin reflected, showing superficial structures.

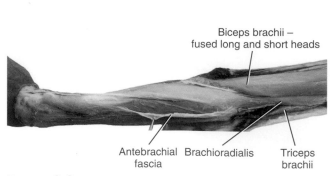

Biceps brachii – fused long and short heads

Antebrachial fascia

Brachioradialis

Triceps brachii

FIGURE 8-9. Posterolateral forearm view with skin removed, revealing fascia and superficial structures.

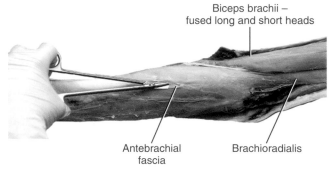

Biceps brachii – fused long and short heads

Antebrachial fascia

Brachioradialis

FIGURE 8-7. Anterior forearm and cubital fossa view with skin removed, revealing fascia.

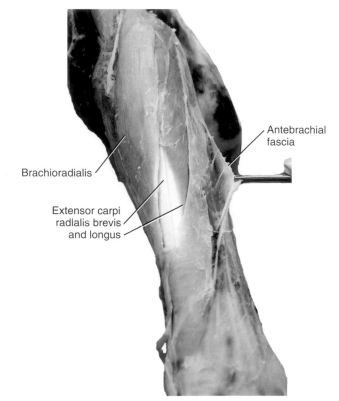

Brachioradialis

Extensor carpi radialis brevis and longus

Antebrachial fascia

FIGURE 8-10. Posterior forearm view with skin reflected, showing fascia and superficial structures.

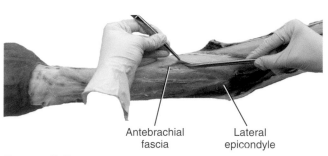

Antebrachial fascia

Lateral epicondyle

FIGURE 8-8. Posterior forearm with skin removed, showing fascia.

superficial branch of the radial nerve just proximal to the lateral side of the wrist (Fig. 8-6).

With a pair of scissors, make a small incision into the antebrachial fascia (deep fascia) near the lateral epicondyle (Fig. 8-7). Reflect the antebrachial fascia, and expose the underlying musculature of the extensor compartment of the forearm (Figs. 8-8 to 8-10). Remove all remnants of deep fascia covering the extensor surface.

> ✎ *DISSECTION TIP:* Take special care when the deep fascia is removed. In the majority of cases, the deep fascia adheres tightly to the muscles of the extensor compartment (Fig. 8-11). To identify the tendinous insertions of the muscles of the extensor compartment, the skin over the dorsum of the hand will also be removed.

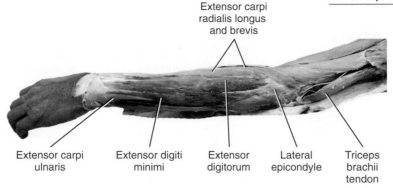

Extensor carpi
radialis longus
and brevis

Extensor carpi
ulnaris

Extensor digiti
minimi

Extensor
digitorum

Lateral
epicondyle

Triceps
brachii
tendon

FIGURE 8-11. Posterior arm and forearm view with skin removed, revealing fascia.

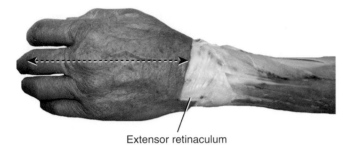

Extensor retinaculum

FIGURE 8-12. Posterior wrist view with skin removed, showing extensor retinaculum.

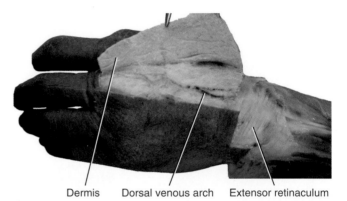

Dermis   Dorsal venous arch   Extensor retinaculum

FIGURE 8-14. Posterior hand view after skin reflection.

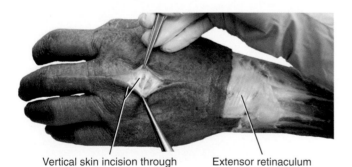

Vertical skin incision through
dermis and subcutaneous tissue

Extensor retinaculum

FIGURE 8-13. Posterior wrist view with skin removed, revealing extensor retinaculum.

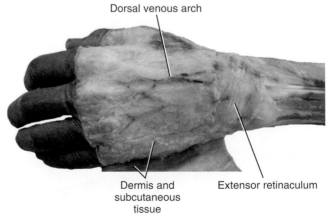

Dorsal venous arch

Dermis and
subcutaneous
tissue

Extensor retinaculum

FIGURE 8-15. Posterior hand and wrist view with skin reflected, revealing superficial structures.

Make a vertical incision at the midpoint of the wrist to the midline of the 3rd digit (Fig. 8-12). With a pair of forceps, lift the skin over the dorsum of the hand, and detach it from the underlying dermis (Fig. 8-13). Reflect the skin laterally without cutting any of the nerves and tributaries of the dorsal venous arch (Figs. 8-14 and 8-15). With a

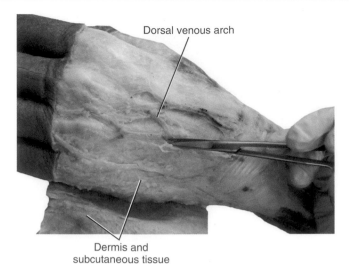

FIGURE 8-16. Posterior hand and wrist view with skin reflected, showing venous arch.

fine pair of scissors, expose the dorsal venous arch (Fig. 8-16). As the subcutaneous tissue is removed, pay special attention to identifying the cutaneous nerves running alongside the dorsal venous arch (Fig. 8-17).

✋ *DISSECTION TIP:* Exposing the dorsal venous arch and the cutaneous nerves on the dorsum of the hand can take some time (Fig. 8-18). If time does not permit, skip this step and remove the subcutaneous tissue, dorsal venous arch, and cutaneous branches en bloc.

FIGURE 8-17. Posterior hand and wrist view with skin reflected, highlighting superficial nerves and veins.

Continue the reflection of the skin over the 3rd digit (Fig. 8-19). Identify the *extensor retinaculum*, a thick fibrous band of the antebrachial fascia that holds the tendons of the extensor compartment in place (Fig. 8-20). Place a probe or scissors underneath the

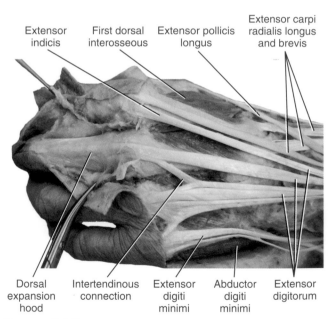

FIGURE 8-19. Posterior hand and wrist with skin reflected, exposing extensor tendons.

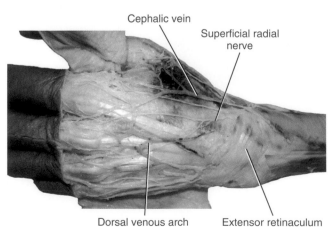

FIGURE 8-18. Posterior hand and wrist with skin reflected, revealing superficial nerves and veins.

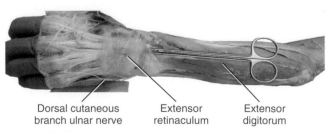

FIGURE 8-20. Posterior hand and forearm with skin removed, revealing superficial structures.

extensor retinaculum (Fig. 8-21), and release it from the underlying tendons. Make a vertical incision, and retract the retinaculum laterally to expose the tendons of the extensor compartment (Fig. 8-22). Identify the extensor digitorum muscle (Fig. 8-22). Lift its tendons and clean away its tendinous sheath (Fig. 8-23). On its ulnar side, identify the extensor digiti minimi muscle, which is seen traveling to the 5th digit. In the majority of specimens, this muscle belly is fused with the extensor digitorum muscle (Fig. 8-24).

On the radial side of the extensor digitorum muscle, identify the tendons of the abductor pollicis longus, extensor pollicis brevis, and extensor pollicis longus muscles (see Fig. 8-23).

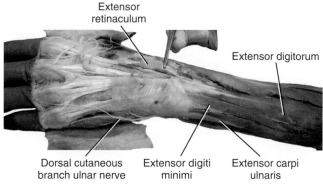

FIGURE 8-21. Posterior hand and forearm view with skin removed, showing superficial structures.

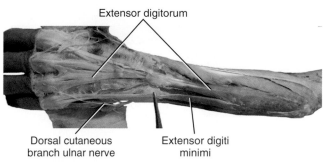

FIGURE 8-22. Posterior hand and forearm with skin removed, highlighting superficial structures.

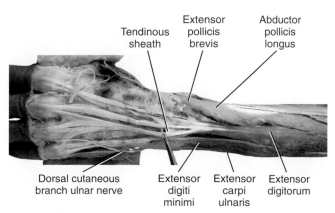

FIGURE 8-23. Posterior hand and forearm with skin reflected, revealing musculotendinous structures.

> ☝ *DISSECTION TIP:* In the majority of specimens, the muscle bellies of the abductor pollicis longus and extensor pollicis brevis muscles are fused. Use your scissors to separate them (Fig. 8-24).

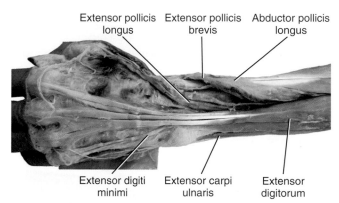

FIGURE 8-24. Posterior hand and forearm with skin reflected, highlighting musculotendinous structures.

Lift the extensor digitorum muscle, and identify the extensor indicis muscle deep to it (Fig. 8-25). The extensor indicis typically runs along the ulnar side of the tendon from the extensor digitorum to the 2nd digit.

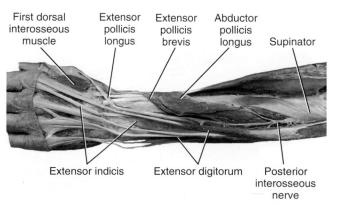

FIGURE 8-25. Posterior forearm view with brachioradialis muscle reflected, revealing muscles and tendons.

At the distal third of the forearm, lift the extensor pollicis longus and extensor pollicis brevis muscles, and underneath them, identify the extensor carpi radialis longus and brevis muscles (Figs. 8-26 and 8-27). Medial to the extensor carpi radialis brevis muscle, palpate Lister's (dorsal radial) tubercle (Fig. 8-28).

On the ulnar side of the extensor digitorum, identify the extensor digiti minimi and the extensor carpi ulnaris muscles (Fig. 8-29). Follow the extensor carpi ulnaris to the wrist. Cut the extensor retinaculum (Fig. 8-30), and release the tendons underneath it (Fig. 8-31). Retract the extensor carpi ulnaris muscle, and separate it from the adjacent extensor digiti minimi muscle (Figs. 8-32 and 8-33).

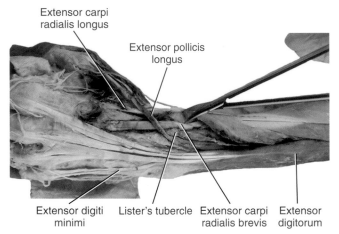

FIGURE 8-26. Posterior hand and forearm view with skin reflected.

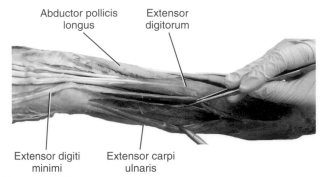

FIGURE 8-29. Anteromedial forearm view, revealing ulnar artery and nerves.

FIGURE 8-27. Posterior hand and forearm with skin reflected.

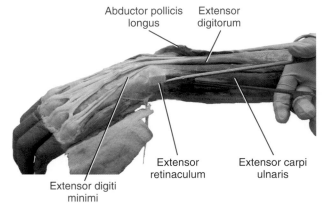

FIGURE 8-30. Medial posterior view of wrist revealing superficial structures.

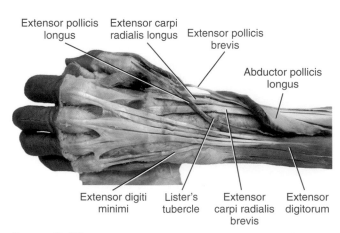

FIGURE 8-28. Posterior hand and forearm with skin reflected.

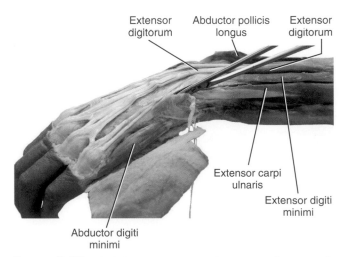

FIGURE 8-31. Medial posterior view of wrist revealing superficial structures.

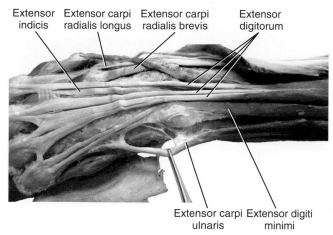

Extensor indicis Extensor carpi radialis longus Extensor carpi radialis brevis Extensor digitorum

Extensor carpi ulnaris Extensor digiti minimi

FIGURE 8-32. Posteromedial view of wrist showing muscle tendons.

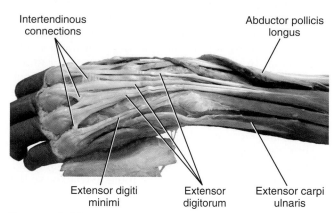

Intertendinous connections Abductor pollicis longus

Extensor digiti minimi Extensor digitorum Extensor carpi ulnaris

FIGURE 8-33. Posteromedial view of wrist exposing muscle tendons.

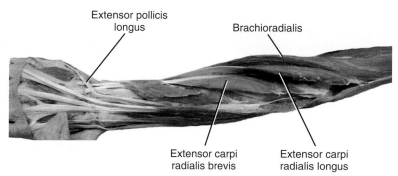

Extensor pollicis longus Brachioradialis

Extensor carpi radialis brevis Extensor carpi radialis longus

FIGURE 8-34. Posterior view of upper forearm, highlighting musculature.

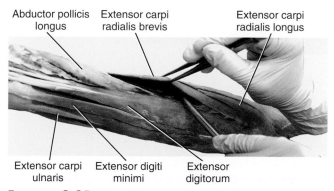

Abductor pollicis longus Extensor carpi radialis brevis Extensor carpi radialis longus

Extensor carpi ulnaris Extensor digiti minimi Extensor digitorum

FIGURE 8-35. Posterior upper forearm view, revealing musculature.

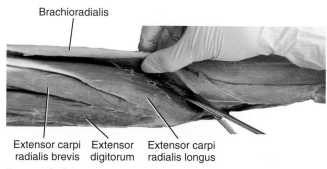

Brachioradialis

Extensor carpi radialis brevis Extensor digitorum Extensor carpi radialis longus

FIGURE 8-36. Posterior upper forearm showing musculature.

On the radial aspect of the proximal part of the forearm, identify and separate the brachioradialis, extensor carpi radialis longus, extensor carpi radialis brevis, and extensor digitorum muscles (Fig. 8-34).

Lift the brachioradialis from the underlying extensor carpi radialis longus muscle. Use a probe or scissors to complete the separation of these two muscles (Figs. 8-35 and 8-36).

Reflect or lift the brachioradialis muscle anteriorly, and identify the radial nerve (Fig. 8-37). Lift the brachioradialis muscle to allow maximum exposure of the radial nerve. Clean the radial nerve and identify its division into superficial and deep branches. The superficial branch runs beneath the brachioradialis to reach the dorsum of the hand. The deep branch of the radial nerve runs through the supinator muscle.

With a pair of scissors, cut between the fibers of the extensor carpi radialis brevis and extensor digitorum muscles, and expose the supinator muscle lying underneath (Fig. 8-38). Reflect the extensor digitorum away from the supinator muscle to expose the supinator's borders (Fig. 8-39). At the inferior border

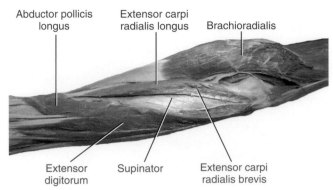

FIGURE 8-38. Posterior view of forearm showing musculature.

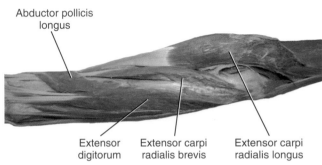

FIGURE 8-37. Posterior view of forearm revealing musculature.

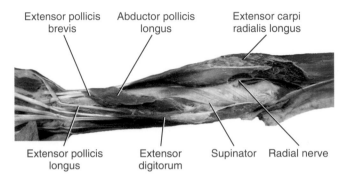

FIGURE 8-39. Posterior view with brachioradialis muscle cut, revealing radial nerve and supinator muscle.

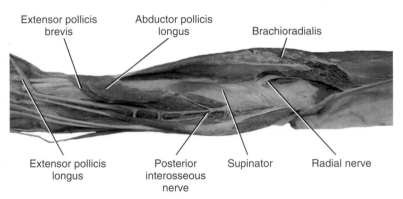

FIGURE 8-40. Posterior view with brachioradialis muscle cut, showing radial nerve and supinator muscle.

of the supinator, trace and expose the deep radial nerve (Fig. 8-40). With a scalpel, make an incision in the supinator where the deep branch of the radial nerve first enters it (Fig. 8-41). Reflect the supinator, and expose the deep radial nerve (Fig. 8-42).

Make an incision on the posterior border of the ulna, and detach the extensor carpi ulnaris muscle. Look for the emergence of the posterior interosseous artery running parallel to the deep branch of the radial nerve between the radius and the ulna.

☞ *DISSECTION TIP:* The recurrent interosseous artery can be found between the anconeus and supinator muscles. Remove the anconeus, which travels from the lateral epicondyle to the lateral aspect of the olecranon process. Just beneath it, on the anterior surface of the supinator, identify the recurrent interosseous artery. This artery is usually small and is often cut during routine dissection.

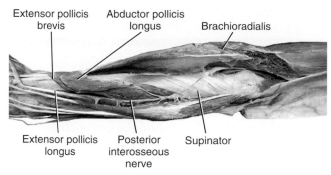

Extensor pollicis
brevis

Abductor pollicis
longus

Brachioradialis

Extensor pollicis
longus

Posterior
interosseous
nerve

Supinator

FIGURE 8-41. Posterior view with brachioradialis cut, revealing supinator muscle.

After completion of the dissection of the extensor compartment, rotate the upper limb and visualize the flexor compartment (Fig. 8-43). Make a vertical incision across the length of the forearm toward the wrist. Make an encircling incision around the cubital fossa and the wrist (Fig. 8-43). Reflect the skin medially and laterally from the flexor compartment, and expose the antebrachial fascia and the flexor retinaculum (Fig. 8-44). Continue the vertical midline incision toward the 3rd digit. Chapter 9 details the dissection of the hand.

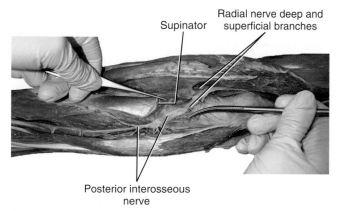

Supinator

Radial nerve deep and
superficial branches

Posterior interosseous
nerve

FIGURE 8-42. Posterior forearm view with brachioradialis cut, revealing radial nerve branches, supinator muscle, and posterior interosseous nerve.

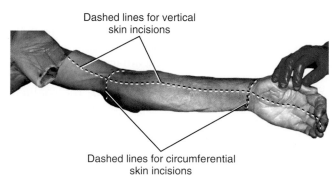

Dashed lines for vertical
skin incisions

Dashed lines for circumferential
skin incisions

FIGURE 8-43. Anterior view of arm, forearm, and hand, with dashed lines for incisions.

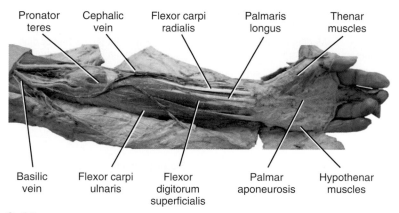

Pronator
teres

Cephalic
vein

Flexor carpi
radialis

Palmaris
longus

Thenar
muscles

Basilic
vein

Flexor carpi
ulnaris

Flexor
digitorum
superficialis

Palmar
aponeurosis

Hypothenar
muscles

FIGURE 8-44. Anterior view of forearm and hand with skin reflected, revealing superficial structures.

Identify the venous network in the flexor compartment and in the cubital fossa. Trace the tributaries of the basilic vein. Identify the median cubital vein connecting the basilic and cephalic veins (Fig. 8-45). Once you identify the cephalic vein, trace it proximally to the arm. Lateral to the cephalic vein, identify the lateral cutaneous nerve to the forearm, or lateral antebrachial cutaneous nerve. This nerve is the cutaneous branch of musculocutaneous nerve and supplies the lateral aspect of the forearm (Fig. 8-45). Notice the thick, flat connective tissue aponeurosis of the biceps brachii muscle, the *bicipital aponeurosis.*

An easy way to identify the muscles of the forearm is to expose them from the wrist toward the cubital fossa. At the wrist, the tendons of each muscle are fairly evident and require minimal dissection. On the radial side of the forearm, identify the flexor carpi radialis muscle (Fig. 8-46). The flexor carpi radialis attaches to the second metacarpal bone, and some of its fibers may radiate to the adjacent 3rd metacarpal. Medial to the flexor carpi radialis, note the palmaris longus muscle inserting into the palmar aponeurosis. On the ulnar side of the forearm, identify the flexor carpi ulnaris muscle. These three muscles occupy the superficial layer of the muscles of the flexor compartment.

> ✒ *DISSECTION TIP:* The palmaris longus muscle is absent in about 10% of the population.

Dissect out the deep fascia and the connective tissue over the tendons and the muscles of the flexor compartment (Figs. 8-47 and 8-48). Expose the tendon insertions of the flexor carpi ulnaris and flexor carpi radialis muscles (Fig. 8-49). Deep to the palmaris longus muscle, note the flexor digitorum superficialis muscle. Retract the flexor carpi ulnaris, and in the space between it and the flexor digitorum superficialis, identify a thick bundle of connective tissue encircling the ulnar artery and nerve (Fig. 8-50). With the aid of scissors, separate the connective tissue over the ulnar artery and nerve (Fig. 8-51). Further retract the flexor digitorum superficialis muscle, and clean and expose the ulnar artery and nerve along the entire length of the forearm (Figs. 8-52 and 8-53).

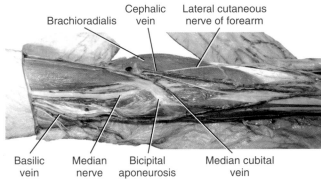

FIGURE 8-45. Anterior cubital fossa revealing superficial structures.

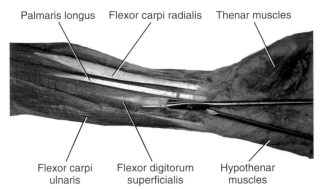

FIGURE 8-47. Anterior forearm and hand revealing muscle-tendon units.

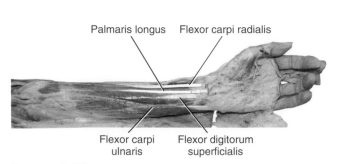

FIGURE 8-46. Anterior view of forearm and hand showing muscle-tendon units.

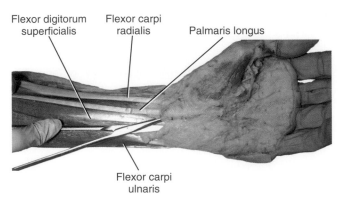

FIGURE 8-48. Anterior forearm and hand, highlighting muscle-tendon units.

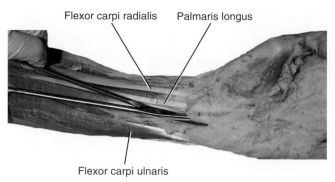

Flexor carpi radialis   Palmaris longus

Flexor carpi ulnaris

FIGURE 8-49. Anterior view of forearm and hand showing muscle-tendon units.

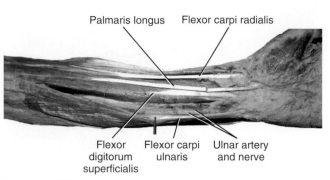

Palmaris longus   Flexor carpi radialis

Flexor digitorum superficialis   Flexor carpi ulnaris   Ulnar artery and nerve

FIGURE 8-50. Anterior forearm and hand view, revealing muscle-tendon units, with traction of flexor carpi ulnaris.

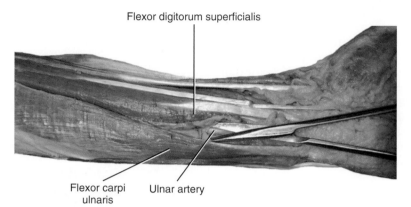

Flexor digitorum superficialis

Flexor carpi ulnaris   Ulnar artery

FIGURE 8-51. Anterior view of forearm and wrist revealing muscle-tendon units.

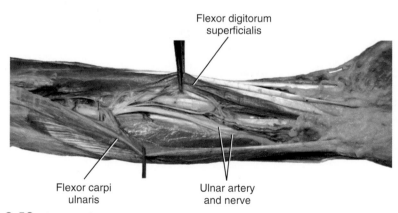

Flexor digitorum superficialis

Flexor carpi ulnaris   Ulnar artery and nerve

FIGURE 8-52. Anterior forearm with traction to flexor digitorum superficialis muscle, showing intermediate layer.

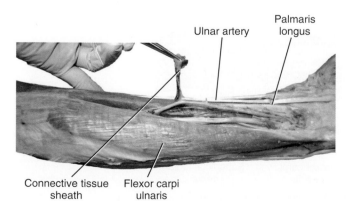

Ulnar artery   Palmaris longus

Connective tissue sheath   Flexor carpi ulnaris

FIGURE 8-53. Anterior forearm noting the flexor carpi ulnaris and palmaris longus muscles.

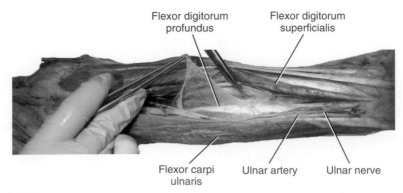

FIGURE 8-54. Anterior forearm view with traction to flexor digitorum superficialis muscle, exposing intermediate level.

Underneath the flexor digitorum superficialis, indentify the flexor digitorum profundus muscle. Clean the loose connective tissue over the flexor digitorum profundus (Fig. 8-54). Identify the radial artery between the brachioradialis and flexor carpi radialis muscles (Fig. 8-55). Further retract the brachioradialis muscle, and expose the radial artery in the forearm (Figs 8-56 and 8-57). Parallel to the radial artery, identify and expose the superficial branch of the radial nerve (Fig. 8-58).

> **DISSECTION TIP:** Note the following landmarks in the course of the radial artery:
> • Passes superficial to the pronator teres muscle.
> • Travels deep to the brachioradialis muscle.
>   At the wrist, the radial artery is found between the tendons of the flexor carpi radialis and the brachioradialis muscles. This point is used to feel the radial pulse or to perform arterial catheterization.

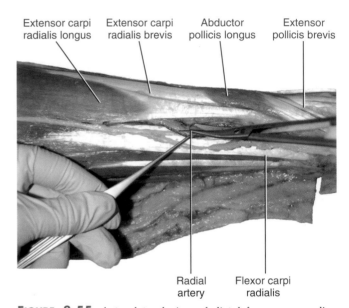

FIGURE 8-55. Anterolateral view of distal forearm, revealing radial neurovascular bundle.

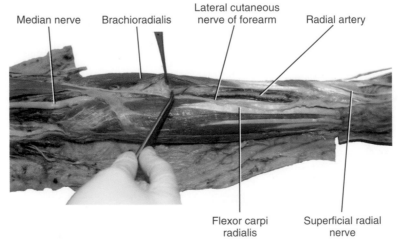

FIGURE 8-56. Anteromedial view of forearm with skin reflected, revealing radial artery and vein.

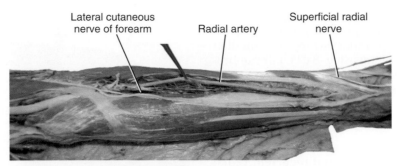

FIGURE 8-57. Anterior forearm view with skin reflected, revealing radial artery and vein.

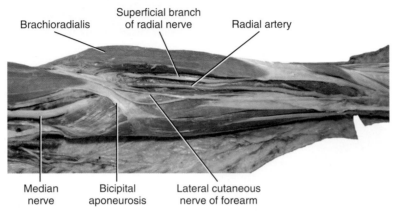

FIGURE 8-58. Anterior forearm view, showing radial artery, vein, and nerve.

The flexor digitorum profundus muscle inserts onto the bases of the distal phalanx of each of the medial four digits. A common variation of the flexor digitorum profundus is that its tendon to the 2nd digit may form an independent muscle. The flexor pollicis longus muscle inserts onto the distal phalanx of the 1st digit.

DISSECTION TIP: The flexor digitorum superficialis muscle inserts onto the base of the middle phalanx of digits 2 to 5. However, the tendon to the 5th digit may be absent.

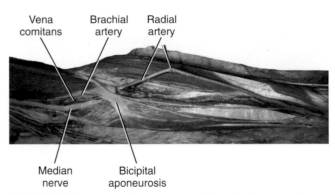

FIGURE 8-59. Anterior forearm view with radial artery and traction revealing musculature.

Expose the radial artery (Fig. 8-59).

Cut the bicipital aponeurosis (Fig. 8-60) to trace the radial artery to its branch point from the brachial artery. Also, identify the ulnar artery, the median nerve, and the vena comitans (Fig. 8-61). Lift the brachial and radial arteries, and expose the ulnar artery with its branches (Fig. 8-62). At this point, use a retractor between the brachioradialis and the flexor digitorum superficialis muscles to expose deeper structures (Fig. 8-63).

Follow the course of the ulnar and radial arteries, and identify the recurrent ulnar and recurrent radial arteries. Identify the pronator teres and its two heads; the humeral (superficial) head is attached to the medial epicondyle and the ulnar (deep) head to

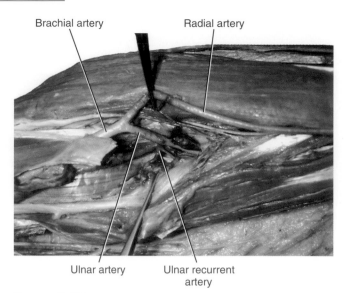

FIGURE 8-62. Anterior view of cubital fossa with bicipital aponeurosis cut, revealing the bifurcation of the brachial artery.

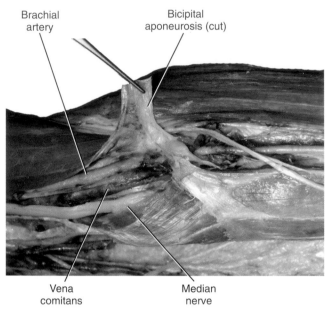

FIGURE 8-60. Anterior view of cubital fossa with bicipital aponeurosis reflected, revealing brachial artery and median nerve.

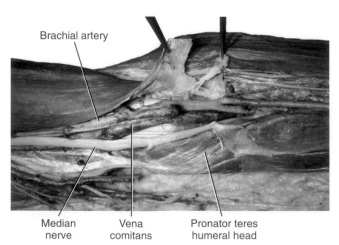

FIGURE 8-61. Anterior cubital fossa view with bicipital aponeurosis reflected, highlighting brachial artery and median nerve.

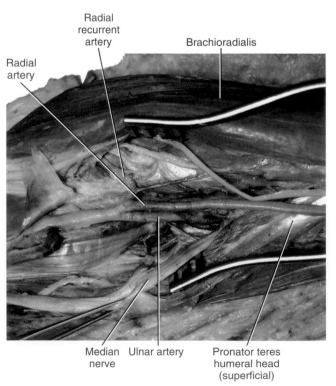

FIGURE 8-63. Anterior cubital fossa view with bicipital aponeurosis reflected, exposing neurovascular structures.

the coronoid process of the ulna. Trace the course of the medial nerve as it travels from the cubital fossa and then enters the forearm between the two heads of the pronator teres (Fig. 8-63). Note the ulnar artery entering the forearm deep to the ulnar (deep) head of the pronator teres muscle (Fig. 8-63). Lift up the median nerve, and identify its muscular branches (Fig. 8-64).

> **DISSECTION TIP:** To continue the dissection, the vena comitans must be removed (Fig. 8-65). Cut the veins in the cubital fossa and as distal as possible in the forearm (Fig. 8-66). Use paper towels to absorb any fluid that issues from the cut veins.

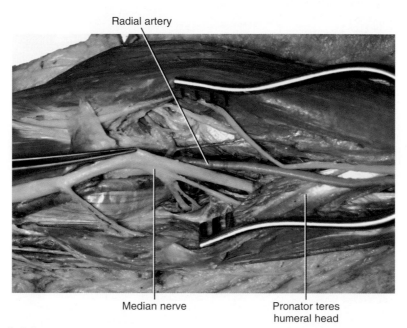

Radial artery

Median nerve

Pronator teres
humeral head

FIGURE 8-64. Anterior cubital fossa view with bicipital aponeurosis reflected, revealing neurovascular structures.

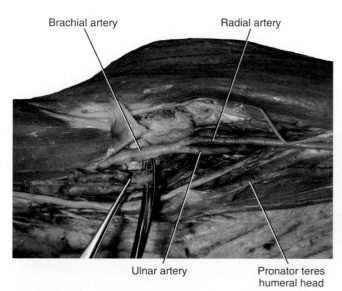

Brachial artery   Radial artery

Ulnar artery   Pronator teres
humeral head

FIGURE 8-65. Anterior view of cubital fossa with bicipital aponeurosis reflected, highlighting neurovascular structures.

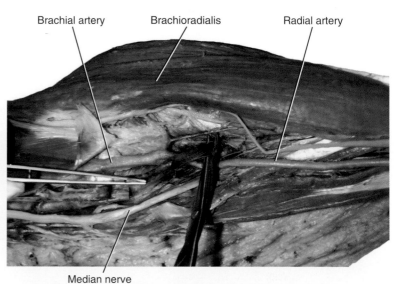

Brachial artery   Brachioradialis   Radial artery

Median nerve

FIGURE 8-66. Anterior cubital fossa view with bicipital aponeurosis reflected, revealing neurovascular structures.

Expose the borders of the pronator teres, and retract the radial artery (Fig. 8-67). Carefully split the humeral head of the pronator teres (Fig. 8-68) from the underlying ulnar (deep) head and flexor digitorum superficialis muscle (Figs. 8-69 and 8-70). Lift the median nerve and expose its course in the deep

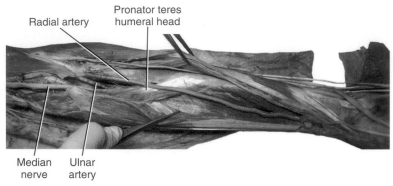

FIGURE 8-67. Anterolateral forearm view with skin reflected, revealing radial artery and musculature.

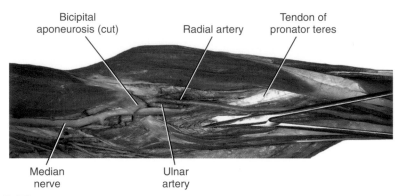

FIGURE 8-68. Anterior cubital fossa with bicipital aponeurosis cut, exposing median nerve, radial artery, and pronator teres muscle.

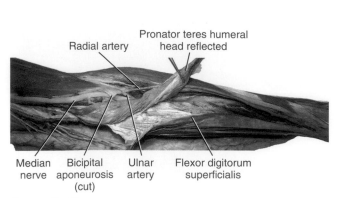

FIGURE 8-69. Anterior view of lateral cubital fossa and forearm with reflected pronator teres, revealing musculature.

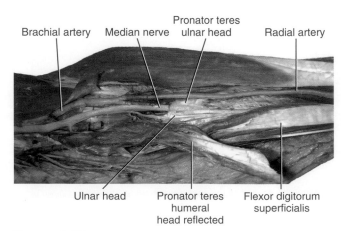

FIGURE 8-70. Anterior cubital fossa view with pronator teres muscle reflected, revealing deeper structures.

flexor compartment of the forearm (Fig. 8-71). Dissect distally the ulnar artery and identify the common interosseous artery (Fig. 8-72). The common interosseous artery arises from the ulnar artery and then divides into the anterior and posterior interosseous branches (Fig. 8-73). The posterior interosseous artery passes through the interosseous membrane to reach the extensor compartment of the forearm. As the median nerve is lifted, identify the anterior interosseous nerve, which arises from the median nerve just proximal to the pronator teres muscle (Figs. 8-72 and 8-73).

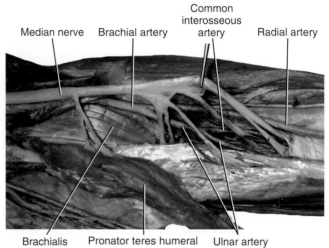

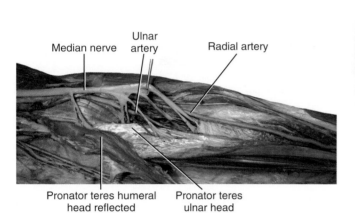

FIGURE 8-71. Anterior cubital fossa view with superficial (humeral) head of pronator teres muscle reflected, and median nerve traction revealing deep (ulnar) head of pronator teres.

FIGURE 8-72. Anterior cubital fossa view with superficial pronator teres head reflected, and median nerve traction revealing deep pronator teres head, and radial and ulnar arteries.

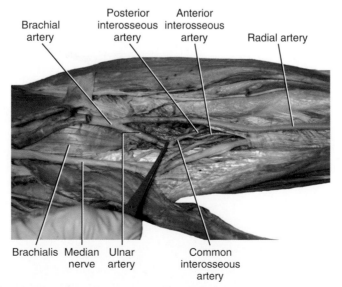

FIGURE 8-73. Anterior cubital fossa view with superficial head of pronator teres reflected, and median nerve traction revealing deep head of pronator teres and radial and ulnar arteries.

Cut the tendons of the flexor digitorum superficialis, or widely retract them, and identify the flexor digitorum profundus and flexor pollicis longus muscles (Fig. 8-74). Finally, identify the *pronator quadratus,* which connects the distal portions of the ulna and radius (Fig. 8-75). In the space between the flexor pollicis longus and flexor digitorum profundus muscles, trace the course of the anterior interosseous artery and anterior interosseous nerve, a branch of the median nerve (Figs. 8-74 and 8-75).

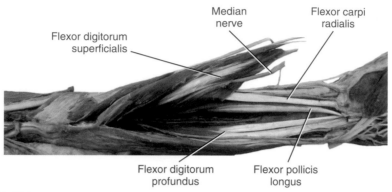

FIGURE 8-74. Anterior forearm view with superficial and intermediate muscle layers cut and reflected, exposing deeper structures.

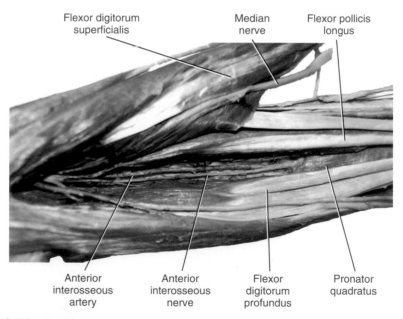

FIGURE 8-75. Anterior view of forearm with superficial and intermediate muscle layers cut and reflected, revealing deeper structures.

LABORATORY IDENTIFICATION CHECKLIST

Nerves
❏ Musculocutaneous
❏ Lateral antebrachial cutaneous
❏ Median
❏ Anterior interosseous
❏ Medial brachial cutaneous
❏ Medial antebrachial cutaneous
❏ Ulnar
❏ Radial
❏ Posterior interosseous

Arteries
❏ Brachial
❏ Radial
❏ Radial recurrent
❏ Interosseous recurrent
❏ Ulnar
❏ Common interosseous
❏ Anterior interosseous
❏ Posterior interosseous
❏ Ulnar anterior recurrent
❏ Ulnar posterior recurrent

Veins
Superficial
❏ Cephalic
❏ Basilic
❏ Cubital
Deep
❏ Brachial
❏ Radial
❏ Ulnar

Muscles
Anterior compartment of arm
❏ Coracobrachialis
❏ Biceps brachii
  ❏ Long head
  ❏ Short head
❏ Brachialis
Posterior compartment of arm
❏ Triceps brachii
  ❏ Long head
  ❏ Lateral head
  ❏ Medial head
❏ Anconeus
Anterior compartment of forearm
SUPERFICIAL LAYER
  ❏ Pronator teres
    ❏ Humeral (superficial) head
    ❏ Ulnar (deep) head
  ❏ Flexor carpi radialis
  ❏ Palmaris longus
  ❏ Flexor carpi ulnaris
INTERMEDIATE LAYER
  ❏ Flexor digitorum superficialis
DEEP LAYER
  ❏ Flexor digitorum profundus
  ❏ Flexor pollicis longus
  ❏ Pronator quadratus

Muscles—cont'd
Posterior compartment of forearm
SUPERFICIAL LAYER
  ❏ Brachioradialis
  ❏ Extensor carpi radialis longus
  ❏ Extensor carpi radialis brevis
  ❏ Extensor digitorum
  ❏ Extensor digiti minimi
  ❏ Extensor carpi ulnaris
DEEP LAYER
  ❏ Supinator
  ❏ Abductor pollicis longus
  ❏ Extensor pollicis longus
  ❏ Extensor pollicis brevis
  ❏ Extensor indicis

Ligaments
❏ Ulnar collateral
❏ Radial collateral
❏ Annular

Connective Tissue
❏ Bicipital aponeurosis
❏ Antebrachial fascia
❏ Flexor retinaculum
❏ Extensor retinaculum

Bones
❏ Scapula
❏ Humerus
❏ Radius
❏ Ulna
❏ Carpal bones
❏ Metacarpals
❏ Phalanges

CHAPTER 9

HAND

Netter: 440–459, 463–464

McMinn: 161–173

Gray's Atlas: 392–395, 406–422

PALPATION

Flex and extend your digits, noting the movements of the tendons beneath the skin. On the dorsal side of your hand, identify the tendons of the extensor digitorum muscle. At the flexor aspect of the palm, note the distal skin crease (crease between wrist and forearm), marking the proximal edge of the flexor retinaculum (transverse carpal ligament) (Fig. 9-1). At the ulnar side of the distal skin crease, palpate the pisiform bone. At the radial side of the distal skin crease, palpate the scaphoid bone. Immediately beneath the radial and ulnar sides of the distal skin crease, palpate the radial and ulnar styloid processes, respectively.

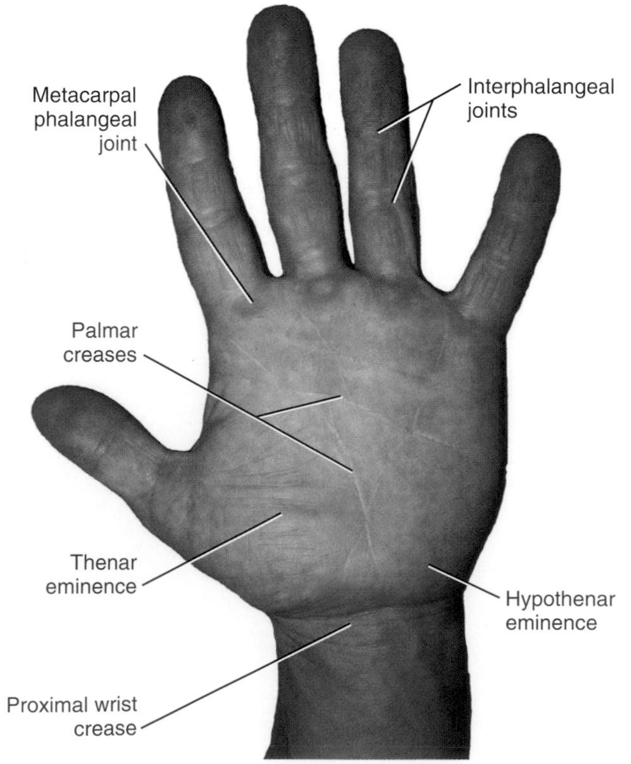

By flexing the closed fist against resistance, you should be able to indentify several tendons at the anterior wrist, from medial to lateral: the flexor carpi ulnaris, flexor digitorum superficialis, palmaris longus, and flexor carpi radialis. However, the most prominent tendons are those of the palmaris longus, lying at the midline, and the flexor carpi radialis, lying in the radial side. Lateral to the tendon of the flexor carpi radialis, you can palpate the radial artery. The pulsations of the ulnar artery are much more difficult to detect and are usually felt about 3 cm proximal to the pisiform bone, medial to the flexor carpi ulnaris muscle. Note the thenar and hypothenar eminences, which contain muscles of the 1st digit and the 5th digit, respectively.

On the dorsum surface of the hand, extend the 1st digit, noting the tendons of the abductor pollicis longus (to base of 1st metacarpal bone), the extensor pollicis brevis (to base of 1st phalanx), and the extensor pollicis longus muscles (to base of distal phalanx of 1st digit) forming the "anatomic snuffbox" (Fig. 9-2). This anatomic area is important because the radial artery lies on the scaphoid bone and passes to reach the dorsum of the 1st digit.

FIGURE 9-1. Anterior view of palmar surface of hand. Note positioning of interphalangeal and metacarpal phalangeal joints, palmar and wrist creases, and thenar and hypothenar eminences.

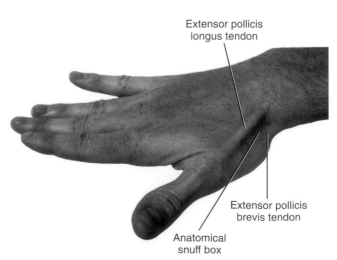

FIGURE 9-2. Dorsolateral view of wrist, noting "anatomic snuffbox," which is bordered by the underlying extensor pollicis longus and brevis tendons.

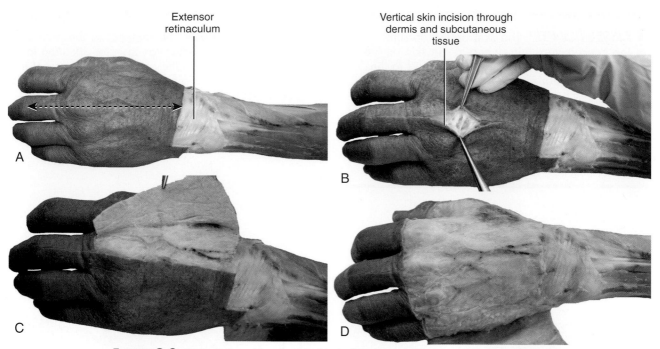

FIGURE 9-3. Dorsal view of hand, with skin incisions exposing the subcutaneous layer.

DISSECTION

Make a midline incision on the dorsal surface of the hand as indicated in Chapter 8 (Figs. 8-12 to 8-16) (Fig. 9-3). Make a similar midline incision on the palmar surface, starting from the distal palmar crease to the base of the 3rd digit (Fig. 9-4). Make a second midline incision on the palmar surface of each digit. Join these with transverse incisions at the bases of the digits. With additional incisions as necessary, reflect and remove the skin from the hand (Fig. 9-5).

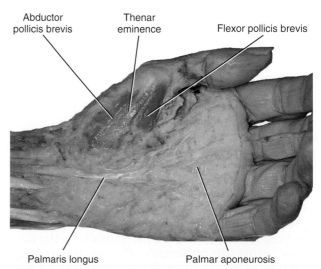

FIGURE 9-4. Anterior view of palmar hand, with dashed lines showing skin incision sites.

FIGURE 9-5. Anterior view of hand with skin reflected, noting superficial structures, including muscles of thenar eminence and the palmar aponeurosis. Note palmaris longus muscle inserting into palmar aponeurosis.

> ☝ *DISSECTION TIP:* The skin on the dorsum of the hand is very thin, whereas the skin on the palmar surface is thick and tightly bound to the underlying palmar aponeurosis. Make a shallow incision on the dorsum of the hand, and with the aid of dissecting scissors, separate the skin from the underlying tissues. Make a deeper incision on the palmar surface of the hand, using the palmaris longus muscle as a guide to remove the skin with sharp dissection.

> ☝ *DISSECTION TIP:* The removal of the palmar aponeurosis takes time. Pay special attention to using the scalpel as little as possible so as not to injure the palmar digital nerves and the superficial palmar arch. These structures travel deep to the palmar aponeurosis.

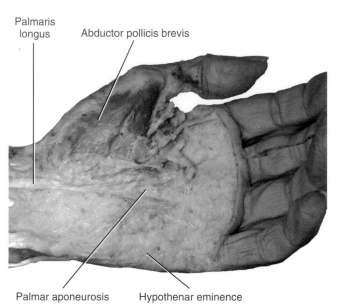

FIGURE 9-6. Anterior view of hand with skin reflected, illustrating subcutaneous fat covering muscles that make up the hypothenar eminence.

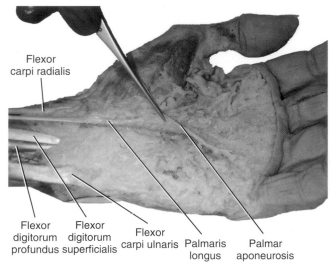

FIGURE 9-7. Anterior hand with skin reflected and traction on the palmar aponeurosis. The aponeurosis will be reflected to reveal deeper structures.

After removal of the skin on the palmar surface of the hand, trace the continuation of the palmaris longus muscle to the palmar aponeurosis (Fig. 9-5). Note the thenar eminence with the flexor pollicis brevis and abductor pollicis muscles (Fig. 9-6). Lift the palmar aponeurosis (Fig. 9-7) and with the aid of dissecting scissors separate it from the underlying structures (Fig. 9-8). The *palmar aponeurosis* is composed of longitudinal and transversely oriented fibers of dense connective tissue. The longitudinal fibers form digital bands that attach to the bases of the proximal phalanges and become continuous with the fibrous digital sheaths (ligamentous tubes enclosing synovial sheaths). With scissors, cut the attachments of the longitudinal bands from the bases of the proximal phalanges. Reflect the palmaris longus muscle and the palmar aponeurosis toward the forearm (Fig. 9-9).

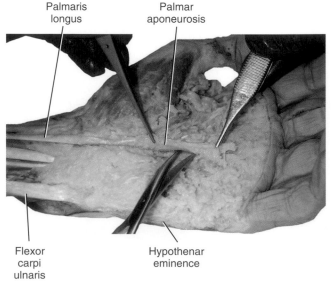

FIGURE 9-8. Anterior hand with skin reflected, revealing palmar aponeurosis. Constant tension of the aponeurosis will allow scissors to be inserted deep to it.

After removal of the palmar aponeurosis, start exposing the superficial palmar arch (Figs. 9-10 and 9-11). The *superficial palmar arch* is the termination of the superficial branch of the ulnar artery, which gives rise to three common palmar digital arteries. These arteries anastomose with the palmar metacarpal branches from the deep palmar arterial arch. The common palmar digital arteries then divide into a pair of proper digital arteries, supplying the adjacent sides of the 2nd to 4th digits.

☝ *DISSECTION TIP:* The superficial palmar arch is related to the superficial venous arch, as well as with common palmar digital branches of the median nerve. With scissors, separate the nerves from the superficial palmar arch (Figs. 9-10 to 9-12). Also, remove any venous structures from this area.

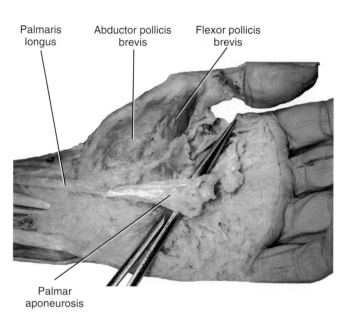

FIGURE 9-9. Anterior hand with skin reflected, revealing palmar aponeurosis. Once the aponeurosis is cut distally, it can be reflected to demonstrate deeper structures.

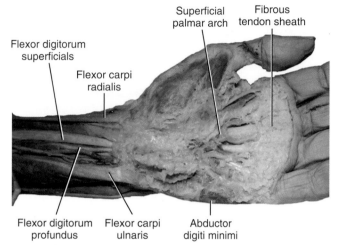

FIGURE 9-11. Anterior view of hand with skin and aponeurosis reflected, showing tendon sheaths and neurovascular structures such as superficial palmar arch.

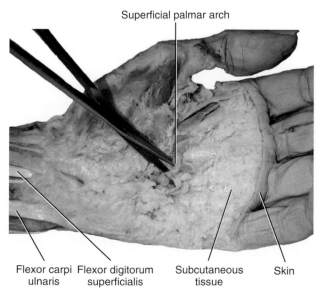

FIGURE 9-10. Anterior view of hand with skin and aponeurosis reflected, revealing deeper structures such as the superficial palmar arch.

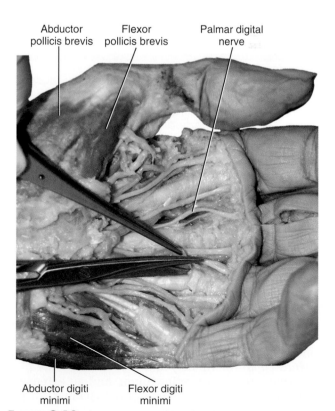

FIGURE 9-12. Anterior view of hand with skin and aponeurosis reflected, revealing tendon sheaths and adjacent neurovascular structures.

Immediately after its passage through the carpal tunnel, the median nerve gives rise to several smaller branches: the recurrent branch of the median nerve (motor) and the common palmar digital branches (cutaneous). At this point in the dissection, identify the common palmar digital branches of the median nerve running alongside the common palmar digital arteries (Fig. 9-13).

Continue the dissection toward the phalanges, and expose the separation of the common palmar digital branches of the median nerve into proper palmar digital nerves of the digits. Similarly, expose the site at which the common palmar digital arteries give rise to palmar digital arteries (Fig. 9-14). Clean away the fascia investing the abductor and flexor digiti minimi muscles over the hypothenar region.

> ☝ *DISSECTION TIP:* In about 65% of the specimens, a communication between the ulnar and median nerves exists distal to the flexor retinaculum.

Continue the removal of fat and remnants of the palmar aponeurosis at the medial aspect of the palm, the *hypothenar eminence* (see Fig. 9-8). Identify the flexor digiti minimi and the abductor digiti minimi muscles (see Fig. 9-12). Expose the palmar digital branches to the 5th digit and medial half of the 4th digit (see Fig. 9-14).

> ☝ *DISSECTION TIP:* The most superficially placed muscle in the hypothenar eminence is the *palmaris brevis*. This muscle is extremely thin and often blended with adipose tissue, arising from the palmar aponeurosis to insert into the skin. It is rather difficult to expose the palmaris brevis because it is detached during removal of the palmar aponeurosis and skin.

Trace the palmar digital branches to the 5th digit and medial half of the 4th digit toward their origin from the superficial branch of the ulnar nerve (Fig. 9-15). Remove the deep fascia at the ulnar side of the wrist, and using scissors (Fig. 9-16), expose the superficial branch of the ulnar nerve (Fig. 9-17). The ulnar artery and nerve travel lateral to the pisiform bone to enter the palm. This point is referred as *Guyon's canal* (or tunnel) and is formed by the pisiform bone, the flexor retinaculum, and an extension of the deep fascia of the forearm (palmar carpal ligament).

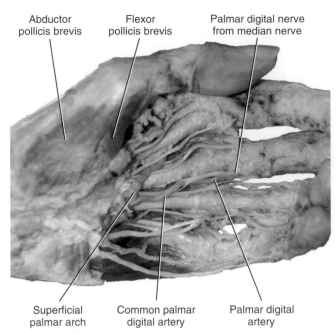

Abductor pollicis brevis   Flexor pollicis brevis   Palmar digital nerve from median nerve

Superficial palmar arch   Common palmar digital artery   Palmar digital artery

FIGURE 9-13. Anterior view of hand with skin and aponeurosis reflected, highlighting tendon sheaths and neurovascular structures such as palmar digital nerves and arteries.

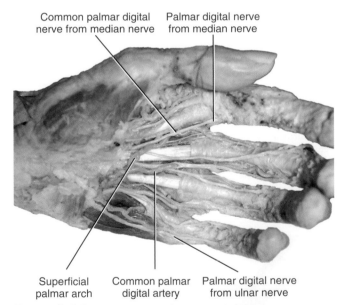

Common palmar digital nerve from median nerve   Palmar digital nerve from median nerve

Superficial palmar arch   Common palmar digital artery   Palmar digital nerve from ulnar nerve

FIGURE 9-14. Anterior view of hand with skin and aponeurosis reflected, revealing tendon sheaths and neurovascular structures. Note common palmar arteries arising from superficial palmar arch.

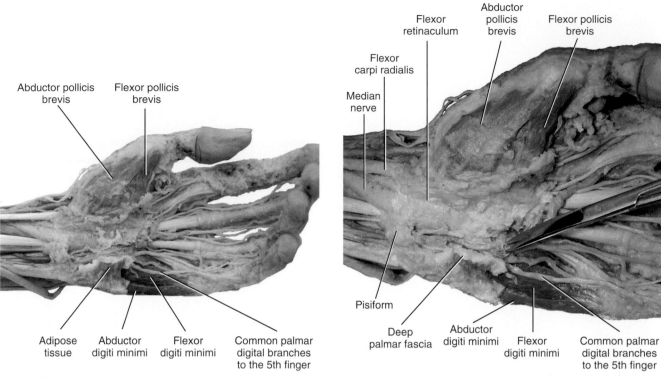

FIGURE 9-15. Anterior hand with skin and aponeurosis reflected, revealing thenar and hypothenar muscles.

FIGURE 9-16. Anterior hand with skin and aponeurosis reflected, revealing thenar and hypothenar muscles. Note median nerve traveling deep to flexor retinaculum within the carpal tunnel.

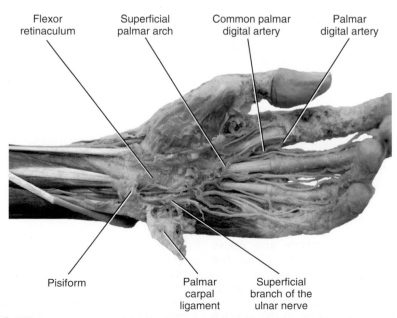

FIGURE 9-17. Anterior hand with skin and aponeurosis reflected, revealing thenar and hypothenar muscles. Note the palmar carpal ligament that has been reflected to better illustrate the deeper flexor retinaculum.

> **DISSECTION TIP:** The tendons of the flexor digitorum superficialis and flexor digitorum profundus muscles are enclosed by a synovial sheath, the *ulnar bursa*. The tendon of the flexor pollicis longus is also enclosed by a synovial sheath, the *radial bursa*. To free up the superficial palmar arch and nerve structures from the underlying long flexor tendons, incise the fibrous tendinous sheaths longitudinally (Fig. 9-20)

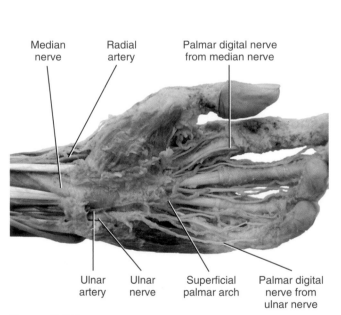

FIGURE 9-18. Anterior hand with skin and aponeurosis removed, revealing superficial palmar arch. Note that the primary contributor to the superficial palmar arch is the ulnar artery.

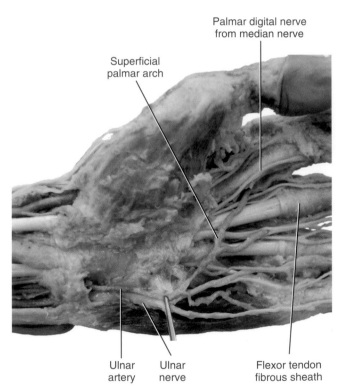

FIGURE 9-19. Anterior hand with skin and aponeurosis removed, revealing superficial palmar arterial arch and branches to the digits.

Expose the superficial ulnar artery and nerve toward the pisiform bone (Fig. 9-18). Clean the adipose tissue and remnants of the palmar aponeurosis surrounding the superficial palmar arch distally to the carpal tunnel and flexor retinaculum (Fig. 9-18). Expose the ulnar artery and clean the surface of the flexor retinaculum (Fig. 9-19).

Immediately distal to the pisiform bone and lateral to the flexor retinaculum, expose the division of the ulnar artery and nerve into deep and superficial branches (Figs. 9-21 and 9-22). The deep branches dive deeply between the abductor and flexor digiti minimi muscles of the 5th digit.

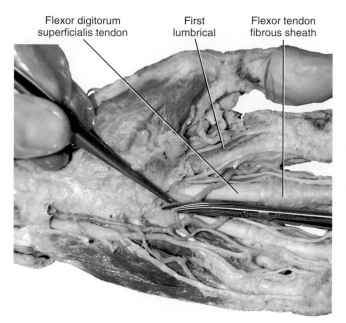

Flexor digitorum superficialis tendon   First lumbrical   Flexor tendon fibrous sheath

FIGURE 9-20. Anterior hand with skin and aponeurosis removed. Use scissors to open the fibrous tendon sheaths to identify tendons of flexor digitorum superficialis and profundus muscles.

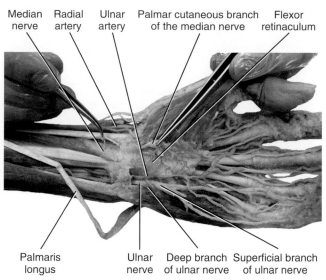

Median nerve   Radial artery   Ulnar artery   Palmar cutaneous branch of the median nerve   Flexor retinaculum

Palmaris longus   Ulnar nerve   Deep branch of ulnar nerve   Superficial branch of ulnar nerve

FIGURE 9-22. Anterior hand with skin and aponeurosis removed, revealing palmar cutaneous branch of median nerve, which passes superficial to the flexor retinaculum to supply skin over the thenar eminence.

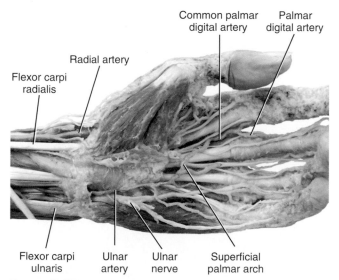

Flexor carpi radialis   Radial artery   Common palmar digital artery   Palmar digital artery

Flexor carpi ulnaris   Ulnar artery   Ulnar nerve   Superficial palmar arch

FIGURE 9-21. Anterior hand with skin and aponeurosis removed, revealing digital arteries and nerves and superficial branches of ulnar nerve and artery (superficial palmar arch).

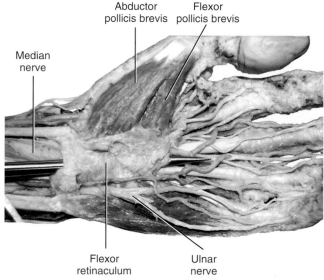

Median nerve   Abductor pollicis brevis   Flexor pollicis brevis

Flexor retinaculum   Ulnar nerve

FIGURE 9-23. Anterior hand with removed skin and aponeurosis showing flexor retinaculum. Note that the ulnar nerve and artery travel superficial to the flexor retinaculum but deep to the palmar carpal ligament.

Carefully expose the flexor retinaculum and identify its borders. Look for the palmar cutaneous branch of the median nerve (Fig. 9-22). This nerve is often cut during routine dissection. The median nerve is seen at the distal forearm between the tendons of the palmaris longus and flexor carpi radialis and supplies the skin over the central portion of the palm.

The *flexor retinaculum* is a dense connective tissue band that helps create a tunnel *(carpal tunnel)* for the tendons of the flexor digitorum superficialis, flexor digitorum profundus, flexor pollicis longus, and the median nerve to reach the palm. Pass a probe or scissors underneath the flexor retinaculum in the carpal tunnel (Fig. 9-23). Leave the probe within the carpal tunnel and with scissors divide

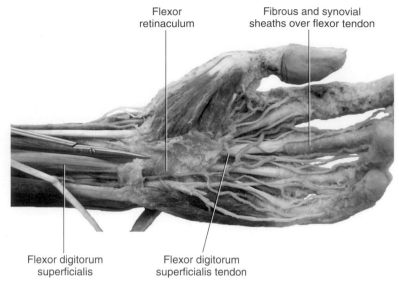

FIGURE 9-24. Anterior hand with removed skin and aponeurosis revealing the flexor retinaculum. This retinaculum is transected by inserting the scissors into the carpal tunnel upwardly, cutting in a proximal-to-distal manner.

the flexor retinaculum on top of the probe (Fig. 9-24). Remove the probe, and retract the flexor retinaculum to expose the median nerve and tendons of the flexor digitorum superficialis (Figs. 9-25 and 9-26).

> ✍ *DISSECTION TIP:* Remove the connective tissue sheath over the median nerve and the underlying flexor digitorum superficialis muscle (Figs. 9-27 and 9-28).

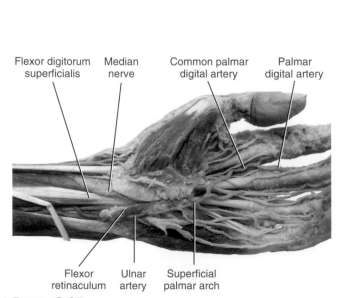

FIGURE 9-25. Anterior hand with transection of the flexor retinaculum. Deeper dissection will reveal the nine tendons and one nerve that course through the carpal tunnel.

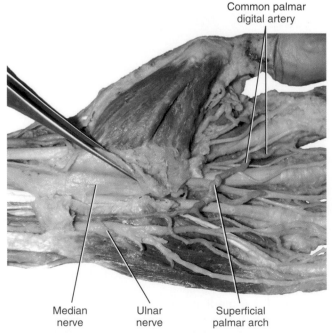

FIGURE 9-26. Anterior hand with flexor retinaculum reflected. Median nerve can be traced from distal forearm to the hand through exposed carpal tunnel. Distal to the flexor retinaculum, note branching pattern of the median nerve.

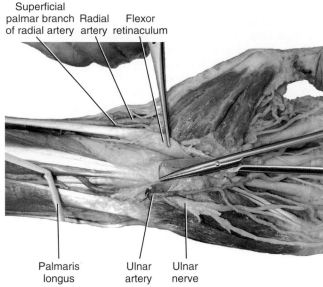

Superficial palmar branch of radial artery   Radial artery   Flexor retinaculum

Palmaris longus   Ulnar artery   Ulnar nerve

FIGURE 9-27. Anterior view of hand after transection of the flexor retinaculum revealing the carpal tunnel.

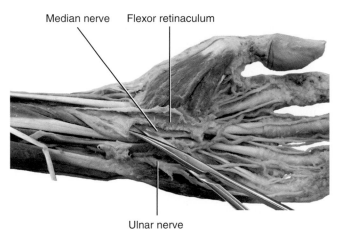

Median nerve   Flexor retinaculum

Ulnar nerve

FIGURE 9-28. Anterior hand demonstrating the carpal tunnel. Connective tissues enveloping tendons of the carpal tunnel can be removed.

Continue exposing the median nerve within the carpal tunnel. Identify the recurrent branch of the median nerve (Fig. 9-29). Finish the exposure of the common palmar digital branches of the median nerve.

> **DISSECTION TIP:** The recurrent branch of the median nerve travels deep to the thenar muscles, and tracing its course anteriorly may be difficult. In such cases, gently retract the median nerve (within exposed carpal tunnel) laterally, and identify the recurrent branch of the median nerve. You may also dissect between the flexor pollicis brevis and the underlying adductor pollicis muscle to trace the recurrent branch of the median nerve.

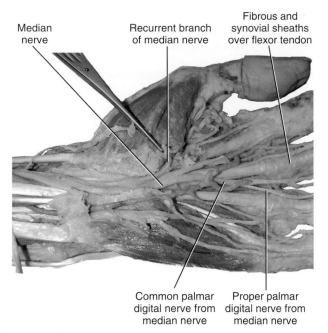

Median nerve   Recurrent branch of median nerve   Fibrous and synovial sheaths over flexor tendon

Common palmar digital nerve from median nerve   Proper palmar digital nerve from median nerve

FIGURE 9-29. Anterior hand with cut flexor retinaculum revealing the carpal tunnel. The median nerve can be traced through the tunnel and its recurrent branch identified near the distal end of the flexor retinaculum.

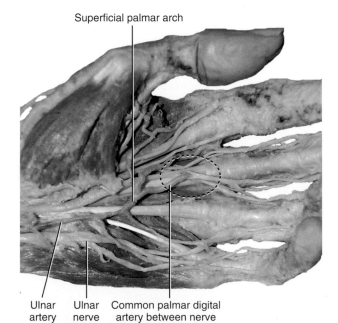

Superficial palmar arch

Ulnar artery   Ulnar nerve   Common palmar digital artery between nerve

FIGURE 9-30. Anterior hand with removed aponeurosis, cut flexor retinaculum, and opened carpal tunnel. Note relationship between common palmar digital arteries and nerves *(circled)*.

> **DISSECTION TIP:** In some cases, branches of the superficial palmar arch travel close to the common palmar digital branches or penetrate them. Use special care when you dissect these structures (Fig. 9-30).

With forceps, retract the abductor digiti minimi muscle laterally, and expose the flexor digiti minimi and the opponens digiti minimi muscles (Fig. 9-31).

> ☝ *DISSECTION TIP:* In the majority of the specimens, the flexor digiti minimi muscle is difficult to be separated from the abductor digiti minimi muscle. Follow the deep branch of the ulnar nerve to the hypothenar muscles. This nerve runs between the flexor digiti minimi and abductor digiti minimi muscles, facilitating their identification. The deepest of the hypothenar muscles is the opponens digiti minimi muscle. You may cut and reflect the abductor digiti minimi near its origin to expose the underlying opponens digiti minimi muscle.

Trace the superficial palmar arch laterally in the space between the 1st digit and the 2nd digit. There is usually an anastomosis between the superficial palmar arch and a branch of the radial artery, the *radialis indicis,* and a branch to the 1st digit, the *princeps pollicis* (Fig. 9-32).

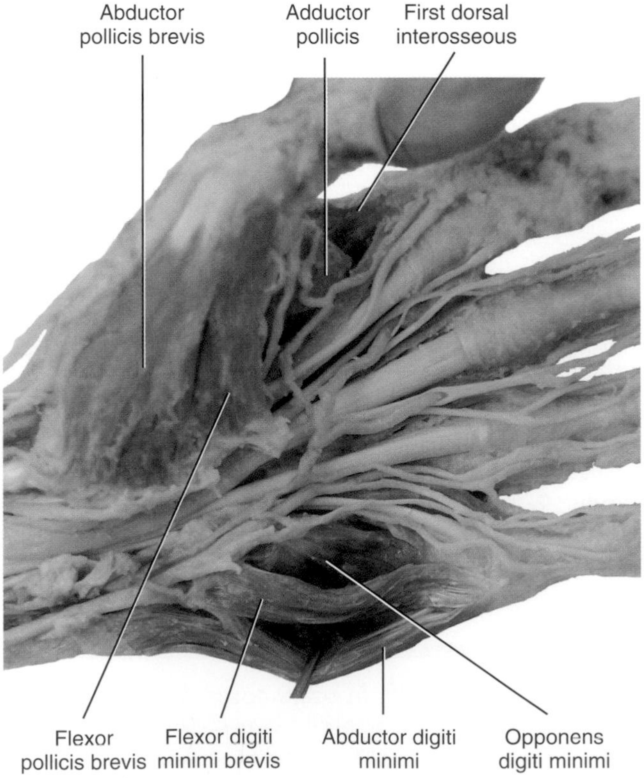

Identify the *abductor pollicis brevis muscle,* lying at the lateral side of the base of the 1st phalanx of the 1st digit (Fig. 9-32). Medial and next to the abductor pollicis brevis muscle, identify the flexor pollicis brevis muscle, which is passing along the radial side of the tendon of the flexor pollicis longus muscle. Retract the abductor pollicis brevis muscle laterally from the flexor pollicis brevis muscle, and identify the opponens pollicis muscle (Fig. 9-33). Finally, identify the adductor pollicis muscle, which can be seen between the base of the 2nd and 1st digits.

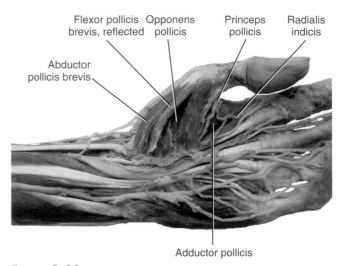

FIGURE 9-32. Anterior hand with removed skin and aponeurosis and cut flexor retinaculum revealing carpal tunnel. With separation, muscles of the thenar eminence are seen.

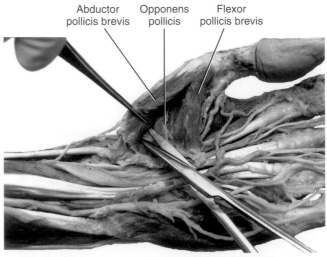

FIGURE 9-31. Anterior hand with removed skin and aponeurosis and cut flexor retinaculum revealing carpal tunnel. With separation, muscular components of hypothenar eminence are seen.

FIGURE 9-33. Anterior hand with skin and aponeurosis removed and flexor reticulum cut revealing thenar muscles. Scissors are used to transect the origin of the abductor pollicis brevis muscle.

DISSECTION TIP: You may also transect the abductor pollicis brevis and identify the opponens pollicis muscle just underneath it (Fig. 9-34). Another way to distinguish the opponens pollicis brevis muscle from the abductor pollicis brevis and the flexor pollicis muscles is its insertion point. The opponens pollicis brevis muscle inserts alongside the 1st metacarpal.

On the dorsum of the hand, clean and expose the tendinous insertions of abductor pollicis longus, the extensor pollicis brevis, and the extensor pollicis longus (Fig. 9-35). The tendons of these three muscles form the boundaries of the anatomic snuffbox, through which the radial artery passes to reach the dorsum of the 1st digit. Identify the radial artery and trace it as it passes between the two heads of the 1st dorsal interosseous muscle (Fig. 9-35).

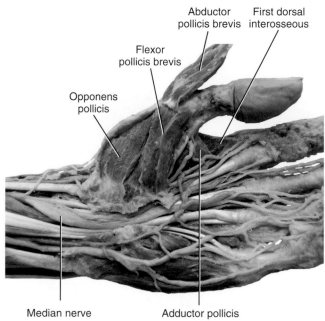

FIGURE 9-34. Anterior hand with skin and aponeurosis removed and flexor reticulum cut revealing thenar structures. With abductor pollicis brevis reflected, the deeper-lying opponens pollicis is visualized.

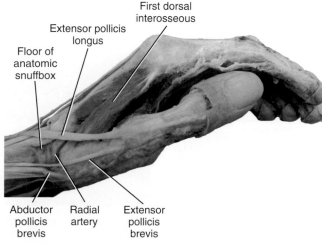

FIGURE 9-35. Region of "anatomic snuffbox," with borders and contents, including radial artery. Note 1st dorsal interosseous muscle between 1st and 2nd digits.

Observe the radial side of the 2nd digit. At the level of the proximal interphalangeal joint, note the extensor mechanism splitting into three parts. Note that one of these parts, the lateral bands, to which the extensor tendons contribute, eventually unite with the transverse metacarpal ligament (Fig. 9-36). At the palmar side of the digits, observe the fibrous synovial sheaths surrounding the tendons of the long flexor muscles (Fig. 9-37). These fibrous sheaths are thin at the interphalangeal joints (cruciate fibers) and thick over the phalanges (annular fibers/ligament). With a scalpel, cut at the midline the fibrous synovial sheath, and expose the tendon of the flexor digitorum superficialis and flexor digitorum profundus (Figs. 9-38 and 9-39).

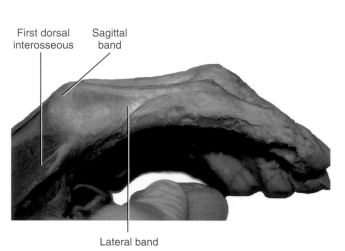

FIGURE 9-36. Dorsal view of 1st and 2nd digits with skin removed, revealing superficial structures. Note components of dorsal expansion, including sagittal and lateral bands.

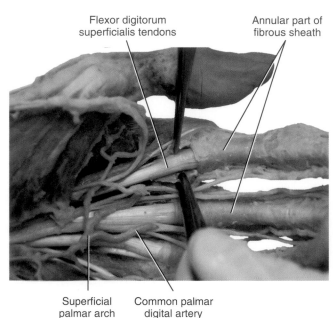

FIGURE 9-38. Anterior view of palm after partial opening of flexor digital sheaths of the 2nd and 3rd digits. Note annular components of fibrous sheaths and internally located flexor tendons.

FIGURE 9-37. Anterior view of palm illustrating fibrous digital sheaths and related structures (e.g., palmar digital nerves).

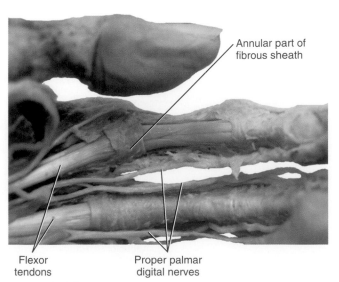

FIGURE 9-39. Anterior view of 1st to 3rd digits. Note annular component of fibrous digital sheath and deeper-lying flexor tendons.

Extend the distal interphalangeal joint. Observe the tendon of the flexor digitorum superficialis dividing before inserting at the base of the middle phalanx. In addition, the tendon of the flexor digitorum profundus passes through the divided tendon of the flexor digitorum superficialis to insert onto the distal phalanges (Figs. 9-40 and 9-41). Note the vinculum *longum*, a thin ligament that adds support for the attachments of the flexor digitorum superficialis and flexor digitorum profundus.

Once all muscles, nerves, and arteries of the hand have been identified (Fig. 9-42), pass a probe or a pair of scissors underneath the flexor digitorum superficialis tendons (Fig. 9-43) and transect them at the level of the carpal tunnel (Fig. 9-44). Lift the flexor digitorum superficialis and expose the median nerve. Clean the median nerve and its surrounding muscles from any loose connective tissue (Figs. 9-45 and 9-46). Transect the median, ulnar, and radial nerves, as well as the ulnar artery at the same level (Fig. 9-47).

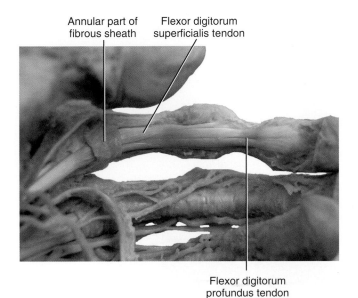

FIGURE 9-40. Anterior view of 1st to 4th digits with portions of fibrous digital sheaths removed. Note the deeper-lying flexor tendons of flexor digitorum superficialis and profundus muscles.

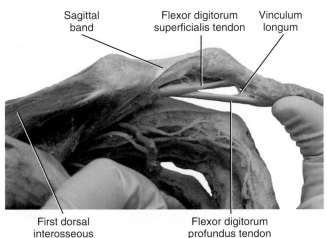

FIGURE 9-41. Lateral view of interspace between 1st and 2nd digits. Note the flexor digitorum profundus tendon passing through the split tendon of flexor digitorum superficialis muscle.

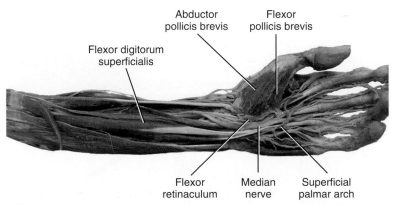

FIGURE 9-42. Anterior forearm and hand view with aponeurosis removed revealing superficial and intermediate musculature.

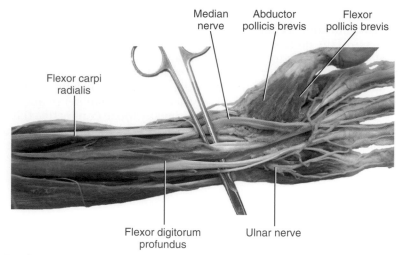

FIGURE 9-43. Anterior view of forearm and hand with aponeurosis removed revealing superficial and intermediate musculature. The median nerve is pulled from between flexor digitorum superficialis and profundus muscles; these muscles are pulled forward and scissors placed deep to them.

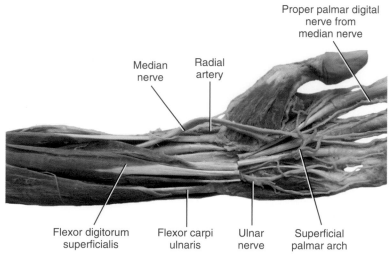

FIGURE 9-44. Anterior forearm and hand with skin and aponeurosis removed; superficial and intermediate muscles are cut at the wrist. Median nerve is retracted.

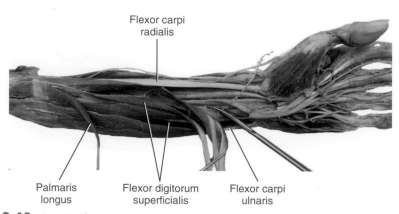

FIGURE 9-45. Anterior forearm and hand with skin and aponeurosis removed and superficial and intermediate muscles reflected, revealing neurovascular structures.

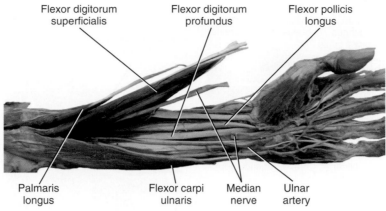

Flexor digitorum superficialis   Flexor digitorum profundus   Flexor pollicis longus

Palmaris longus   Flexor carpi ulnaris   Median nerve   Ulnar artery

FIGURE 9-46. Anterior hand with skin and aponeurosis removed and flexor retinaculum cut, revealing tendons and muscles. Median nerve has been transected in the distal forearm.

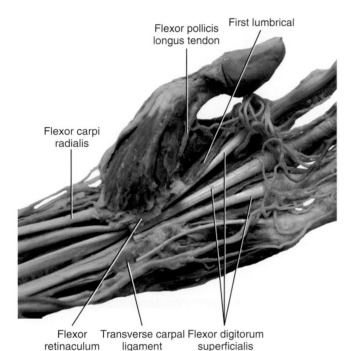

Flexor pollicis longus tendon   First lumbrical

Flexor carpi radialis

Flexor retinaculum   Transverse carpal ligament   Flexor digitorum superficialis

FIGURE 9-47. Anterior hand with skin and aponeurosis removed and flexor retinaculum cut, revealing tendons and muscles. Flexor pollicis longus tendon is exposed, and superficial neurovascular structures are reflected distally.

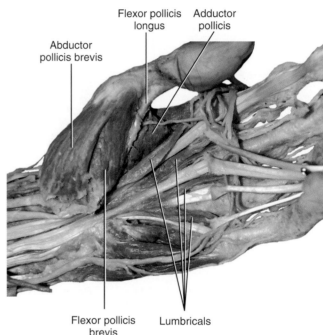

Abductor pollicis brevis   Flexor pollicis longus   Adductor pollicis

Flexor pollicis brevis   Lumbricals

FIGURE 9-48. Anterior hand with skin and aponeurosis removed, revealing deeper muscles (e.g., adductor pollicis, lumbricals).

Retract the neurovascular bundles distally to expose the tendons of the flexor digitorum superficialis. Lift the tendons of the flexor digitorum superficialis and expose all four lumbrical muscles (Fig. 9-48). The lumbricals arise from the tendons of the flexor digitorum profundus muscle and travel to the radial side of the medial four digits to insert into the extensor expansion of each digit.

Clamp the tendons of the flexor digitorum superficialis with a hemostat and retract the tendons distally. Pass a probe or scissors underneath the flexor digitorum profundus (Fig. 9-49) and transect it at the level of the carpal tunnel (Fig. 9-50). Lift this part of the flexor digitorum profundus within the palm, and separate it from the underlying structures with scissors (Fig. 9-51). Identify the adductor pollicis muscle, and at the center of the palm, observe the loose connective tissue covering the underlying structures (Fig. 9-52).

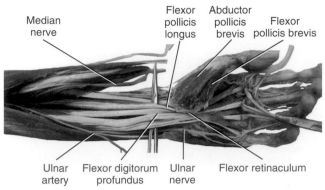

Median nerve — Flexor pollicis longus — Abductor pollicis brevis — Flexor pollicis brevis

Ulnar artery — Flexor digitorum profundus — Ulnar nerve — Flexor retinaculum

FIGURE 9-49. Anterior forearm and hand with skin and aponeurosis removed; superficial and intermediate muscles reflected, revealing deep muscles. Tendon of flexor pollicis longus can be seen entering and exiting carpal tunnel. Scissors placed deep to nine tendons that travel through the carpal tunnel.

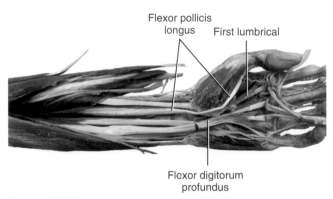

Flexor pollicis longus — First lumbrical

Flexor digitorum profundus

FIGURE 9-50. Anterior view of hand and wrist with skin and aponeurosis removed and flexor retinaculum cut revealing carpal tunnel tendons.

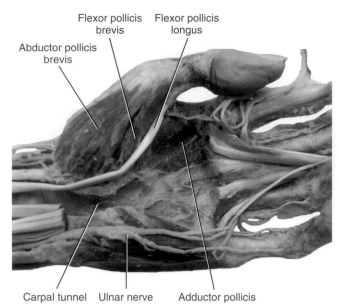

Flexor pollicis brevis — Flexor pollicis longus

Abductor pollicis brevis

Carpal tunnel — Ulnar nerve — Adductor pollicis

FIGURE 9-52. Anterior hand with skin and aponeurosis removed; tendons reflected from carpal tunnel revealing thenar and palmar muscles.

With sharp scissors, clean the connective tissue, and expose the deep palmar arch and the deep branch of the ulnar nerve (Fig. 9-53). The radial artery enters the deep portion of the hand between the two heads of the adductor pollicis and anastomoses with the deep branch of the ulnar artery.

Continue exposing the deep palmar arch and the ulnar nerve and identify the interossei muscles. Identify four dorsal and three palmar interossei muscles (Fig. 9-54).

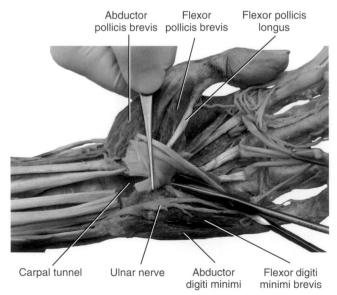

Abductor pollicis brevis — Flexor pollicis brevis — Flexor pollicis longus

Carpal tunnel — Ulnar nerve — Abductor digiti minimi — Flexor digiti minimi brevis

FIGURE 9-51. Anterior hand with skin and aponeurosis removed; superficial and deep tendons cut and reflected, revealing carpal tunnel and its contents. Tendons of flexor digitorum superficialis and profundus are cut and reflected.

✋ DISSECTION TIP: The dorsal and palmar interossei muscles insert partially on the base of the 1st phalanx of each of the medial four digits and into their extensor expansions:

- 1st dorsal interosseous muscle inserts on radial side of 2nd digit.
- 2nd and 3rd dorsal interossei insert on either side of 3rd digit.
- 4th dorsal interosseous muscle inserts on ulnar side of 4th digit.
- 1st palmar interosseous muscle inserts on ulnar side of 2nd digit.
- 2nd palmar interosseous muscle inserts on radial side of 4th digit.
- 3rd palmar interosseous muscle inserts on radial side of 5th digit.

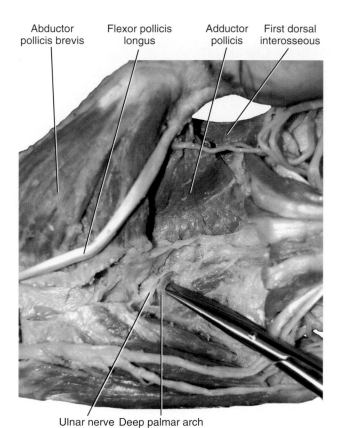

Abductor pollicis brevis Flexor pollicis longus Adductor pollicis First dorsal interosseous

Ulnar nerve Deep palmar arch

FIGURE 9-53. Anterior hand with skin and aponeurosis removed; tendons cut and reflected to reveal the deep palmar arch, with its blood flow contributed to primarily by the radial artery.

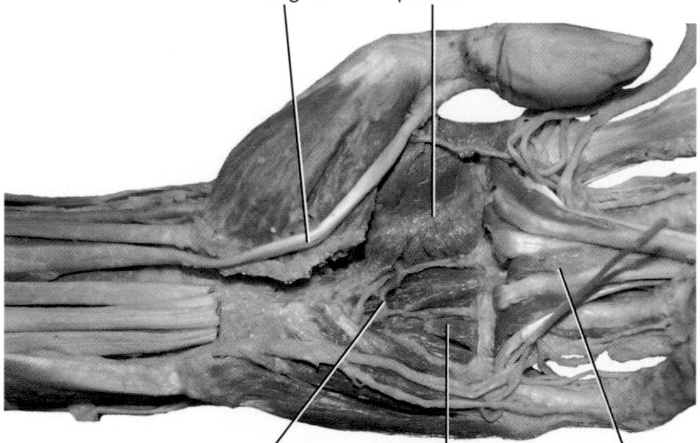

Reflect the flexor digitorum profundus and superficialis, and note the pronator quadratus muscle. This muscle requires no dissection (Fig. 9-55).

At the end of the dissection, place all structures back to their original anatomic position (Fig. 9-56). By following this dissection technique, you will be able to examine the specimen with all the structures in their original position.

> ✴ *DISSECTION TIP:* The palmar fascial spaces are *potential spaces*, which are clinically important as routes of infection spread. These are not dissected in routine dissection.

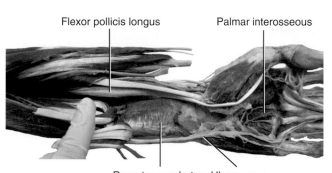

Flexor pollicis longus Palmar interosseous

Pronator quadratus Ulnar nerve

FIGURE 9-55. Anterior hand and wrist with skin and aponeurosis removed and tendons cut revealing deeper structures such as pronator quadratus muscle.

Flexor pollicis longus Adductor pollicis

Deep palmar arch Palmar interosseous Third lumbrical

FIGURE 9-54. Anterior forearm and hand with skin and aponeurosis removed; superficial and intermediate muscles reflected, revealing deep structures, including deep palmar arch and interosseous muscles.

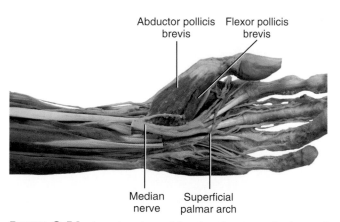

Abductor pollicis brevis Flexor pollicis brevis

Median nerve Superficial palmar arch

FIGURE 9-56. Anterior view of hand and wrist with skin and aponeurosis removed. Median nerve is transected in distal anterior forearm. Note palmar cutaneous branch of median nerve crossing superficial to flexor retinaculum.

LABORATORY IDENTIFICATION CHECKLIST

Nerves
- ❒ Median
  - ❒ Superficial branch
  - ❒ Recurrent branch
- ❒ Common palmar digital
  - ❒ Palmar digital
- ❒ Ulnar
  - ❒ Superficial branch
- ❒ Common palmar digital
  - ❒ Palmar digital nerve
  - ❒ Dorsal branch
  - ❒ Dorsal digital nerve
- ❒ Radial
  - ❒ Superficial branch
  - ❒ Dorsal digital branches

Arteries
- ❒ Ulnar
  - ❒ Superficial palmar arterial arch
    - ❒ Common palmar digital
    - ❒ Palmar digital
- ❒ Radial
  - ❒ Deep arterial arch
- ❒ Princeps pollicis
- ❒ Radialis indicis
- ❒ Palmar metacarpal
  - ❒ Palmar digital
  - ❒ Dorsal arterial arch
- ❒ Dorsal metacarpal
  - ❒ Dorsal digital

Veins
- ❒ Dorsal digital
- ❒ Dorsal metacarpal
- ❒ Dorsal venous arch
  - ❒ Cephalic
  - ❒ Basilic
- ❒ Palmar digital

Muscles
Thenar muscles
- ❒ Abductor pollicis brevis
- ❒ Flexor pollicis brevis
- ❒ Opponens pollicis brevis

Hypothenar muscles
- ❒ Abductor digiti minimi brevis
- ❒ Flexor digiti minimi
- ❒ Opponens digiti minimi
- ❒ Palmaris brevis

Palmar muscles
- ❒ Adductor pollicis
- ❒ Palmar interosseous
- ❒ Dorsal interosseous
- ❒ Lumbricals

Ligaments
- ❒ Ulnar collateral ligament
- ❒ Radial collateral ligament
- ❒ Palmar carpal ligament

Connective Tissue
- ❒ Digital fibrous sheath with annular and cruciate regions
- ❒ Palmar aponeurosis
- ❒ Flexor retinaculum
- ❒ Extensor retinaculum
- ❒ Vinculum longum

Bones
Carpal bones
- ❒ Scaphoid
- ❒ Lunate
- ❒ Triquetrum
- ❒ Hamate
- ❒ Capitate
- ❒ Trapezium
- ❒ Trapezoid
- ❒ Pisiform
- ❒ Metacarpals
- ❒ Phalanges
  - ❒ Proximal
  - ❒ Middle
  - ❒ Distal

SUBACROMIAL BURSITIS INJECTION

Gray's Anatomy for Students: 672

Netter: 410

Clinical Application

Provides relief for frequently inflamed bursa lying beneath the acromion near the supraspinatus tendon.

Anatomic Landmarks (Fig. IV-1)

- Anterior acromion
- Lateral acromion
- Posterior acromion
- Scapular spine
- Humeral head

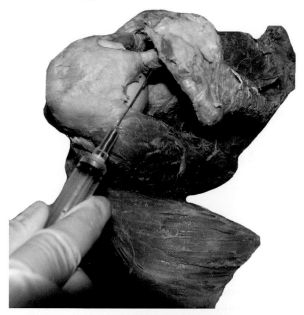

FIGURE IV-1.

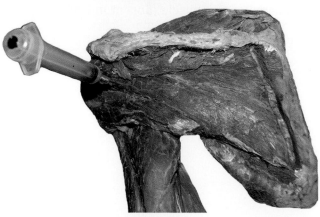

FIGURE IV-2.

ACROMIOCLAVICULAR JOINT INSPECTION

Gray's Anatomy for Students: 669

Netter: 410

Clinical Application

Relieve pain from acromioclavicular joint irritation.

Anatomic Landmarks

- Anterior acromion
- Lateral acromion
- Acromioclavicular joint

GLENOHUMERAL JOINT INJECTION

Gray's Anatomy for Students: 670

Netter: 410

Clinical Application

Relieve pain from glenohumeral joint irritation.

Anatomic Landmarks
(Figs. IV-2 and IV-3) (Posterior Approach)

- Skin
- Subcutaneous tissue
- Infraspinatus
- Joint capsule
- Glenoid cavity
- Humeral head
- Posterior cord of brachial plexus and its branches

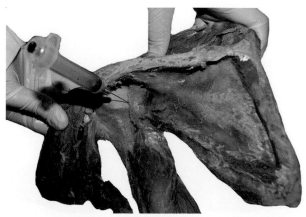

FIGURE IV-3.

STERNOCLAVICULAR JOINT INJECTION

Gray's Anatomy for Students: 668

Netter: 180

Clinical Application

Relieve pain from sternoclavicular joint irritation.

Anatomic Landmarks

- Skin
- Subcutaneous tissue
- Anterior sternoclavicular ligament
- Articular disc
- Medial clavicle
- Manubrium
- Brachiocephalic vein
- Subclavian artery
- Medial branch of supraclavicular nerve
- Nerve to subclavius muscle

BICIPITAL TENOSYNOVITIS INJECTION

Gray's Anatomy for Students: 670

Netter: 410

Clinical Application

Acute trauma or chronic overuse of the biceps brachii tendon (usually long head); relieves pain and may prevent further shoulder pathology.

Anatomic Landmarks (Fig. IV-4)

- Supinated upper limb
- Inferior border of pectoralis major muscle
- Biceps brachii long head
- Humerus

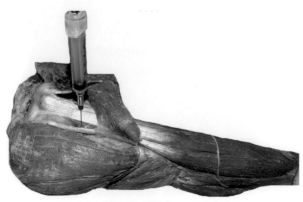

FIGURE IV-4.

ULNAR NERVE BLOCK FOR CUBITAL TUNNEL SYNDROME

Gray's Anatomy for Students: 706–707

Netter: 433, 464

Clinical Application

For relief of pain caused by irritation of the ulnar nerve.

Anatomic Landmarks

- Externally rotated upper limb
- Medial epicondyle of humerus
- Ulnar sulcus of humerus
- Olecranon process of ulna
- Flexor carpi ulnaris
- Tendinous arch connecting two heads of flexor carpi ulnaris

Needle is advanced parallel to the ulnar nerve.

MEDIAN NERVE BLOCK (INJECTION AT WRIST)

Gray's Anatomy for Students: 772–773

Netter: 442

Clinical Application

Median nerve block anesthetizes the lateral palmar 3½ digits.

Anatomic Landmarks (Figs. IV-5 and IV-6)

- Skin
- Proximal palmar skin crease
- Subcutaneous tissue
- Flexor retinaculum
- Palmaris longus muscle (absent in ~20%)
- Flexor carpi radialis muscle
- Median nerve

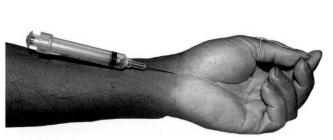

FIGURE IV-5.

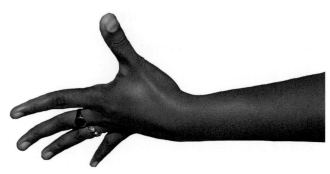

FIGURE IV-7.

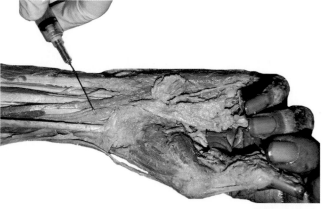

FIGURE IV-6.

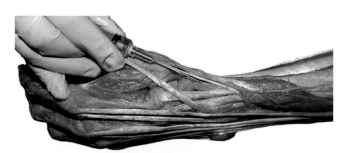

FIGURE IV-8.

DE QUERVAIN DISEASE INJECTION

Gray's Anatomy for Students: 748–749

Netter: 458

Clinical Application

Relieve pain associated with stenosing tenosynovitis of the extensor pollicis brevis muscle.

Anatomic Landmarks (Figs. IV-7 and IV-8)

- Skin
- Subcutaneous tissue
- 1st dorsal compartment retinaculum
- Cephalic vein
- Radial artery branches
- 1st metacarpal base
- 1st metacarpophalangeal joint
- Extensor pollicis brevis

MEDIAL EPICONDYLITIS INJECTION

Gray's Anatomy for Students: 728

Netter: 430, 431, 434

Clinical Application

Relief of pain caused by strain to the attachment of the forearm flexors at the medial epicondyle region.

Anatomic Landmarks

- Skin
- Subcutaneous tissue
- Common tendon of forearm flexors at medial epicondyle
- Medial epicondyle

LATERAL EPICONDYLITIS INJECTION

Gray's Anatomy for Students: 728

Netter: 429, 432–433

Clinical Application

Relief of pain caused by strain to the attachment of the forearm flexors at the lateral epicondyle region.

Anatomic Landmarks (Figs. IV-9 and IV-10)

- Skin
- Subcutaneous tissue
- Common tendon of forearm extensors at the lateral epicondyle
- Lateral epicondyle

DIGITAL NERVE BLOCK (HAND)

Gray's Anatomy for Students: 772

Netter: 454–457

Clinical Application

Anesthetize the palmar or dorsal side of a single or multiple digits to perform invasive procedures.

Anatomic Landmarks (Figs. IV-11 and IV-12)

- Skin
- Subcutaneous tissue
- Common digital nerves/arteries
- Palmar digital nerves/arteries
- Dorsal digital nerves/arteries
- Metacarpophalangeal joints
- Proximal interphalangeal joints

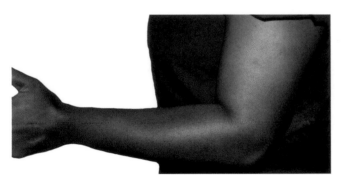

FIGURE IV-9.

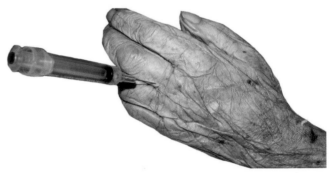

FIGURE IV-11.

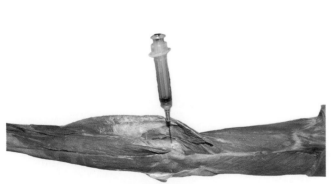

FIGURE IV-10.

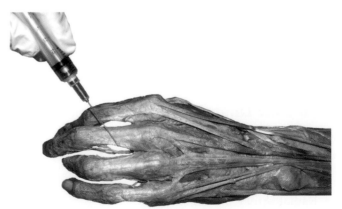

FIGURE IV-12.

VENIPUNCTURE OR PHLEBOTOMY

Gray's Anatomy for Students: 664

Netter: 400, 403–405

Clinical Application

To withdraw venous blood through needle penetration, or to insert intravenous (IV) cannula.

Anatomic Landmarks (Fig. IV-13)

- Skin
- Subcutaneous tissue
Elbow:	Antecubital vein
Forearm:	Cephalic vein
	Basilic vein
Hand dorsum:	Cephalic vein
	Basilic vein
	Dorsal venous arch
	Metacarpal veins

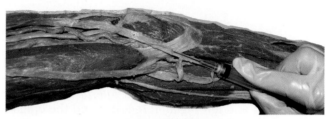

FIGURE IV-13.

ANTERIOR ABDOMINAL WALL

Netter: 240–246, 251–255, 367–370

McMinn: 221–225, 228, 266

Gray's Atlas: 124–140, 224–225

BEFORE DISSECTION

The anterior abdominal wall can be divided into regions: the right and left *hypochondriac* regions; the right and left *lateral* regions; the right and left *inguinal* regions; and the epigastric, umbilical, and pubic regions (Fig. 10-1).

Less specifically, the abdomen can be divided into right and left superior quadrants and right and left inferior quadrants. This division in based on drawing vertical and horizontal lines through the umbilicus (Fig. 10-2).

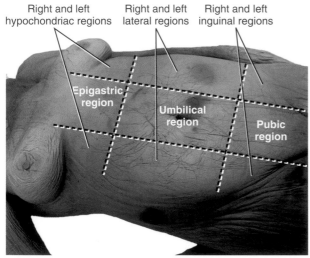

FIGURE 10-1. Anterior view of abdomen showing division into regions.

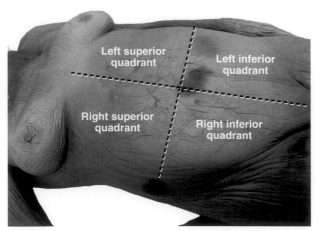

FIGURE 10-2. Anterior view of abdomen showing simplified division into quadrants.

PALPATION

Identify and palpate the umbilicus (typically located at the level of 4th lumbar vertebra), the anterior superior iliac spines, the pubic symphysis, and the pubic and iliac crests. Also, palpate the lower costal margins, which form the subcostal plane, and tubercles of the iliac crests, which form the intertubercular plane. This latter plane is located at the L5 level just inferior to the bifurcation of the abdominal aorta (Fig. 10-2).

DISSECTION

Palpate the xiphoid process, and make a midline vertical skin incision from the xiphoid process to the pubic symphysis. Do not cut through the umbilicus; make a circumferential incision around it. Palpate the costal margins, and make a second incision following this margin, from the midaxillary line to the xiphoid process. Finally, make an incision from the anterior superior iliac spine to the pubic symphysis (Fig. 10-3).

> *DISSECTION TIP:* An alternate method is to make a vertical incision from the midaxillary line to 5 cm (2 inches) inferior to the anterior superior iliac spine. Make a transverse incision inferior to the inguinal ligament. Reflect the skin inferiorly to the level of the anterior superior iliac spine to expose the inguinal region.

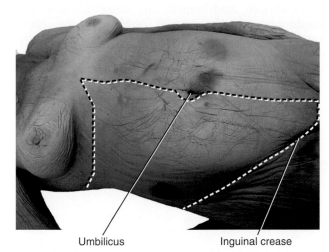

Umbilicus   Inguinal crease

FIGURE 10-3. Anterior view of abdomen showing the skin incisions *(dashed lines)* used to begin dissection.

> ✦ *DISSECTION TIP:* Reflect the superficial fatty layer similar to the previously made skin incision. Make a shallow incision with the scalpel and place your index finger into the incision so that lateral traction can be applied and reflection performed. Continue with blunt dissection to identify the deep membranous fascia over the abdominal muscles. Once this is achieved, continue the dissection using a scalpel.

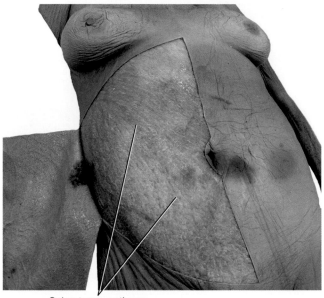

Subcutaneous tissue
(superficial fascia of abdomen)

FIGURE 10-5. Anterior view of abdomen showing skin reflection with underlying subcutaneous tissues.

Dissect the skin from the midline and reflect it laterally (Fig. 10-4).

Expose the superficial fascia (fatty layer) beneath the skin (Fig. 10-5). As the superficial fascia is reflected (Fig. 10-6), note a superficial fatty layer and a deeper membranous layer. The fatty layer of the superficial fascia is also known as *Camper's fascia,* while the membranous layer is known as *Scarpa's fascia.*

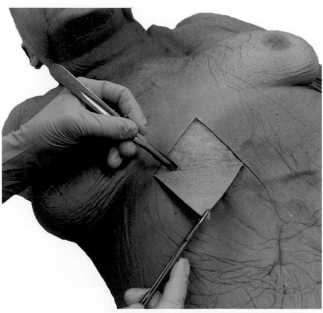

FIGURE 10-4. Method used to reflect skin from underlying fascia. Note tension placed on corner of skin flap as scalpel liberates this layer from underlying fascia.

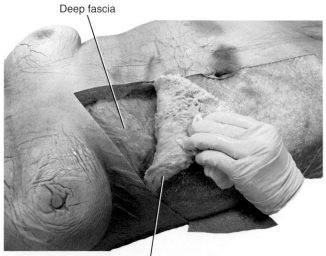

Deep fascia

Subcutaneous tissue
(superficial fascia of abdomen)

FIGURE 10-6. Anterior view of abdomen with skin and fascia reflected from the midline on right side.

Continue the dissection by reflecting the superficial fatty layer and expose the muscles of the anterior abdomen (covered with deep fascia) and the outer layer of the rectus sheath (Fig. 10-7). At the level of the midaxillary line, remove the deep fascia and expose the external abdominal oblique muscle (Fig. 10-8). Clean the deep fascia over the external abdominal oblique and outer layer of the rectus sheath, and identify the linea alba and linea semilunaris (at the lateral border of the rectus sheath) (Figs. 10-9 and 10-10). Once the external abdominal oblique muscle is exposed at the midabdomen, continue the reflection of the deep fascia over the pubic symphysis and inguinal ligament to further expose the external abdominal oblique muscle (Fig. 10-11).

Outer rectus sheath covered with membranous layer of superficial fascia

External abdominal oblique

FIGURE 10-7. With additional dissection, the external abdominal oblique muscle is identified with its contribution to the outer rectus sheath.

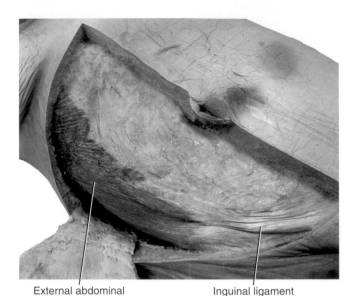

External abdominal oblique

Inguinal ligament

FIGURE 10-9. Anterior view of abdomen noting exposed external abdominal oblique muscle and contributions medially into outer rectus sheath.

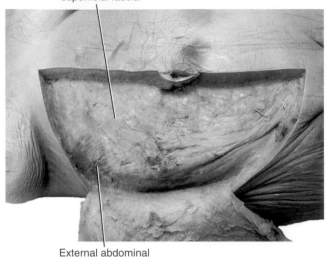

Outer rectus sheath

External abdominal oblique

FIGURE 10-8. Anterior view of abdomen noting exposed external abdominal oblique muscle and contributions medially into outer rectus sheath.

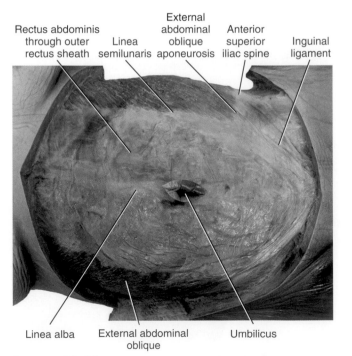

Rectus abdominis through outer rectus sheath

Linea semilunaris

External abdominal oblique aponeurosis

Anterior superior iliac spine

Inguinal ligament

Linea alba

External abdominal oblique

Umbilicus

FIGURE 10-10. Anterior view of full abdominal exposure showing anatomic landmarks. Note linea alba traveling in the midline with interposed umbilicus.

With forceps, lift the outer layer of the rectus sheath (anterior lamina) at the level of the xiphoid process. With scissors, make a small incision into the rectus sheath (Figs. 10-12 and 10-13). Lift the rectus sheath upward and identify the rectus abdominis muscle underneath it (Fig. 10-14).

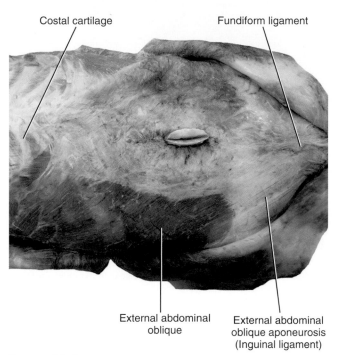

Costal cartilage   Fundiform ligament

External abdominal oblique   External abdominal oblique aponeurosis (Inguinal ligament)

FIGURE 10-11. Anterior view of abdomen noting upper attachments of external abdominal oblique muscle along costal margin and inferiorly with specialization of its aponeurosis, the inguinal ligament.

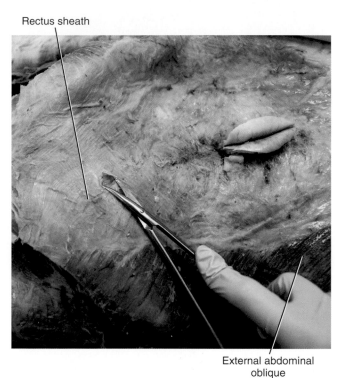

Rectus sheath

External abdominal oblique

FIGURE 10-13. Anterior view of abdomen showing expansion of outer rectus fascia.

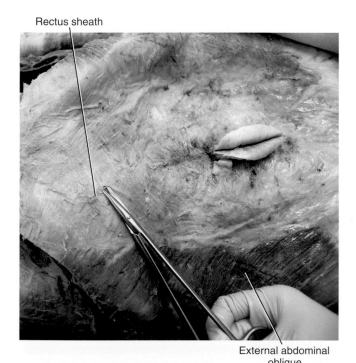

Rectus sheath

External abdominal oblique

FIGURE 10-12. Note method of entering outer rectus sheath to begin exposure of rectus abdominis muscle.

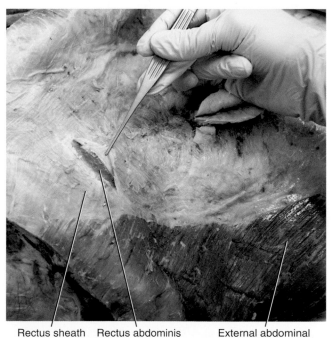

Rectus sheath   Rectus abdominis   External abdominal oblique

FIGURE 10-14. Anterior view of abdomen noting continued opening of outer rectus sheath.

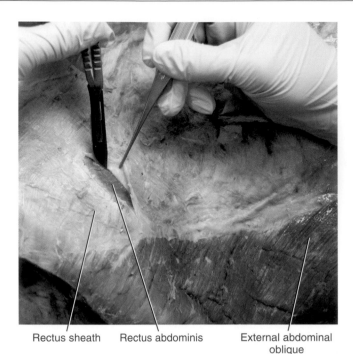

Rectus sheath   Rectus abdominis   External abdominal oblique

FIGURE 10-15. Anterior view of abdomen showing continued opening of outer rectus sheath.

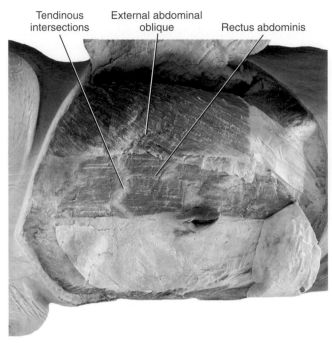

Tendinous intersections   External abdominal oblique   Rectus abdominis

FIGURE 10-17. Rectus abdominis muscle is exposed more or less along its entirety.

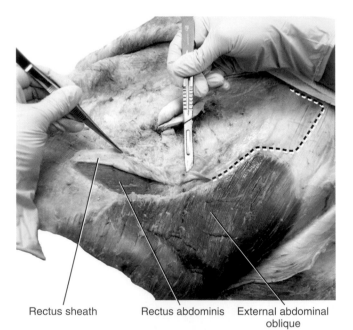

Rectus sheath   Rectus abdominis   External abdominal oblique

FIGURE 10-16. Outer sheath is exposed along lateral edge of the junction of external abdominal oblique muscle with its aponeurosis.

With your scalpel, detach the outer layer of the rectus sheath (anterior lamina) (Fig. 10-15) alongside its border with the external abdominal oblique muscle (Fig. 10-16).

Reflect the outer layer of the rectus sheath (anterior lamina) from the pubic symphysis to the xiphoid process, and completely expose the rectus abdominis muscle. Leave a small part of the rectus sheath intact (Fig. 10-17). Identify the tendinous intersections, formed by the tendinous inscriptions of the rectus abdominis muscle and its segmentation, and the *linea alba,* the avascular fusion point of the aponeuroses of the muscles of the anterior abdominal wall at the midline extending from the xiphoid process to the pubic symphysis.

> ☝ *DISSECTION TIP:* The tendinous intersections attach firmly to the anterior lamina of the rectus sheath. Employ sharp dissection when necessary to remove the anterior lamina. Observe the linea alba becoming wider and thicker above the umbilicus.

At the inferior portion of the rectus abdominis muscle and anterior to it, identify the pyramidalis muscle (Fig. 10-18).

> ☝ *DISSECTION TIP:* The pyramidalis muscle is absent in about 20% of cases.

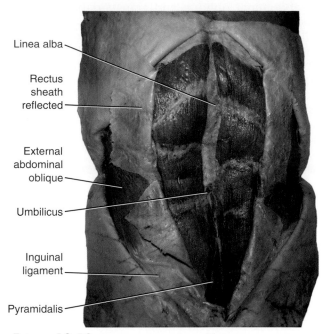

Linea alba

Rectus
sheath
reflected

External
abdominal
oblique

Umbilicus

Inguinal
ligament

Pyramidalis

FIGURE 10-18. Continued exposure of outer rectus sheath.

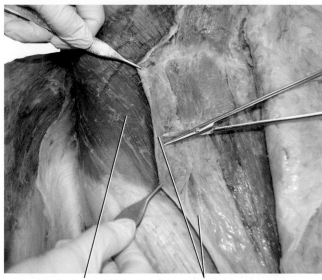

External abdominal   External abdominal
oblique   oblique aponeurosis

FIGURE 10-19. Continued exposure of outer rectus sheath.

During the dissection of the anterior abdominal wall, note the anterior primary rami of the 7th to 12th thoracic nerves (T7 to T12) supplying the muscles of the anterior abdominal wall.

> ✋ *DISSECTION TIP:* There are five important nerves in this region:
> - T7, usually found just inferior to xiphoid process.
> - T10, at the level of the umbilicus.
> - T12, at the level just above the pubis.
> - Ilioinguinal nerve, at the level of the anterior superior iliac spine, underneath the external abdominal oblique muscle.
> - Iliohypogastric nerve, 3 to 4 cm above the ilioinguinal nerve at the level of the anterior superior iliac spine.

At the level of the linea semilunaris, make a small incision between the external abdominal oblique and rectus abdominis muscles. Retract the external abdominal oblique muscle laterally, and expose the fibers of the underlying internal abdominal oblique muscle (Figs. 10-19 and 10-20). Note the difference

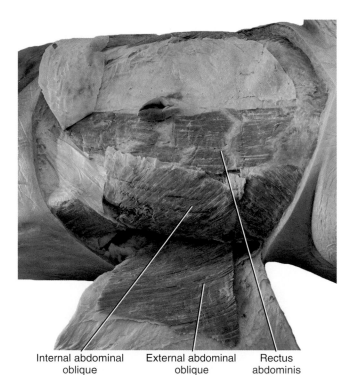

Internal abdominal   External abdominal   Rectus
oblique   oblique   abdominis

FIGURE 10-20. After reflecting part of the external abdominal oblique muscle, the deeper layer composed of the internal abdominal oblique muscle is visualized.

Rectus   Transversus   Internal abdominal   Anterior primary
abdominis   abdominis   oblique   rami

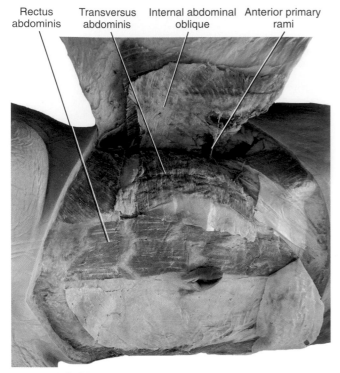

FIGURE 10-21. After reflecting part of the internal abdominal oblique, the deeper transversus abdominis muscle is seen.

Transversalis   Transversus   Anterior primary
fascia   abdominis   rami

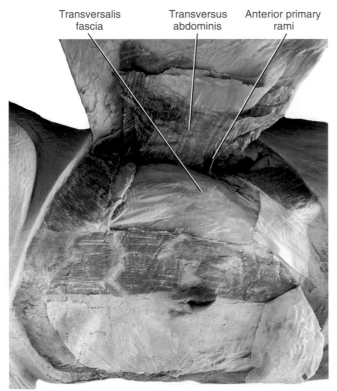

FIGURE 10-22. After reflecting part of the transversus abdominis muscle, the deeper transversalis fascia is observed.

in the muscle fiber orientation between the external abdominal oblique and transversus abdominis muscles.

Similarly, cut the internal abdominal oblique muscle at the level of the linea semilunaris, and expose the underlying transversus abdominis muscle (Fig. 10-21). Cut the transversus abdominis muscle and reflect it to expose the underlying transversalis fascia (Fig. 10-22).

> ✎ *DISSECTION TIP:* Between the internal oblique and transversus abdominis muscles, identify anterior primary rami from T7 to T12. The three muscles of the external abdominal wall—external abdominal oblique, internal abdominal oblique, and transversus abdominis—are covered by a superficial fascia and a deep fascia. The outermost fascia covering the external abdominal oblique muscle (deep) is called the *fascia of Gallaudet.* The fascia that lies deep to the transversus abdominis (at its deepest surface) is the *transversalis fascia* (Fig. 10-22).

An alternate method is to make a vertical incision at the external abdominal oblique muscle on the midaxillary line, where the underlying internal abdominal oblique and transversus abdominis muscles are usually the thickest. Reflect the external abdominal oblique muscle, and identify the internal abdominal oblique muscle. Continue the same process with the internal abdominal oblique, and identify the transversus abdominis muscle (Figs. 10-23 and 10-24).

At the level of the xiphoid process, make a shallow transverse incision at the rectus abdominis muscle (Fig. 10-25). Lift the rectus abdominis from its posterior lamina of the rectus sheath, and reflect it downward (Fig. 10-26). Identify the primary rami of T7 to T12 penetrating the posterior lamina of the rectus sheath.

> ✎ *DISSECTION TIP:* The superior epigastric artery may be difficult to identify.

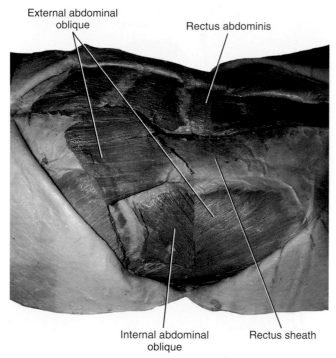

External abdominal oblique

Rectus abdominis

Internal abdominal oblique

Rectus sheath

FIGURE 10-23. Anterior view showing external abdominal oblique and rectus abdominis muscles.

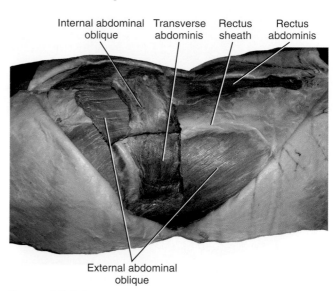

Internal abdominal oblique   Transverse abdominis   Rectus sheath   Rectus abdominis

External abdominal oblique

FIGURE 10-24. Additional view after muscular flap cuts showing outermost external abdominal oblique muscle and reflected, deeper-lying internal abdominal oblique muscle. Deep to reflected internal abdominal oblique, the transversus abdominis muscle is seen.

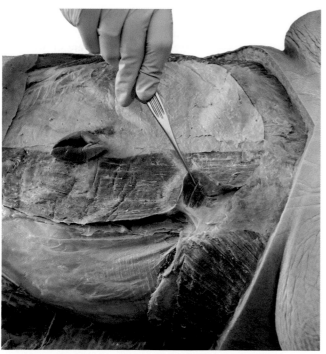

FIGURE 10-25. The rectus abdominis muscle is reflected inferiorly.

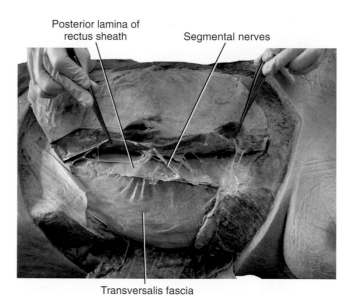

Posterior lamina of rectus sheath   Segmental nerves

Transversalis fascia

FIGURE 10-26. With reflection of the rectus abdominis muscle, the segmental nerves of this region are appreciated.

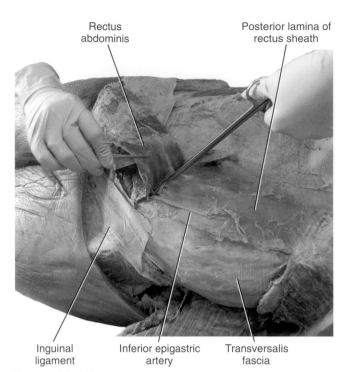

FIGURE 10-27. With continued reflection of the rectus abdominis muscle, the inferior epigastric vessels are seen.

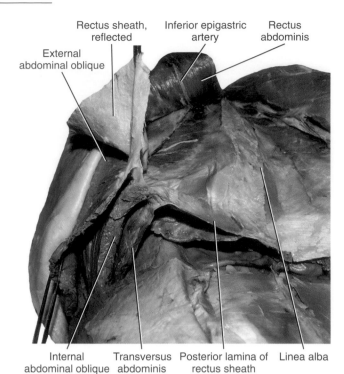

FIGURE 10-29. Anterior view of the left abdominal wall muscles. Note that rectus abdominis muscle is reflected inferiorly and shown laterally are the external and internal oblique and transversus abdominis muscles.

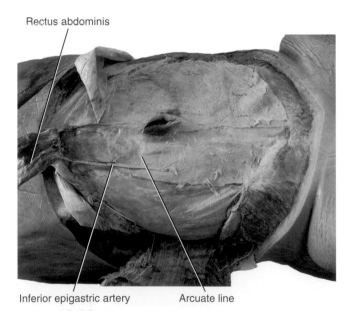

FIGURE 10-28. Rectus abdominis muscle is reflected superiorly, and inferior epigastric vessels are seen. Note the arcuate line.

Reflect the rectus abdominis muscle superiorly from the posterior lamina of the rectus sheath, and identify, on its deep surface, the superior and inferior epigastric arteries (Fig. 10-27). Just inferior to the umbilicus, identify the arcuate line of the rectus sheath, where the posterior lamina of the sheath is formed only by transversalis fascia (Figs. 10-28 and 10-29).

Dissection Preferably on One Side Only

Identify the inferior edge of the aponeurosis of the external abdominal oblique muscle, the *inguinal ligament* (Fig. 10-30). Reflect part of the skin over the superior portion of the thigh, and identify the great saphenous vein (Fig. 10-31).

Extend the skin flap medially (Fig. 10-32), and expose the inferior border of the inguinal ligament (Fig. 10-33). Clean the adipose tissue and identify the superficial (external) inguinal ring and the spermatic cord covered by the external spermatic fascia. Identify the superomedial part of the inguinal ligament, the *superior crus,* and the inferolateral part, the *inferior crus* (Fig. 10-34).

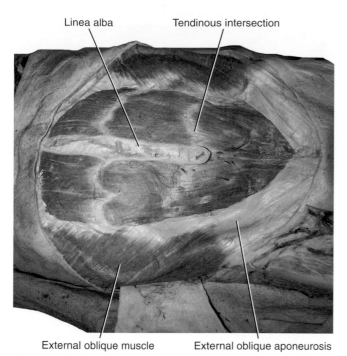

Linea alba   Tendinous intersection

External oblique muscle   External oblique aponeurosis

FIGURE 10-30. Anterior view of anterior abdominal wall. With muscles intact, note the linea alba and external abdominal oblique muscle and its aponeurosis.

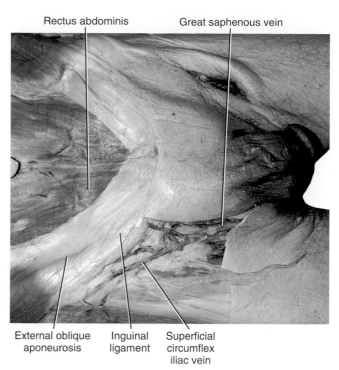

Rectus abdominis   Great saphenous vein

External oblique aponeurosis   Inguinal ligament   Superficial circumflex iliac vein

FIGURE 10-31. Anterior view of the inguinal region in the male.

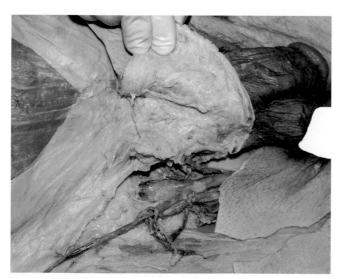

FIGURE 10-32. Anterior view of the inguinal region in the male with skin reflection.

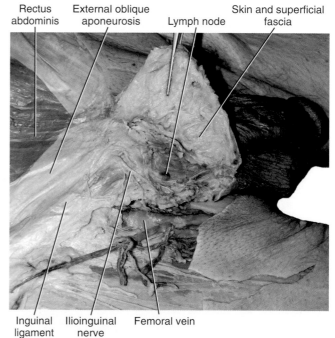

Rectus abdominis   External oblique aponeurosis   Lymph node   Skin and superficial fascia

Inguinal ligament   Ilioinguinal nerve   Femoral vein

FIGURE 10-33. Anterior view of the inguinal region in the male showing the ilioinguinal nerve.

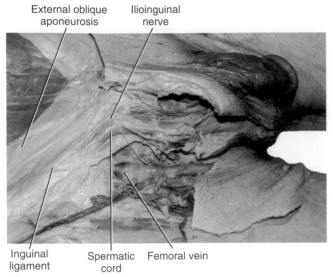

FIGURE 10-34. Anterior view of the inguinal region in the male.

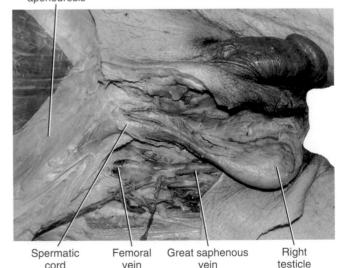

FIGURE 10-36. The inguinal region noting the inguinal ligament.

Just superior and anterior to the superior crus, identify the ilioinguinal nerve. Look for the genital branch of the genitofemoral nerve as it travels through both the internal and the external inguinal rings within the spermatic cord. Cut the skin covering the spermatic cord inferiorly toward the testis, and remove the skin over the penis (Figs. 10-35 and 10-36). Retract the testis laterally (Fig. 10-37).

With scissors, cut the aponeurosis of the external oblique muscle between the two crura at the external inguinal ring (Fig. 10-38). Place the scissors underneath the external spermatic fascia, and make a small incision (Fig. 10-39) to expose the contents of the spermatic cord (Fig. 10-40).

FIGURE 10-37. Inguinal region, noting superficial ring of inguinal canal and spermatic cord and right testicle.

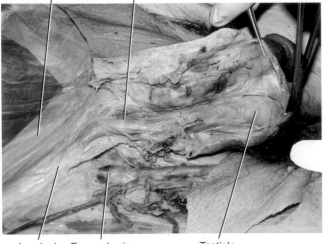

FIGURE 10-35. Anterior view of inguinal region in the male, showing relationship between aponeurosis of external abdominal oblique muscle and inguinal ligament.

> ✎ DISSECTION TIP: Place your index finger in the opening of the superficial ring to appreciate the oblique course of the *spermatic cord* through the body wall toward the internal ring. In the female, the *round ligament* replaces the spermatic cord in the inguinal canal. The fascia covering the spermatic cord, and specifically its superolateral aspect, is named the *cremasteric fascia*.

External spermatic fascia

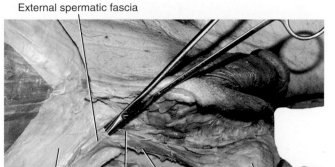

External oblique aponeurosis Ilioinguinal nerve Spermatic cord Right testicle

FIGURE 10-38. Inguinal and proximal femoral regions.

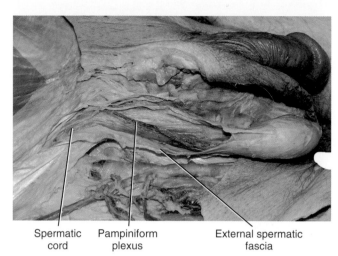

Spermatic cord Pampiniform plexus External spermatic fascia

FIGURE 10-41. Note pampiniform plexus of veins.

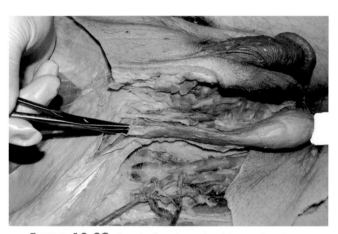

FIGURE 10-39. Inguinal and proximal femoral regions.

Incise the external spermatic fascia, formed by the external abdominal oblique muscle. Trace the pampiniform venous plexus, and incise the cremasteric fascia, derived from the internal oblique muscle (Fig. 10-41). Dissect the deepest fascial layer of the spermatic cord, the *internal spermatic fascia,* formed from the fascia of the transversus abdominis muscle, and identify the vas deferens (Fig. 10-42).

Ilioinguinal nerve   Genital branch of genitofemoral nerve

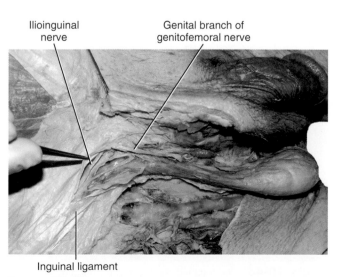

Inguinal ligament

FIGURE 10-40. Inguinal region. Note the genital branch of the genitofemoral nerve.

Vas deferens

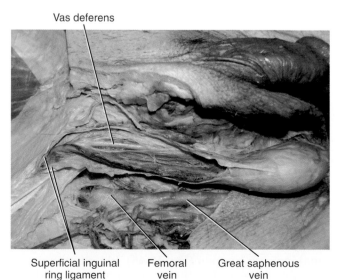

Superficial inguinal ring ligament   Femoral vein   Great saphenous vein

FIGURE 10-42. With deeper dissection within spermatic cord, note the vas deferens.

Vas deferens

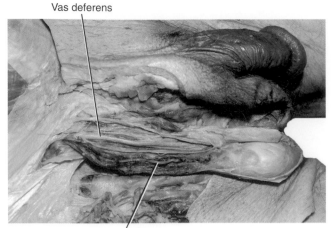

Cremasteric artery

FIGURE 10-43. Inguinal region in the male showing cremasteric artery.

Vas deferens

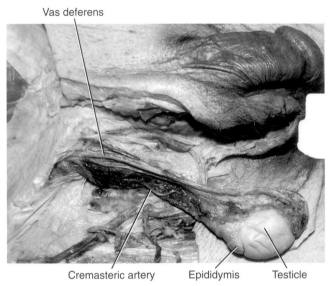

Cremasteric artery   Epididymis   Testicle

FIGURE 10-44. Inguinal region showing epididymis and its relationship to vas deferens.

Identify the cremasteric artery (Fig. 10-43).

Continue the incision of the external spermatic fascia to the scrotum and expose the testis in the scrotal sac. Lift the spermatic cord and liberate the testis from the scrotum (Fig. 10-44). Identify a double serous membrane, the *tunica vaginalis,* which covers the anterior part and the sides of the testis and epididymis. Note the outermost layer the parietal layer and the visceral layer of the tunica vaginalis connecting the epididymis to the testis (with a distinct fold). Identify the epididymis, and note its head, body, and tail (Fig. 10-44).

Hold the testis and with a scalpel make a longitudinal incision to open (Fig. 10-45). Identify the dense capsule of the testis, the *tunica albuginea,* and the septae, which arise from the capsule and divide the testis into several compartments.

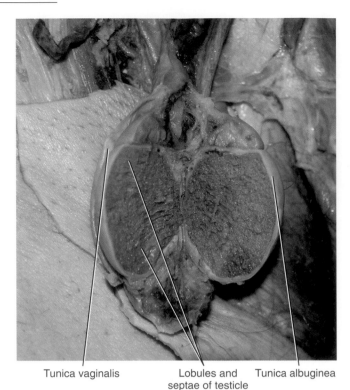

Tunica vaginalis   Lobules and   Tunica albuginea
septae of testicle

FIGURE 10-45. Coronal section through proximal penis noting its layers and components.

If you dissect a female cadaver, identify the round ligament of the uterus. The round ligament (ligamentum teres) of the uterus is a fibrous cord traveling from the uterus through the inguinal canal to attach to the labia majora. Identify the round ligament at the superficial ring, and follow it toward the labia majora.

Continue to remove fat and skin over the pubic symphysis and the penis (Figs. 10-46 and 10-47).

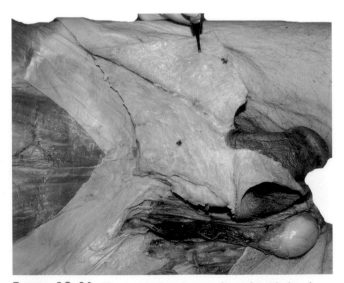

FIGURE 10-46. The inguinal region on the right side has been dissected; on the left side, fascia and the underlying layers are exposed.

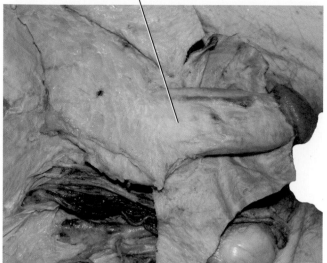

Superficial penile fascia

FIGURE 10-47. Dorsal view of penis with its superficial fascia exposed.

Identify the superficial dorsal vein of the penis embedded in the superficial fascia of the penis (Fig. 10-48). Dissect out and reflect the superficial fascia of the penis laterally (Fig. 10-49). Notice the deep fascia, *Buck's fascia,* of the penis deep to the superficial fascia (Fig. 10-50). On the dorsal surface of the penis, note the separation between the superficial and deep dorsal veins of the penis by Buck's fascia (Fig. 10-51). Separate Buck's fascia and identify the

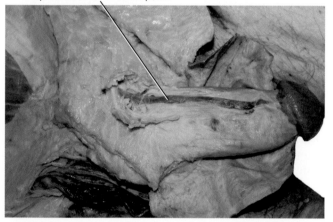

Superficial dorsal vein of penis

FIGURE 10-48. Deeper dissection of dorsal penis shows superficial dorsal vein of penis.

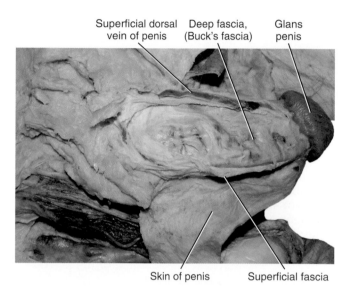

Superficial dorsal vein of penis   Deep fascia, (Buck's fascia)   Glans penis

Skin of penis   Superficial fascia

FIGURE 10-50. Deeper dissection of dorsal penis reveals deep fascia of penis.

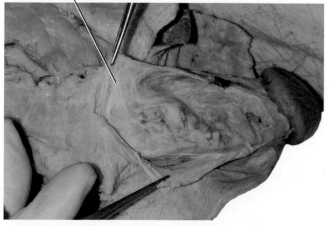

Superficial penile fascia

FIGURE 10-49. Dorsal view of penis and its related fascia.

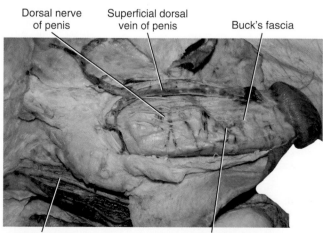

Dorsal nerve of penis   Superficial dorsal vein of penis   Buck's fascia

Vas deferens   Deep dorsal vein of penis

FIGURE 10-51. Dorsal view of penis showing relationship between superficial and deep fasciae. Note position of superficial dorsal vein of penis.

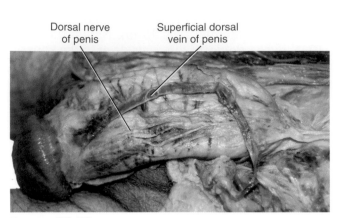

FIGURE 10-52. Dorsal view of penis with deeper dissection, showing underlying dorsal nerve of penis and its branches.

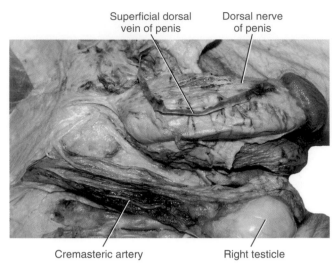

FIGURE 10-54. Dorsal view of penis showing left dorsal nerve of penis and its relationship to surrounding fasciae.

dorsal artery of the penis, which is located bilaterally on the dorsum of the penis medial to the dorsal nerves of the penis (Fig. 10-52). Continue the removal of the fat toward the pubic symphysis and expose the fundiform ligament of the penis arising from the superficial fascia (Figs. 10-53 and 10-54).

Insert scissors or a probe into the superficial ring just underneath the tendon of the external abdominal oblique muscle, directed toward the anterior superior iliac spine (Fig. 10-55). Incise the inguinal ligament over the probe or scissors that was previously inserted, and reflect its borders laterally (Fig.

10-56). Pull the spermatic cord laterally and expose the lacunar ligament (Gimbernat's ligament), which represents the medial triangular expansion of the inguinal ligament to the pectineal line of the pubis (Figs. 10-57 and 10-58). Locate the pectineal ligament (Cooper's ligament), which is a strong fibrous band that extends laterally from the lacunar ligament along the pectineal line of the pubis (Figs. 10-57 and 10-58).

Lift the spermatic cord upward and locate the inferior epigastric artery. Try to identify the cremasteric artery a branch of the inferior epigastric artery, which accompanies the spermatic cord (Fig. 10-59).

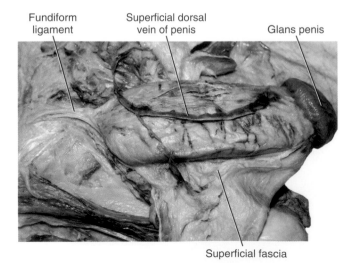

FIGURE 10-53. Dorsal view of penis showing relationship between fundiform ligament and penis.

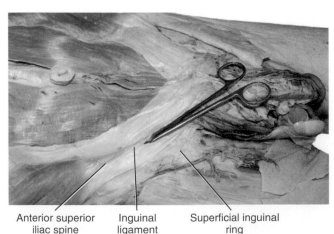

FIGURE 10-55. The superficial inguinal ring is opened, revealing deeper structures of the inguinal canal.

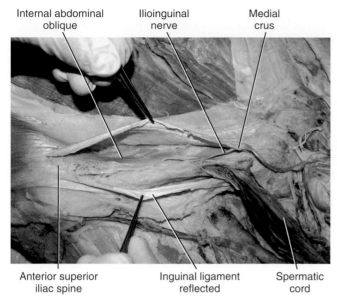

Internal abdominal oblique   Ilioinguinal nerve   Medial crus

Anterior superior iliac spine   Inguinal ligament reflected   Spermatic cord

FIGURE 10-56. Inguinal region on right side, showing exposed inguinal canal and its contents.

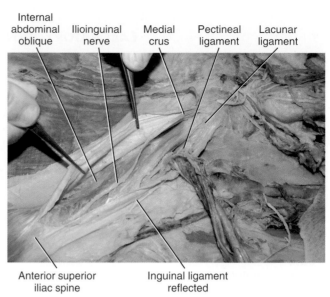

Internal abdominal oblique   Ilioinguinal nerve   Medial crus   Pectineal ligament   Lacunar ligament

Anterior superior iliac spine   Inguinal ligament reflected

FIGURE 10-57. Inguinal region on right side. Note specializations of inguinal ligament—the lacunar and pectineal ligaments.

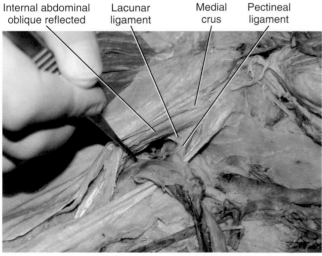

Internal abdominal oblique reflected   Lacunar ligament   Medial crus   Pectineal ligament

FIGURE 10-58. Inguinal region on right side, showing specializations of inguinal ligament, the lacunar and pectineal ligaments.

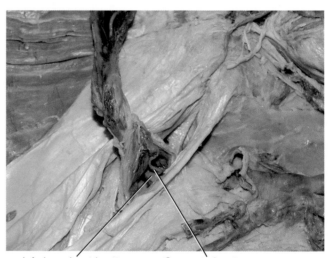

Inferior epigastric artery   Cremasteric artery

FIGURE 10-59. Inguinal region on right side, highlighting cremasteric and inferior epigastric arteries.

LABORATORY IDENTIFICATION CHECKLIST

Nerves
❏ Iliohypogastric
❏ Ilioinguinal
❏ Genitofemoral
  ❏ Genital branch
  ❏ Femoral branch
❏ Dorsal, of penis
❏ Femoral

Artery
❏ Cremasteric

Veins
❏ Inferior epigastric
❏ Superficial external pudendal
❏ Superficial dorsal, of penis

Muscles
❏ External oblique
  ❏ External oblique
    aponeurosis
❏ Internal oblique
❏ Cremasteric
❏ Transversus abdominis
❏ Rectus abdominis
  ❏ Tendinous intersections
  ❏ Linea alba

Bones
❏ Pubis
❏ Ischium
❏ Ilium

Ligaments
❏ Inguinal
  ❏ Superficial ring
  ❏ Deep ring
❏ Lacunar
❏ Pectineal
❏ Fundiform

Fascia
❏ Superficial
❏ External spermatic
❏ Cremasteric
❏ Superficial, of penis
❏ Deep, of penis

Other Structures
❏ Spermatic cord
❏ Testes
  ❏ Lobules
  ❏ Septae
❏ Epididymis
❏ Vas deferens
❏ Tunica vaginalis
❏ Tunica albuginea

CHAPTER 11

PERITONEAL CAVITY

Netter: 247, 252, 261, 267, 278

McMinn: 226–227, 230–236, 245

Gray's Atlas: 141–146

DISSECTION

Technique I

After removal of the skin over the anterior abdominal wall, palpate the most inferior costal cartilages and the xiphoid process (Fig. 11-1). With scissors or a scalpel, cut the attachments of the rectus abdominis and external abdominal oblique muscles over the right and left hypochondriac areas (Fig. 11-2). Continue the incision of the muscles from the xiphoid process toward the midaxillary line on both sides of the cadaver (Fig. 11-3).

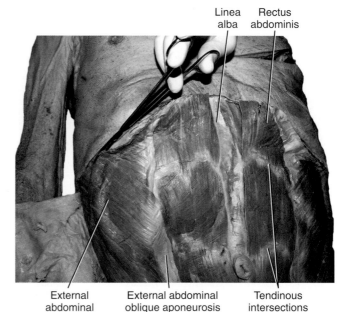

FIGURE 11-2. Attachments of rectus abdominis and external oblique muscles incised over right and left hypochondriac areas.

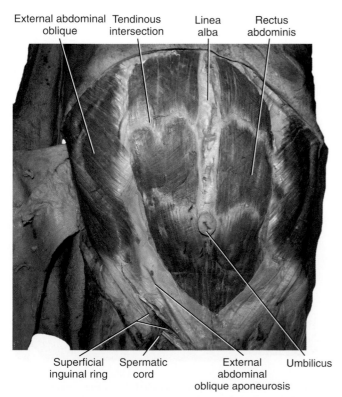

FIGURE 11-1. Anterior abdomen with skin and subcutaneous tissue reflected revealing rectus abdominis and external oblique muscles.

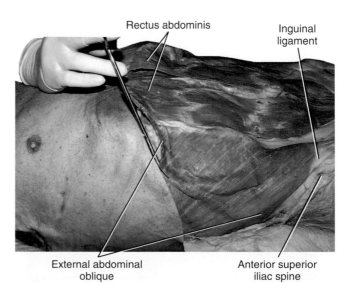

FIGURE 11-3. Incision of the muscles from xiphoid process to midaxillary line on both sides.

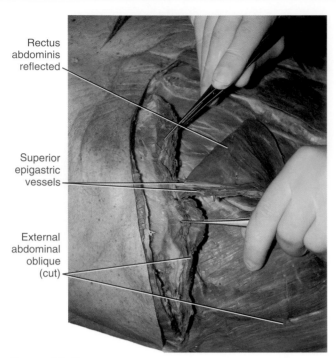

FIGURE 11-4. Rectus abdominis and abdominal oblique muscles reflected inferiorly.

Reflect the rectus abdominis and abdominal oblique muscles inferiorly (Fig. 11-4).

When necessary use blunt dissection to expose the peritoneal cavity (Fig. 11-5). Cut the attachments of the diaphragm, falciform ligament, and ligamentum teres (round ligament) to the abdominal wall. Reflect the anterior abdominal wall toward the pubic symphysis, and observe the contents of the abdominal cavity (Figs. 11-6 and 11-7).

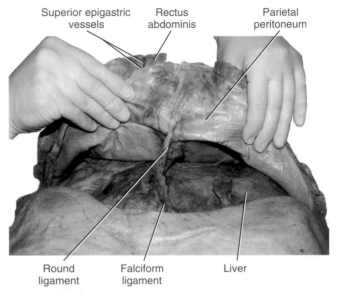

FIGURE 11-6. Attachments of the diaphragm, falciform ligament, and round ligament (ligamentum teres) incised at abdominal wall, with anterior abdominal wall reflected toward pubic symphysis.

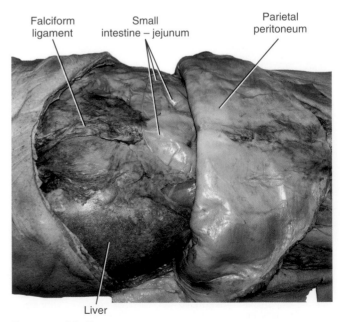

FIGURE 11-7. Peritoneum reflected showing contents of abdomen and abdominal wall.

FIGURE 11-5. Blunt dissection to expose peritoneal cavity.

Technique II

Reflect the rectus sheath and expose the rectus abdominis muscle and the posterior lamina of the rectus sheath (Figs. 11-8 and 11-9). Make a midline vertical incision at the linea alba from the xiphoid process to the pubic symphysis. Make a second horizontal incision from the xiphoid process to the midaxillary line, and reflect the muscle flap laterally (Fig. 11-10). Use the same technique on the contralateral side, and expose the peritoneal cavity (Fig. 11-11).

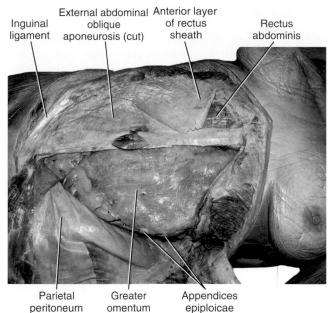

FIGURE 11-10. Xiphoid process to pubic symphysis incision.

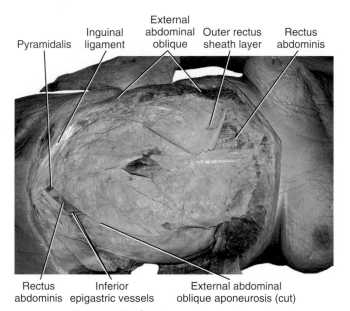

FIGURE 11-8. Rectus sheath reflected.

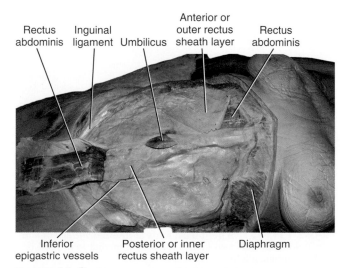

FIGURE 11-9. Observe exposed rectus abdominis muscles and posterior lamina of rectus sheath.

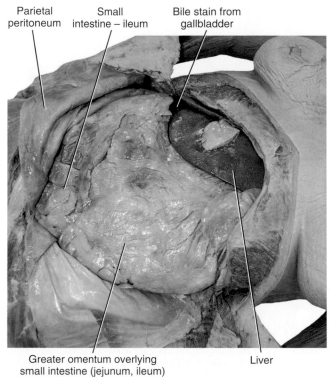

FIGURE 11-11. Second horizontal incision from xiphoid process to midaxillary line on both sides with laterally reflected muscle flap.

Technique III

Make a midline vertical incision on the linea alba from the xiphoid process to the pubic symphysis. Make a second horizontal incision from the right to the left midaxillary line, passing through the umbilicus, and laterally reflect the four muscle flaps (Fig. 11-12).

DISSECTION TIPS: In some specimens the peritoneal cavity is small. To expose it further, with a saw, cut the ribs in the midaxillary line on both sides of the cadaver. You may also extend the cuts with those made previously to expose the thoracic cavity.

All cuts with the scalpel should be carefully made to avoid cutting too deeply into the peritoneal cavity and underlying viscera.

In some cadavers, you will be able to separate the parietal peritoneum from the transversalis fascia. In most, however, these two layers are tightly adherent.

Identify and cut the falciform and round ligaments on the anterior surface of the liver. Trace the round ligament (ligamentum teres) along its pathway from the anterior surface of the liver to the median aspect of the anterior abdominal wall to the umbilicus. At the internal (posterior) surface of the anterior abdominal wall, identify five notable peritoneal folds: the lateral (right and left), the medial (right and left), and the single median umbilical folds (Fig. 11-13).

Make an incision at the posterior layer of the rectus sheath (and peritoneum) and expose the rectus abdominis muscle (Fig. 11-14). Trace the course of the inferior epigastric artery and identify its origin from the external iliac artery (Figs. 11-15 to 11-17). The peritoneal fold covering the inferior epigastric artery and vein is the lateral umbilical peritoneal folds. The medial umbilical folds are formed by an elevation of the peritoneum over the obliterated umbilical arteries. Similarly, the median umbilical fold is an elevation of the peritoneum over the remnants of the urachus (intraabdominal part of allantois). The space between the medial umbilical fold and median umbilical fold is termed the *supravesical fossa.* The depressed region between the medial umbilical fold and the lateral umbilical fold is termed the *medial inguinal fossa.* The lateral inguinal fossa is the area lateral to the lateral inguinal fold.

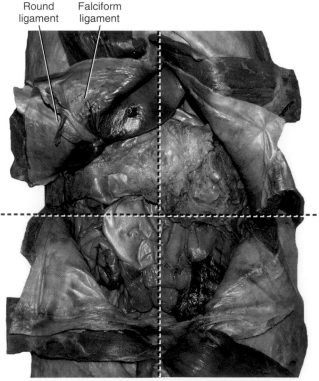

FIGURE 11-12. Midline vertical incision at linea alba from xiphoid process to pubic symphysis, with second horizontal incision from right to left midaxillary lines through umbilicus, with four muscle flaps reflected laterally.

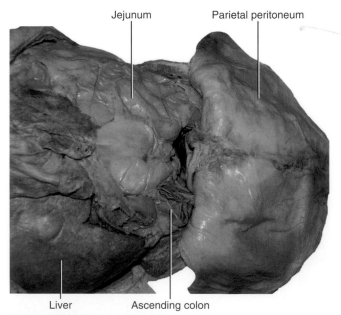

FIGURE 11-13. Five peritoneal folds at internal surface of anterior abdominal wall: two lateral folds, two medial folds, and one median umbilical fold.

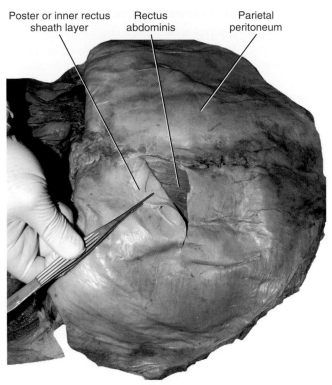

FIGURE 11-14. Posterior layer of rectus sheath cut exposing rectus abdominis muscle.

Poster or inner rectus sheath layer
Rectus abdominis
Parietal peritoneum

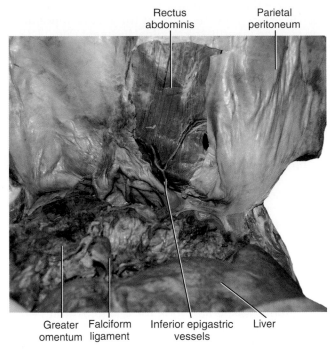

Rectus abdominis
Parietal peritoneum
Greater omentum
Falciform ligament
Inferior epigastric vessels
Liver

FIGURE 11-16. Dissect the inferior epigastric artery and vein.

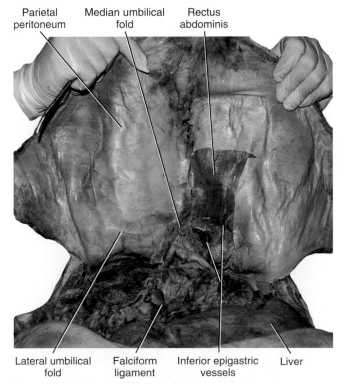

Parietal peritoneum
Median umbilical fold
Rectus abdominis
Lateral umbilical fold
Falciform ligament
Inferior epigastric vessels
Liver

FIGURE 11-15. Appreciate the inferior epigastric artery and vein, as well as medial and lateral umbilical peritoneal folds.

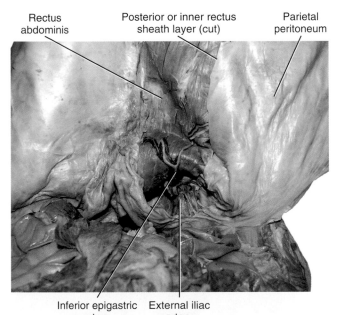

Rectus abdominis
Posterior or inner rectus sheath layer (cut)
Parietal peritoneum
Inferior epigastric artery
External iliac artery

FIGURE 11-17. Dissect the inferior epigastric artery where it arises from the external iliac artery.

DISSECTION TIP: In approximately 30% of cadavers, the inferior epigastric artery will give rise to the obturator artery, which travels medially over the pelvic brim.

Remove the peritoneum covering the inferior epigastric artery and the base of the rectus abdominis muscle, and identify the inguinal ligament (Fig. 11-18). Notice the triangle of Hesselbach formed by the lateral border of the rectus abdominis muscle, the inguinal ligament, and the inferior epigastric vessels. Laterally to the inferior epigastric artery and vein, identify the internal inguinal ring and the ductus deferens (round ligament) passing within it.

Continue the dissection by identifying the pubic tubercle and, lateral to it, a strong ligamentous band running over the periosteum of the pectineal line, the *pectineal ligament* (Cooper's ligament) (Fig. 11-18). Note the medial one third of the inguinal ligament forming an aponeurotic expansion attaching to the pectineal line of the pubis and pectineal ligament, the *lacunar ligament* (Gimbernat's ligament) (Fig. 11-18).

Lateral to the lacunar ligament, expose the femoral vessels, and identify the *femoral ring* (lying medial to femoral vein), the opening to the femoral canal. Clean the adipose tissue and look for a large lymph node, the *lymph node of Cloquet*. Retract the femoral vein medially and note a fascial partition under the inguinal ligament between the femoral vein and the iliopsoas muscle. This partition between the vascular portion (lacuna vasorum) and the muscular portion (lacuna musculorum) is called the *iliopectineal ligament* (Fig. 11-18).

> **✍ DISSECTION TIP:** At the medial part of the femoral ring, look for a small artery, the aberrant obturator artery. This artery is present in at least 50% of specimens.

Inspect the contents of the peritoneal cavity, and identify the liver, stomach (with its greater and lesser curvatures), small and large intestines, and greater omentum (Fig. 11-19). The peritoneal cavity is traditionally divided into two parts, the greater and lesser sacs, or into supracolic and infracolic compartments. The *greater sac* is the entire area of the peritoneal cavity with the exception of the area extending behind the stomach to the diaphragm at the left side, which is the *lesser sac* (omental bursa). Similarly, the *supracolic compartment* is the area of the peritoneal cavity which extends from the transverse mesocolon to the diaphragm. The *infracolic compartment* is the area of the peritoneal cavity extending from the transverse mesocolon below to the pelvic brim.

Identify the greater curvature of the stomach, and lift the greater omentum (Figs. 11-20 and 11-21). Expose the transverse colon with its transverse mesocolon (Fig. 11-22) and identify the ileum, jejunum, cecum, ascending colon, transverse colon, and descending sigmoid colon (Fig. 11-23).

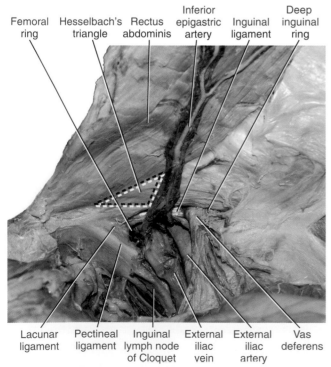

Femoral ring   Hesselbach's triangle   Rectus abdominis   Inferior epigastric artery   Inguinal ligament   Deep inguinal ring

Lacunar ligament   Pectineal ligament   Inguinal lymph node of Cloquet   External iliac vein   External iliac artery   Vas deferens

FIGURE 11-18. Dissect the peritoneum covering over the inferior epigastric artery and base the of rectus abdominis muscle and identify the inguinal ligament. Continue the dissection by locating pubic tubercle and lateral to it identify pectineal ligament.

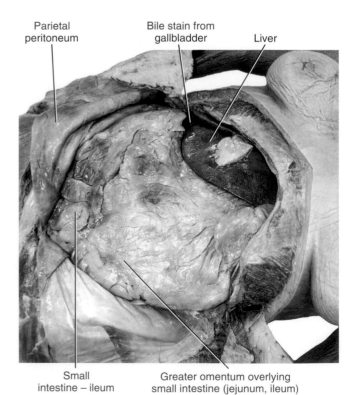

Parietal peritoneum   Bile stain from gallbladder   Liver

Small intestine – ileum   Greater omentum overlying small intestine (jejunum, ileum)

FIGURE 11-19. Appreciate the liver, stomach, small and large intestines, and greater omentum.

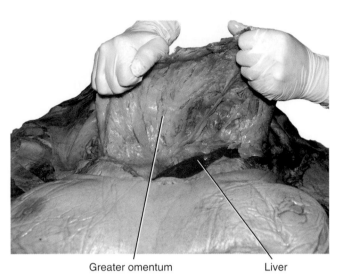

FIGURE 11-20. Lift the greater omentum at the greater curvature of stomach.

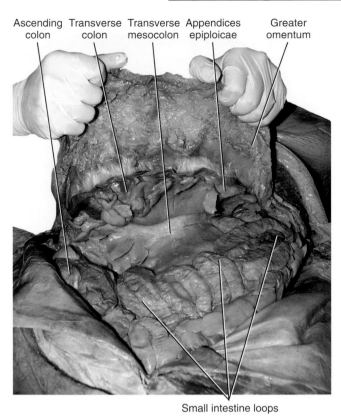

FIGURE 11-21. Appreciate the structures under the greater omentum.

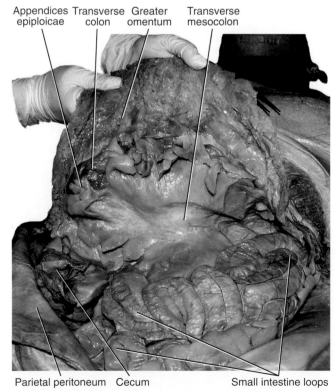

FIGURE 11-22. Expose and locate the transverse colon and mesocolon.

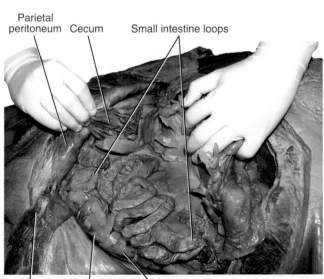

FIGURE 11-23. Identify the ileum, jejunum, cecum, and the ascending, transverse, and descending colon.

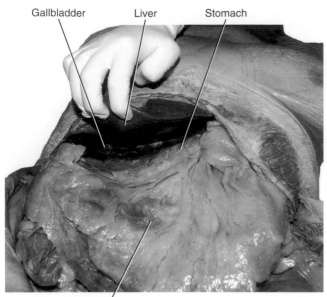

Gallbladder   Liver   Stomach

Greater omentum

FIGURE 11-24. Locate the space between the liver and stomach and identify the gallbladder and lesser omentum.

Observe the space between the liver and the stomach and identify the gallbladder and lesser omentum (Fig. 11-24).

With blunt dissection using your fingertips, separate any adhesions between the stomach and the liver (Figs. 11-25 and 11-26). Cut the greater omentum 3 to 4 cm away from the greater curvature, and leave its attachments from the transverse colon (Fig. 11-27). Pull apart the stomach from the transverse colon, and note the area of the lesser sac. Notice also the pancreas lying directly behind the stomach (Fig. 11-28). Continue the dissection by pulling the stomach inferiorly from the liver, and note the *epiploic foramen* (of Winslow) (Fig. 11-29). Pass a probe or scissors underneath the lesser omentum through the epiploic foramen (Fig. 11-30).

> ✎ *DISSECTION TIP:* Often you will find several adhesions between their contents of the peritoneal cavity. Take some time, and separate these adhesions to restore the normal anatomy and position of the organs.

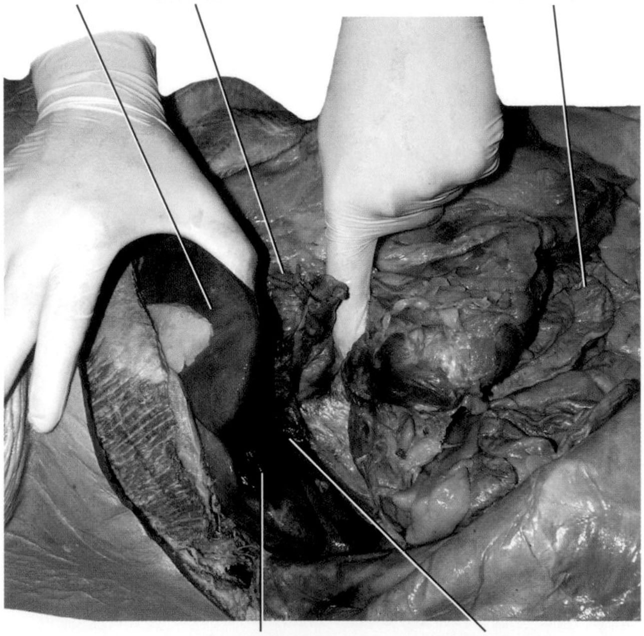

Liver   Stomach   Small intestine

Gallbladder   Epiploic foramen (Winslow)

FIGURE 11-25. With your fingers, bluntly dissect any connections between the stomach and liver.

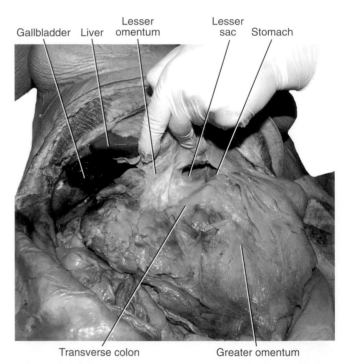

                  Lesser   Lesser
Gallbladder Liver omentum   sac   Stomach

Transverse colon   Greater omentum

FIGURE 11-26. Continue the blunt dissection with your fingers.

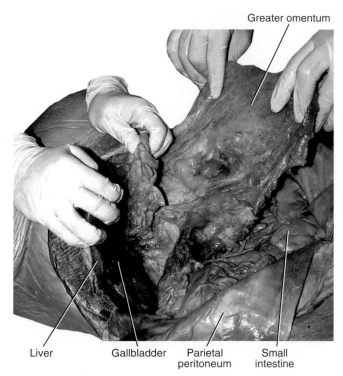

Greater omentum

Liver   Gallbladder   Parietal   Small
                 peritoneum intestine

FIGURE 11-27. Cut the greater omentum approximately 3 cm from the greater curvature of stomach, but do *not* cut its connection with the transverse colon.

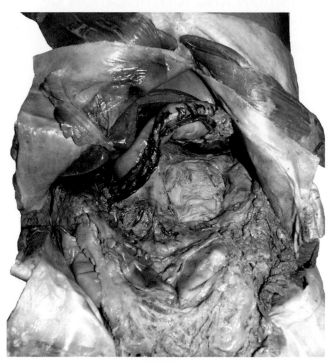

FIGURE 11-28. Pull the stomach from the transverse colon to appreciate the lesser sac and pancreas.

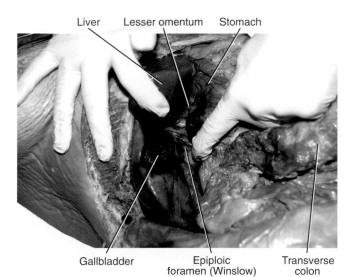

Liver   Lesser omentum   Stomach

Gallbladder   Epiploic   Transverse
           foramen (Winslow)   colon

FIGURE 11-29. Pull the stomach inferiorly from the liver and locate the epiploic foramen.

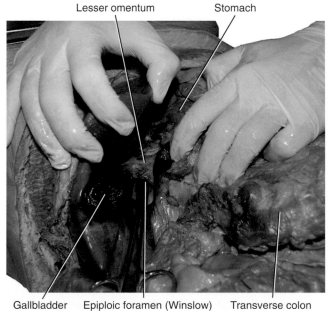

Lesser omentum   Stomach

Gallbladder   Epiploic foramen (Winslow)   Transverse colon

FIGURE 11-30. Pass a probe or scissors posterior to the lesser omentum via the epiploic foramen.

PALPATION AND IDENTIFICATION OF STRUCTURES (WITHOUT DISSECTION)

- Lesser omentum
- Epiploic foramen
- Stomach
- Gallbladder
- Spleen

The *lesser omentum* includes the hepatogastric and hepatoduodenal ligaments. To distinguish them, note that the *hepatogastric* ligament connects the liver to the stomach, whereas the *hepatoduodenal* ligament connects the liver to the duodenum. The hepatoduodenal ligament contains the common bile duct, the hepatic artery, and the hepatic portal vein.

Place your thumb at the *epiploic foramen* and index finger on top of the hepatoduodenal ligament, and feel for these structures. This is called the *Pringel maneuver* and is useful for controlling hemorrhage from the hepatic artery when accidentally injured.

Palpate the anterior surface of the *stomach* and notice the greater and lesser curvatures, the body, the fundus, and the hard and thick pyloric sphincter. Identify the *gallbladder* (if present) at the internal surface of the liver. A surgical landmark to identify the gallbladder is the point of intersection between the 9th costal cartilage and the linea semilunaris.

👆 *DISSECTION TIP:* Note on neighboring cadavers that the stomach exhibits variable shapes and sizes, which is a normal feature.

Palpation

Lift the stomach and pass your fingers posterior to it to reach the spleen. Feel the *gastrosplenic ligament* connecting the greater curvature of the stomach to the spleen. Palpate the *spleen,* and with your palm, try to feel the posterior surface of the spleen up against the body wall. Attempting this maneuver, your palm will come up against the *splenorenal ligament,* which connects the spleen to the body wall. Similarly, if you try to reach the diaphragm, moving your fingertips upward from the spleen, you will feel the *phrenicocolic ligament* connecting the spleen to the diaphragm.

With your fingertips, palpate the *liver,* and identify the falciform, round, and coronary ligaments.

Small Intestine

Palpate the pyloric sphincter and distal to it, feel for the much softer, 1st portion of the duodenum. Lift the greater omentum, and identify the transverse colon with its mesentery, the *transverse mesocolon.* Just behind the transverse mesocolon, the 2nd part of the duodenum is passing vertically on the right side of the cadaver. The mesentery of the ileum and jejunum covers the 3rd (horizontal) part of the duodenum. The final, 4th part of the duodenum can be identified at the *duodenojejunal flexure.* At the duodenojejunal flexure feel for a connective tissue band, the "suspensory ligament of the duodenum" (ligament of Treitz).

Continue palpating the *jejunum,* which makes up approximately two fifths of the small intestine. Identify the mesentery of the ileum and jejunum.

Large Intestine

Palpate the distal part of the *ileum* and in the right lower quadrant of the abdominal cavity and identify the *cecum* and the ileocecal junction. Explore the cecum for an *appendix.* Notice that the appendix has its own mesentery, the *mesoappendix.*

👆 *DISSECTION TIP:* In the majority of cadavers the appendix will originate from the posterior part of the cecum. This is termed *retrocecal appendix.* In addition, the appendix has often been surgically removed; look for the original location of the appendix, if possible.

Continue identifying the ascending, transverse, descending, and sigmoid parts of the colon. The rectum and anus will not be identified during this part of dissection. Palpate the proximal part of the ascending colon, the *ileocecal junction,* as well as its distal part the right colic or hepatic flexure at the level of the liver. At the hepatic flexure, the ascending colon turns left and becomes the transverse colon. Similarly, the transverse colon reaches the splenic flexure or left colic flexure, which turns to the right (inferiorly) to become descending colon. At the lower lever of the left lower quadrant, the descending colon becomes sigmoid colon, exhibiting a characteristic S shape. Notice its mesentery, the *sigmoid mesocolon.* It is difficult to appreciate the entire length of the sigmoid mesocolon and sigmoid colon, because most of it is located within the pelvic cavity. This portion will be identified at a later dissection.

With your hands, lift and medially pull up the ascending colon and descending colon, and identify the longitudinal depressions; they rest in the right and left paracolic gutters.

> ✋ *DISSECTION TIP:* The large intestine exhibits some characteristic morphologic features:
> - *Teniae coli* are three narrow muscular bands of the external longitudinal muscle layer of the large intestine.
> - *Haustra,* or sacculations, are pouches produced by the teniae coli.
> - *Appendices epiploicae* are peritoneum-covered fat-filled sacs, attached in rows along the teniae coli.

LABORATORY IDENTIFICATION CHECKLIST

Ligaments
- ❐ Gastrosplenic
- ❐ Hepatogastric
- ❐ Hepatoduodenal
- ❐ Inguinal (Poupart's)
- ❐ Lacunar (Gimbernat's)
- ❐ Pectineal (Cooper's)
- ❐ Median arcuate
- ❐ Medial arcuate
- ❐ Lateral arcuate
- ❐ Median umbilical (urachus)
- ❐ Medial umbilical

Liver
- ❐ Falciform
- ❐ Round (ligamentum teres)
- ❐ Right triangular
- ❐ Left triangular
- ❐ Coronary
- ❐ Suspensory ligament of duodenum (of Treitz)

Other Connective Tissue
- ❐ Greater omentum
- ❐ Lesser omentum
- ❐ External oblique aponeurosis
- ❐ Linea alba
- ❐ Anterior sheath of rectus abdominis
- ❐ Posterior sheath of rectus abdominis
- ❐ Greater omentum
- ❐ Lesser omentum
- ❐ Transverse mesocolon
- ❐ Sigmoid mesentery
- ❐ Appendicular mesentery
- ❐ Dorsal root mesentery
- ❐ Appendices epiploicae
- ❐ Teniae coli

Organs
- ❐ Esophagus
- ❐ Liver
  - ❐ Left lobe
  - ❐ Right lobe
  - ❐ Caudate
  - ❐ Quadrate
- ❐ Gallbladder
- ❐ Fundus
  - ❐ Body
  - ❐ Neck
- ❐ Pancreas
- ❐ Spleen
- ❐ Stomach
  - ❐ Fundus
  - ❐ Body
  - ❐ Cardia
  - ❐ Pylorus
  - ❐ Greater curvature
  - ❐ Lesser curvature
- ❐ Small intestine
  - ❐ Duodenum
  - ❐ Jejunum
  - ❐ Ileum
- ❐ Large intestine
  - ❐ Cecum
  - ❐ Appendix
  - ❐ Ileocecal junction
    - ❐ Ascending colon
    - ❐ Transverse colon
    - ❐ Descending colon
    - ❐ Sigmoid colon
- ❐ Hepatic flexure
- ❐ Splenic flexure

Muscles
- ❐ External oblique
- ❐ Internal oblique
- ❐ Transversus abdominis
- ❐ Rectus abdominis
- ❐ Pyramidalis
- ❐ Psoas major

Bones
- ❐ Ribs 9-11
- ❐ Xiphoid process of sternum
- ❐ Sacrum
- ❐ Iliac crest of ilium

Spaces
- ❐ Omental foramen (of Winslow)
- ❐ Omental bursa

CHAPTER 12

GASTROINTESTINAL TRACT

Netter: 262–287, 289–291, 293–296

McMinn: 237–239, 244–253

Gray's Atlas: 147–172

In most cadavers, the liver occupies a significant portion of the peritoneal cavity. The gallbladder may be difficult to see at this point but look for its fundus. The gallbladder, if not surgically removed, will be seen as the dissection proceeds.

With a scalpel, make a horizontal incision at the lower edge of the liver, removing 3 to 4 cm (1½ inches) of liver parenchyma (Fig. 12-1). Pull the stomach downward and fully expose the gallbladder and the hepatoduodenal ligament (Figs. 12-2 and 12-3). With scissors or a probe, carefully strip away the hepato-duodenal ligament and expose the common bile duct, proper hepatic artery, and hepatic portal vein (Fig. 12-4). Note the relationships among these three struc-tures; within the hepatoduodenal ligament, the portal vein is located posteriorly, deep to the common bile duct and proper hepatic artery (Figs. 12-5 and 12-6).

> *DISSECTION TIP:* Stripping away the hepatoduodenal ligament, you will see several nerves running alongside the common bile duct and proper hepatic artery. These nerves are part of the autonomic nervous system and are primarily sympathetic fibers (Fig. 12-4).

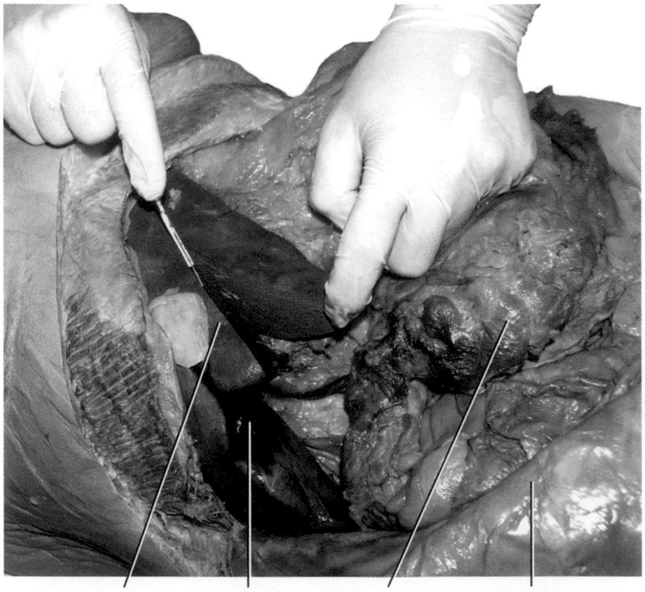

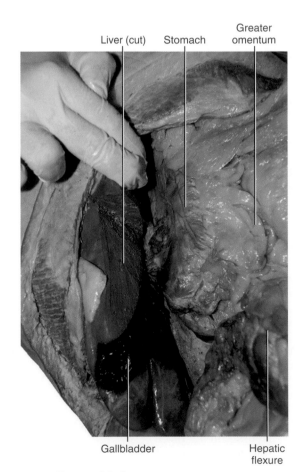

Liver (cut)   Stomach   Greater omentum

Gallbladder   Hepatic flexure

FIGURE 12-2. Identify the gallbladder.

Liver (cut)   Gallbladder   Transverse colon   Parietal peritoneum

FIGURE 12-1. Horizontal incision at lower edge of the liver.

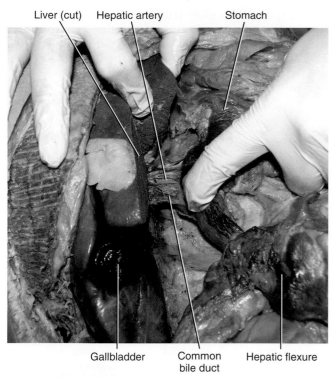

FIGURE 12-3. Pull the stomach downward to expose the gall-bladder and hepatoduodenal ligament.

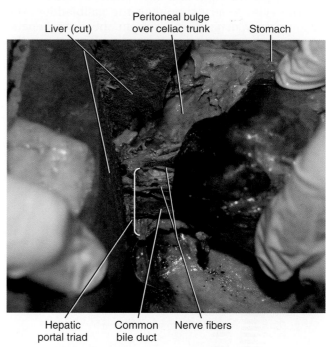

FIGURE 12-4. Cut the hepatoduodenal ligament to expose the common bile duct, proper hepatic artery, portal vein, hepatic portal triad, and autonomic nerve fibers.

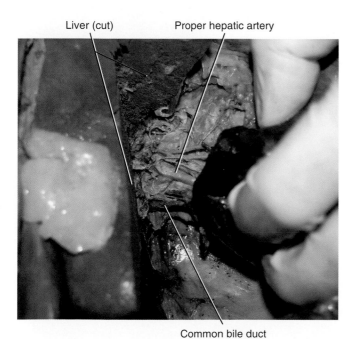

FIGURE 12-5. View shows relationship of proper hepatic artery and common bile duct.

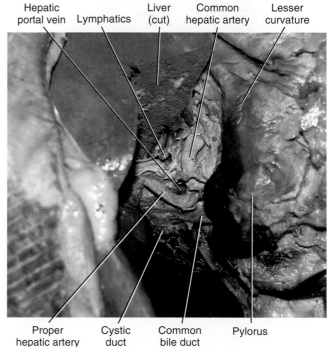

FIGURE 12-6. View demonstrates relationship of proper hepatic artery, common bile duct, and hepatic portal vein.

Clean the proper hepatic artery toward the liver, and identify the right and left hepatic arteries. Look for the *cystic artery* supplying the gallbladder. The cystic artery usually arises from the right hepatic artery or the proper hepatic artery. Dissect out the cystic duct from the gallbladder toward its junction with the common hepatic duct to form the common bile duct (Fig. 12-7). Once these structures are cleaned and identified, observe the *hepatocystic triangle* formed by the common hepatic duct, the cystic duct, and the liver. In the majority of cases, the cystic artery is identified within this triangular region.

To expose the celiac trunk and its branches, with blunt dissection, release the transverse and the descending colon from the gastrocolic ligament (Figs. 12-8 and 12-9). With scissors, cut the gastrocolic ligament at the superior border of the transverse colon and release it from the stomach (Fig. 12-10).

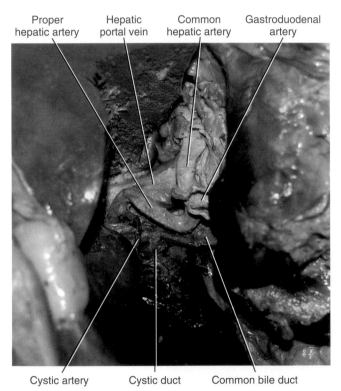

FIGURE 12-7. View shows dissected cystic duct from gallbladder to junction with common hepatic duct.

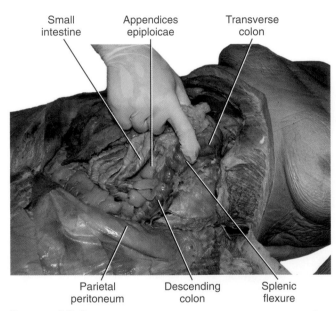

FIGURE 12-8. Identify the transverse colon and descending colon.

▎*DISSECTION TIP:* In about 65% of cases, the cystic artery arises from the right hepatic artery. If you are not able to identify the cystic artery in its typical location, lift the cystic duct and look inferior to it.

To expose the splenic artery and spleen, cut the inferior edge of the costal cartilages with a saw to expose fully the area anterior to the spleen. Place paper towels underneath the costal cartilages (Fig. 12-11). Identify the inferior border of the spleen, hidden by the gastrosplenic and splenorenal ligaments and abundant fat (Fig. 12-12).

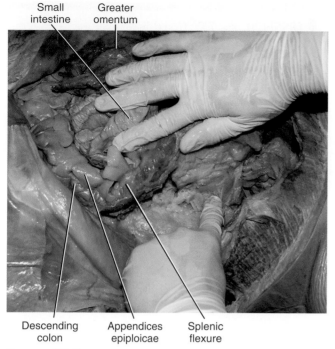

FIGURE 12-9. Blunt dissection of transverse and descending colon from the gastrocolic ligament.

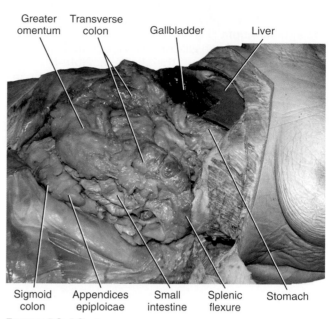

FIGURE 12-10. Cut the gastrocolic ligament at superior border of the transverse colon to release the colon from stomach.

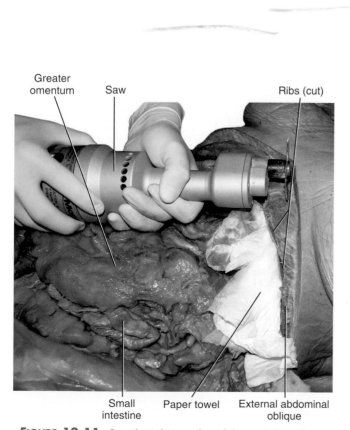

FIGURE 12-11. Saw the inferior edge of the costal cartilage.

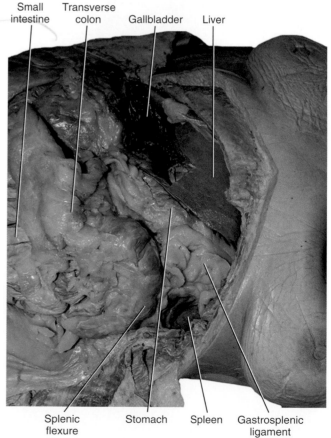

FIGURE 12-12. Identify the superior borders of the spleen.

Clean the fat and the gastrosplenic and splenorenal ligaments, and expose the splenic pedicle receiving the splenic artery and vein (Fig. 12-13). Continue the exposure of the splenic artery and vein and identify the splenic hilum (Fig. 12-14).

Identify the short gastric arteries, which pass to the greater curvature of the stomach. Note the relationship of the spleen with the stomach and the pancreas. Identify the left gastroepiploic artery, which typically derives from the most inferior splenic artery hilar branch (Fig. 12-15).

Pull the stomach upward and expose the tail of the pancreas (Fig. 12-15). Continue the dissection of the splenic artery and vein from the hilum of the spleen toward the celiac trunk. The splenic artery is tortuous and lies hidden at the upper border of the tail and body of the pancreas (Fig. 12-16).

> ☝ *DISSECTION TIP:* The spleen rests on an abundance of adipose tissue. Once the adipose tissue is cleaned away, the spleen will drop inferiorly and posteriorly, and its vessels will be stressed and possibly broken. Place some folded paper towels posterior to the spleen to keep it at the same level as the pancreas. In addition, the paper towels will absorb any embalming fluid that accumulates in this space (see Fig. 12-15).

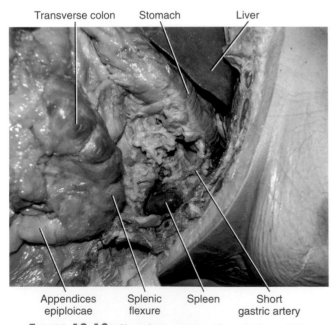

FIGURE 12-13. Clean fat to expose the splenic pedicle.

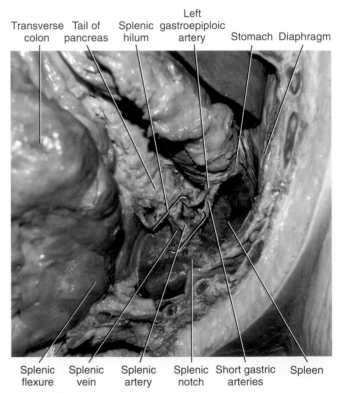

FIGURE 12-14. Expose the splenic artery and vein and identify the splenic hilum.

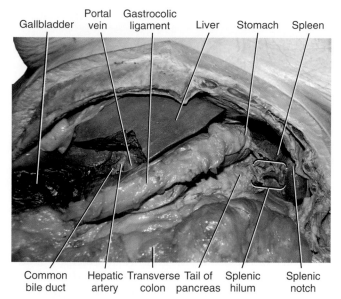

Gallbladder · Portal vein · Gastrocolic ligament · Liver · Stomach · Spleen

Common bile duct · Hepatic artery · Transverse colon · Tail of pancreas · Splenic hilum · Splenic notch

FIGURE 12-15. Identify the left gastroepiploic artery, and pull the stomach upward to expose tail of the pancreas.

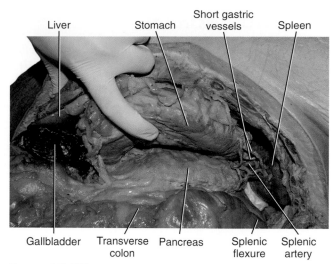

Liver · Stomach · Short gastric vessels · Spleen

Gallbladder · Transverse colon · Pancreas · Splenic flexure · Splenic artery

FIGURE 12-17. Lift the stomach upward to expose body and tail of the pancreas.

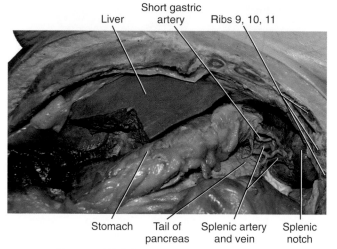

Liver · Short gastric artery · Ribs 9, 10, 11

Stomach · Tail of pancreas · Splenic artery and vein · Splenic notch

FIGURE 12-16. Identify the splenic artery.

Lift the stomach upward and expose the body and tail of the pancreas (Fig. 12-17). Clean out the splenic artery and vein from the adjacent pancreas (Fig. 12-18). Do *not* pull the splenic artery away from the pancreas, because most of its branches are short and can be easily injured.

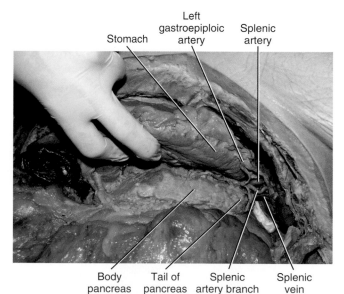

Stomach · Left gastroepiploic artery · Splenic artery

Body pancreas · Tail of pancreas · Splenic artery branch · Splenic vein

FIGURE 12-18. Clean out splenic artery and vein from adjacent pancreas.

The reason for not dissecting the entire celiac trunk from the right side, at this time, is that the view from the gallbladder offers only limited exposure of the area. It is simpler to release the stomach from the gastrocolic ligament and greater omentum, identify the splenic artery at the splenic hilum, and then dissect the middle portion of the celiac trunk.

To visualize the area of the celiac trunk, it is necessary to lift the stomach upward and expose the pancreas. Palpate the upper border of the pancreas, and with your fingers, feel the celiac artery as a prominent bulge covered by the overlying peritoneum.

IDENTIFICATION OF DIFFERENT PARTS OF STOMACH

The stomach is divided into four main regions: the cardia, fundus, body, and pylorus. Identify the *lesser curvature* and the *greater curvature* of the stomach. Identify the *angular notch*, found between the body and pyloric part of the stomach. Look for the cardia and the *cardiac notch* between the esophagus and fundus. The *fundus* is the portion of the stomach above the cardiac notch. The pylorus is further divided into the pyloric antrum and pyloric canal.

Return to the exposed proper hepatic artery, and dissect backward toward its origin from the common hepatic artery (Figs. 12-19 and 12-20). Identify and expose the other branch of the common hepatic artery, the gastroduodenal artery (Fig. 12-20). Dissect out the right side of the lesser curvature of the stomach and identify the *right gastric artery*, a branch of the proper hepatic artery. Next to the right gastric artery, identify the right gastric vein and its connection to the right gastroepiploic vein via the prepyloric vein of Mayo. On the left side of the lesser curvature of the stomach, identify and clean the left gastric artery, then trace it back from its origin from the celiac trunk (Fig. 12-21). Note the esophageal

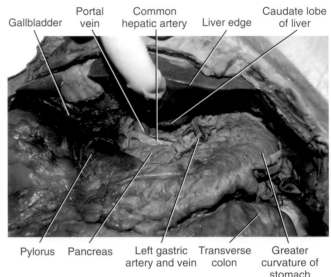

FIGURE 12-20. Dissect the proper hepatic artery backward, toward its origin from the common hepatic artery.

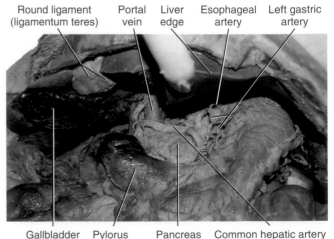

FIGURE 12-21. Identify and clean the left gastric artery.

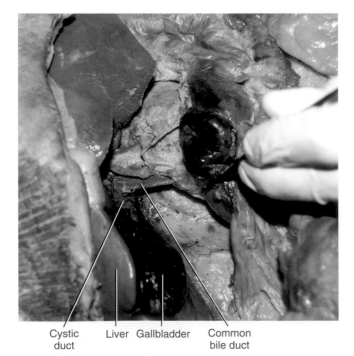

FIGURE 12-19. Identify the common bile duct and cystic duct.

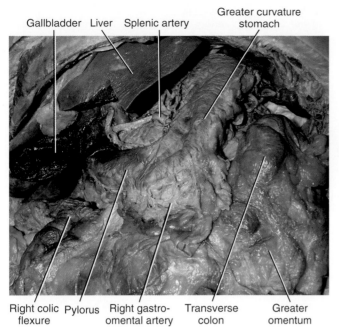

FIGURE 12-22. Identify the greater curvature of the stomach.

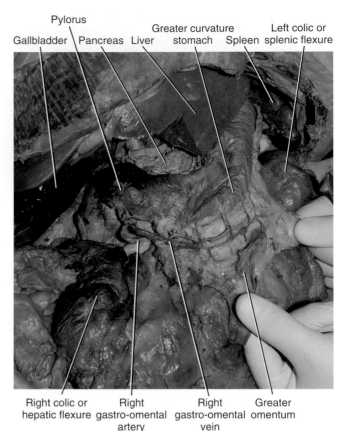

FIGURE 12-23. Dissect out the fat within the gastrocolic ligament and greater omentum and identify the right gastroepiploic artery.

arterial branches of the left gastric artery ascending toward the esophagus. The left gastric artery is accompanied by the left gastric vein. Trace out any esophageal tributaries to the left gastric vein.

In the area between the greater curvature of the stomach and the pylorus, dissect out the fat within the gastrocolic ligament and greater omentum, and identify the right gastroepiploic artery (Figs. 12-22 and 12-23). Similarly, dissect between the left side of the greater curvature of the stomach and spleen and identify the left gastroepiploic artery.

After identifying the right and left gastroepiploic arteries, with scissors, cut along the line marking the junction between the body of the stomach and the pyloric antrum, 4 to 5 cm (~2 inches) proximal to the pylorus (Fig. 12-24).

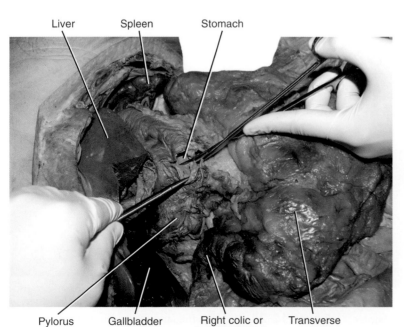

FIGURE 12-24. With scissors, cut along the junction between the body of the stomach and the pyloric antrum.

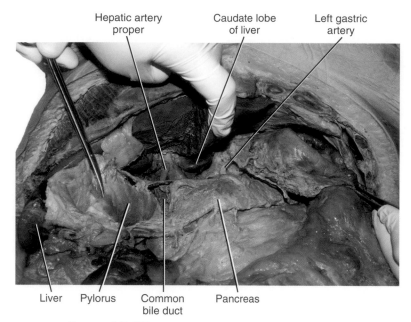

FIGURE 12-25. Expose the celiac trunk and pancreas.

Retract the two parts of the transected stomach laterally and expose the celiac trunk and pancreas (Fig. 12-25). Lift the splenic artery from the upper border of the pancreas and dissect it out (Fig. 12-26). Once the splenic artery is fully exposed, notice its tortuosity (Fig. 12-27). Place the left side of the stomach in such a position that you can visualize all the branches of the celiac trunk and identify the origins and distributions of these branches (Figs. 12-28 and 12-29).

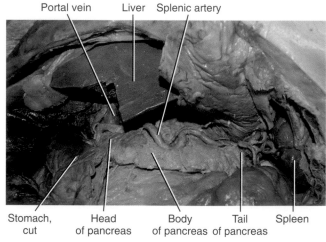

FIGURE 12-27. Note the tortuous route of the splenic artery.

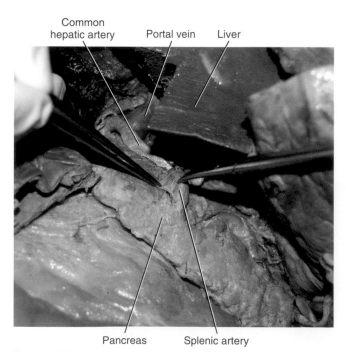

FIGURE 12-26. Dissect the splenic artery from the upper border of the pancreas.

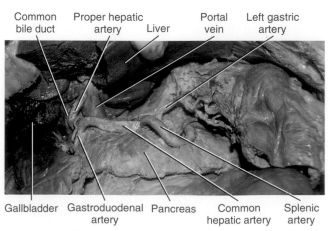

FIGURE 12-28. Displace the stomach in order to visualize the branches of the celiac trunk.

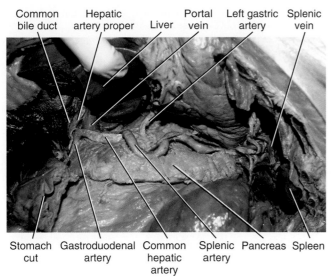

Common bile duct — Hepatic artery proper — Liver — Portal vein — Left gastric artery — Splenic vein

Stomach cut — Gastroduodenal artery — Common hepatic artery — Splenic artery — Pancreas — Spleen

FIGURE 12-29. Identify the origins and distributions of the branches of the celiac artery.

DISSECTION TIP: Note the following common arterial variations of the celiac trunk:
- Celiac artery and superior mesenteric artery arising as a common trunk (celiomesenteric trunk, 2.5% of cases)
- Proper hepatic and superior mesenteric arteries arising as a common trunk (hepatomesenteric trunk)
- Splenic artery and left gastric artery arising as a common trunk (lienogastric [splenogastric] trunk, 5.5%)
- Left gastric and common hepatic artery arising as a common trunk (gastrohepatic or hepatogastric trunk, 1.5%)
- Left gastric artery arising from the left hepatic artery (25%)
- Right hepatic artery arising from the superior mesenteric artery (18%)
- Cystic artery arising from proper hepatic or left hepatic artery
- Aberrant left hepatic artery arising from the left hepatic artery (25%)

BEFORE DISSECTION

The pancreas is typically subdivided into the following parts: head, neck, body, and tail. The head is encircled by the 1st three parts of the duodenum and contains the *uncinate process*, which is located posteroinferiorly to the superior mesenteric artery and vein. Its terminal part, the tail, is related to the hilum of the spleen and left kidney.

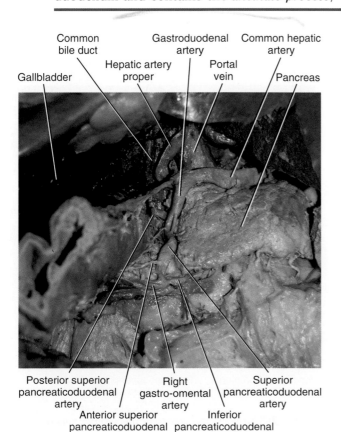

Common bile duct — Hepatic artery proper — Gastroduodenal artery — Portal vein — Common hepatic artery — Pancreas — Gallbladder

Posterior superior pancreaticoduodenal artery — Anterior superior pancreaticoduodenal artery — Right gastro-omental artery — Inferior pancreaticoduodenal artery — Superior pancreaticoduodenal artery

On the right side of the cadaver, dissect out the branches of the gastroduodenal artery anteriorly. Around the head of the pancreas, look for the origin of the two terminal branches of the gastroduodenal artery, the right gastroepiploic and superior pancreaticoduodenal arteries (Fig. 12-30). The right gastroepiploic artery is typically found around the right side of the greater curvature of the stomach. The superior pancreaticoduodenal artery divides into the posterior superior and anterior superior pancreaticoduodenal arteries supplying the head of the pancreas (Fig. 12-30).

FIGURE 12-30. Identify the origin of the two terminal branches of the gastroduodenal artery, the right gastroepiploic artery and superior pancreaticoduodenal artery.

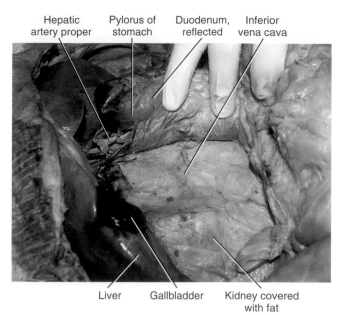

FIGURE 12-31. Reflect the stomach and duodenum to the left, and bluntly dissect the area underneath the duodenum and inferior vena cava.

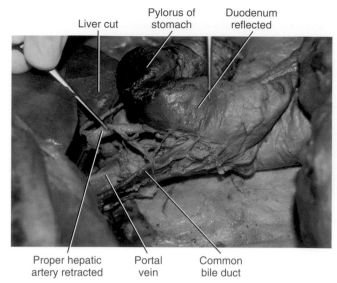

FIGURE 12-32. Follow the gastroduodenal artery posteriorly toward the 1st part of the duodenum, and expose the origin of the posterior superior pancreaticoduodenal artery.

DISSECTION TIP: To expose the arterial branches, as well as the course of the common bile duct down to the duodenum, you will need to reflect the stomach and duodenum to the left. Use your fingers to dissect the area underneath the duodenum and inferior vena cava; this is an avascular plane that is easily reflected to the left. This is called the *Kocher maneuver,* or "kocherizing" (Fig. 12-31).

Follow the gastroduodenal artery posteriorly toward the 1st part of the duodenum and expose the origin of the posterior superior pancreaticoduodenal (PSPD) artery (Figs. 12-32 and 12-33). Trace the course of the anterior superior pancreaticoduodenal artery (Figs. 12-33 and 12-34), and expose its anastomosis with the inferior pancreaticoduodenal artery, a branch of the superior mesenteric artery.

DISSECTION TIP: A good way to trace and expose the PSPD artery is to dissect out the common bile duct from the lateral side (see Fig. 12-31). The artery that crosses over the common bile duct is the PSPD. Furthermore, this artery passes behind the head of the pancreas and the 2nd part of the duodenum.

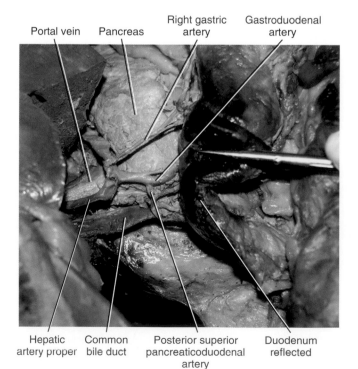

FIGURE 12-33. Trace the course of the anterior superior pancreaticoduodenal artery.

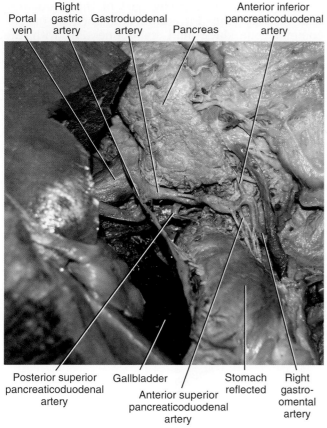

Portal vein — Right gastric artery — Gastroduodenal artery — Pancreas — Anterior inferior pancreaticoduodenal artery

Posterior superior pancreaticoduodenal artery — Gallbladder — Anterior superior pancreaticoduodenal artery — Stomach reflected — Right gastro-omental artery

FIGURE 12-34. Expose the anterior superior pancreaticoduodenal artery's anastomosis with the inferior pancreaticoduodenal artery.

Optional Dissection of Branches of Splenic Artery

Lift the splenic artery up and look for the origin of several branches. The following landmarks help identify these branches:

1. Lift the pancreas and look for the point where the portal vein crosses the pancreas posteriorly (neck of the pancreas). At this point, look for a branch from the splenic artery, the *dorsal pancreatic artery.*
2. The splenic artery will often give off small branches at the superior border of the body and the tail of the pancreas, the *short pancreatic branches.*
3. The largest of these short pancreatic branches is the *great pancreatic artery* (pancreatica magna), often found at the distal one third of the pancreas near its the tail.
4. At the same point of the great pancreatic artery, look for a branch of the splenic artery traveling to the posterior part of the stomach supplying the gastric fundus, the *posterior gastric artery.*
5. Look 1 to 2 cm superior to the inferior border of the pancreas; embedded in its substance is the *transverse pancreatic artery.*

Make a horizontal incision at the pyloric antrum, pylorus, and duodenum and observe the inner surface of these structures (Fig. 12-35).

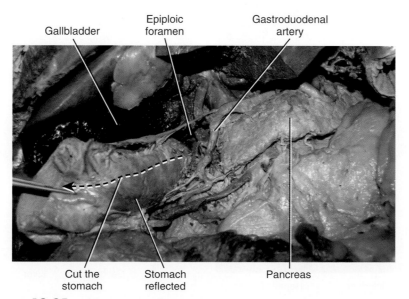

Gallbladder — Epiploic foramen — Gastroduodenal artery

Cut the stomach — Stomach reflected — Pancreas

FIGURE 12-35. Make a horizontal cut at the pyloric antrum, pylorus, and duodenum.

Appreciate the gastric folds at the inner surface of the pyloric antrum and the circular muscle of the pyloric sphincter (Fig. 12-36). Continue the incision at the 1st, 2nd, and 3rd parts of the duodenum, and note the circular folds of Kerckring (Figs. 12-37 and 12-38). Cut the gastroduodenal artery and expose the course of the common bile duct toward the duodenum (Fig. 12-39). The common bile duct is divided into supraduodenal (above duodenum), retroduodenal (behind duodenum), and pancreatic parts (terminal part) (Fig. 12-40).

Open up the descending part of the duodenum and identify the intraduodenal portion of the common bile duct; find its connection with the main pancreatic duct (of Wirsung), forming the hepatopancreatic ampulla (of Vater). Identify the duodenal papilla, which contains the hepatopancreatic ampulla. Expose the main pancreatic duct into the substance of the pancreas by removing pancreatic tissue with your forceps (Fig. 12-40). Look for an accessory pancreatic duct (of Santorini), if present.

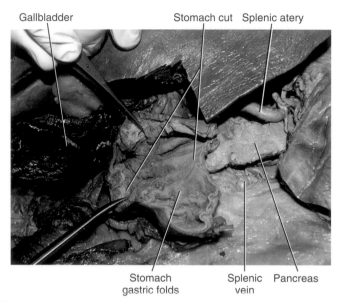

FIGURE 12-36. Note gastric rugae at the inner surface of the pyloric antrum and circular muscle of the pyloric sphincter.

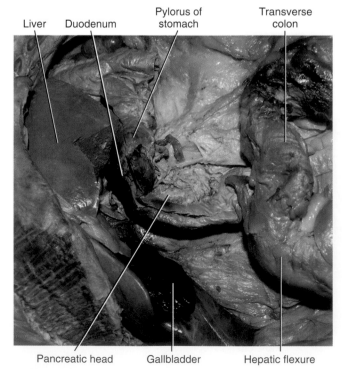

FIGURE 12-37. Continue incision at 1st, 2nd, and 3rd parts of duodenum.

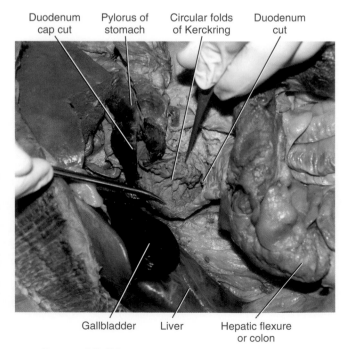

FIGURE 12-38. Note the circular folds of Kerckring.

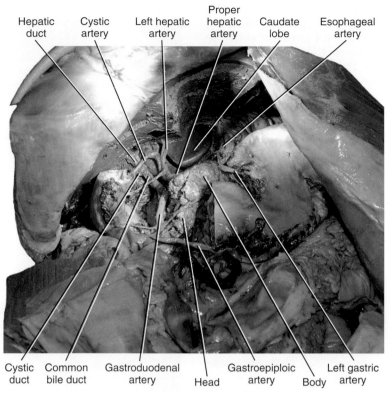

Hepatic duct Cystic artery Left hepatic artery Proper hepatic artery Caudate lobe Esophageal artery

Cystic duct Common bile duct Gastroduodenal artery Head Gastroepiploic artery Body Left gastric artery

FIGURE 12-39. Cut the gastroduodenal artery and expose the course of the common bile duct.

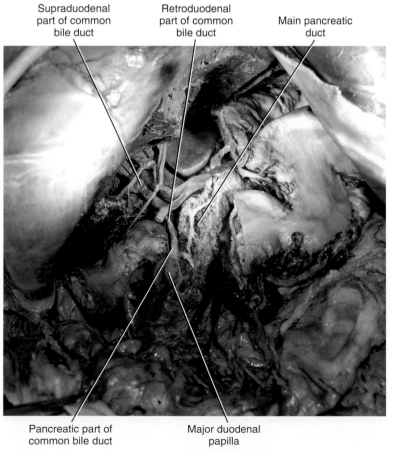

Supraduodenal part of common bile duct Retroduodenal part of common bile duct Main pancreatic duct

Pancreatic part of common bile duct Major duodenal papilla

FIGURE 12-40. Note divisions of the common bile duct: supraduodenal, retroduodenal, and pancreatic parts.

With your forceps, lift the pancreas and identify the *splenic vein* (Fig. 12-41). Expose the splenic vein along its entire length, and trace out its junction with the superior mesenteric vein to form the *portal vein* (Figs. 12-42 and 12-43). Next to the superior mesenteric vein, look for the inferior mesenteric vein, usually draining into the splenic vein. Continue exposing the tributaries of the superior mesenteric vein. Next to its tributaries, expose the arterial branches of the *superior mesenteric artery* (Fig. 12-44). The vast majority of tissue you must remove to expose the branches of the superior mesenteric artery and vein is fat and dense autonomic nerve tissue.

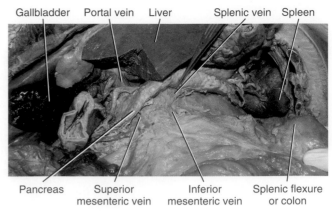

Gallbladder   Portal vein   Liver   Splenic vein   Spleen

Pancreas   Superior mesenteric vein   Inferior mesenteric vein   Splenic flexure or colon

FIGURE 12-42. Expose the splenic vein along its entire length.

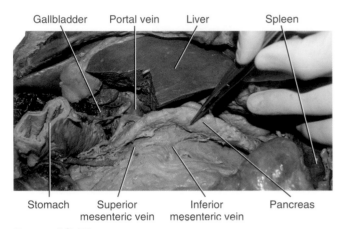

Gallbladder   Portal vein   Liver   Spleen

Stomach   Superior mesenteric vein   Inferior mesenteric vein   Pancreas

FIGURE 12-41. With forceps, lift the pancreas and identify the splenic vein.

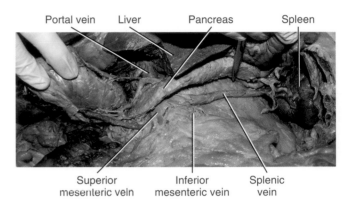

Portal vein   Liver   Pancreas   Spleen

Superior mesenteric vein   Inferior mesenteric vein   Splenic vein

FIGURE 12-43. Trace the splenic vein to its junction with the superior mesenteric vein to form the portal vein.

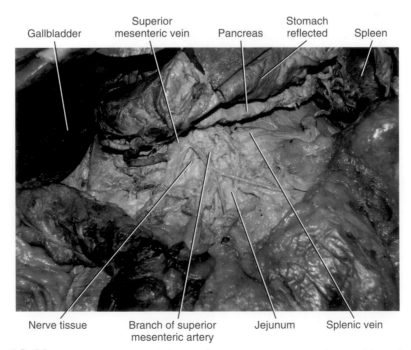

Gallbladder   Superior mesenteric vein   Pancreas   Stomach reflected   Spleen

Nerve tissue   Branch of superior mesenteric artery   Jejunum   Splenic vein

FIGURE 12-44. Expose tributaries of the superior mesenteric vein and arterial branches of the superior mesenteric artery.

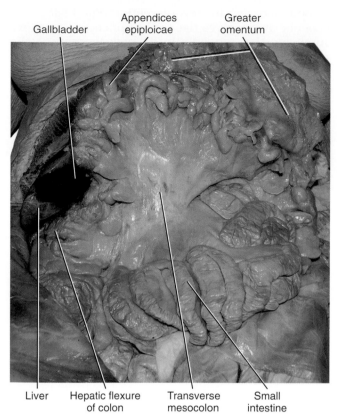

Gallbladder   Appendices epiploicae   Greater omentum

Liver   Hepatic flexure of colon   Transverse mesocolon   Small intestine

FIGURE 12-45. Lift the transverse colon to see the transverse mesocolon.

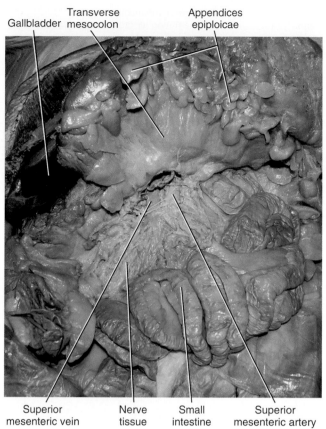

Gallbladder   Transverse mesocolon   Appendices epiploicae

Superior mesenteric vein   Nerve tissue   Small intestine   Superior mesenteric artery

FIGURE 12-46. With your fingertips, penetrate the transverse mesocolon and expose the underlying superior mesenteric artery and vein.

Lift the transverse colon and observe the transverse *mesocolon* (Fig. 12-45). With your fingertips, penetrate the transverse mesocolon and expose the underlying superior mesenteric artery and vein (Fig. 12-46). Continue cleaning the branches of the superior mesenteric artery and the tributaries of the superior mesenteric vein from fat and nerve tissue (Fig. 12-47). Identify the ileocolic artery and trace it to the *ileocecal junction,* between the ileum and the cecum.

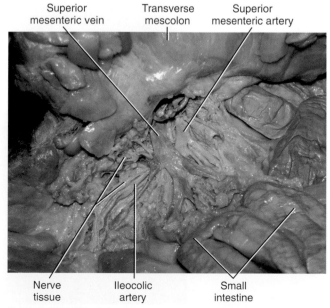

Superior mesenteric vein   Transverse mesocolon   Superior mesenteric artery

Nerve tissue   Ileocolic artery   Small intestine

FIGURE 12-47. Continue separating tributaries of the superior mesenteric vein and branches of the superior mesenteric artery from the fat and nerve tissue.

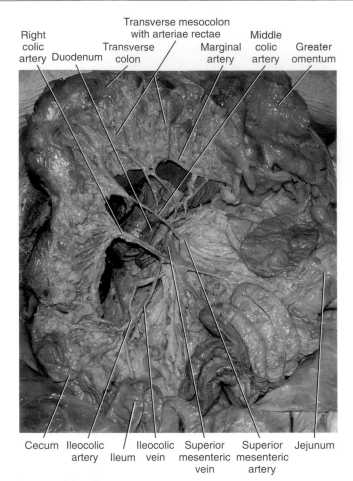

Right colic artery   Duodenum   Transverse mesocolon with arteriae rectae   Transverse colon   Marginal artery   Middle colic artery   Greater omentum

Cecum   Ileocolic artery   Ileum   Ileocolic vein   Superior mesenteric vein   Superior mesenteric artery   Jejunum

FIGURE 12-48. Identify the ileocolic artery and trace it to the ileocecal junction.

The ileocolic artery is fairly constant and provides a good landmark for this dissection (Fig. 12-48). The ileocolic artery gives rise to the appendicular artery supplying the appendix in its own mesentery, the *mesoappendix*. Identify the middle and right colic arteries that supply the transverse and the ascending colon, respectively (Fig. 12-48). Look for a branch of the middle colic artery, the marginal artery (of Drummond), that supplies the ascending, transverse, and descending colon, and anastomose with the left colic artery, a branch of the inferior mesenteric artery (see Fig. 12-52).

Once the main three arterial branches of the *superior mesenteric artery* (middle colic, right colic and ileocolic) are identified, expose the ileal and jejunal arteries from their origin from the superior mesenteric artery to the margin of the ileum and jejunum. Realize that the mesenteric fat is much more abundant in the ileal mesentery than in the jejunal mesentery. Dissect out the vascular arcades, appreciating their greater number in the ileum than in the jejunum (Fig. 12-49). Similarly, the vasa recti are shorter and more numerous in the ileum (Figs. 12-50 and 12-51).

Once the dissection of the superior mesenteric vessels is concluded, lift the transverse colon and review all dissected structures dissected out (Figs. 12-52 and 12-53).

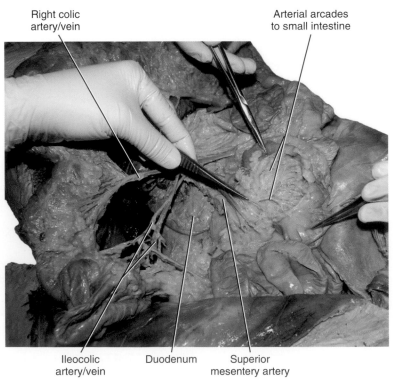

Right colic artery/vein   Arterial arcades to small intestine

Ileocolic artery/vein   Duodenum   Superior mesentery artery

FIGURE 12-49. Dissect out the vascular arcades.

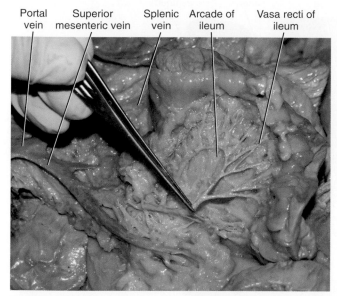

Portal vein | Superior mesenteric vein | Splenic vein | Arcade of ileum | Vasa recti of ileum

FIGURE 12-50. Notice that vasa recti are shorter and more numerous in the ileum than in the jejunum.

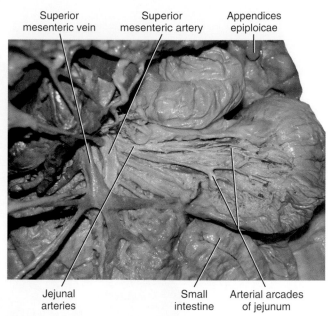

Superior mesenteric vein | Superior mesenteric artery | Appendices epiploicae

Jejunal arteries | Small intestine | Arterial arcades of jejunum

FIGURE 12-51. Note the increased number of arcades in ileum compared with jejunum.

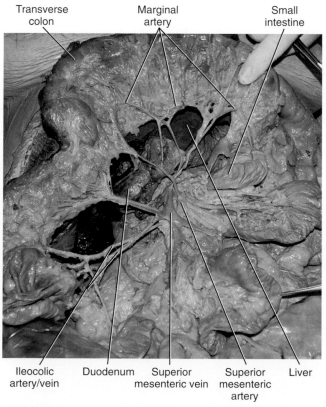

Transverse colon | Marginal artery | Small intestine

Ileocolic artery/vein | Duodenum | Superior mesenteric vein | Superior mesenteric artery | Liver

FIGURE 12-52. Conclude the dissection of the superior mesenteric vessels.

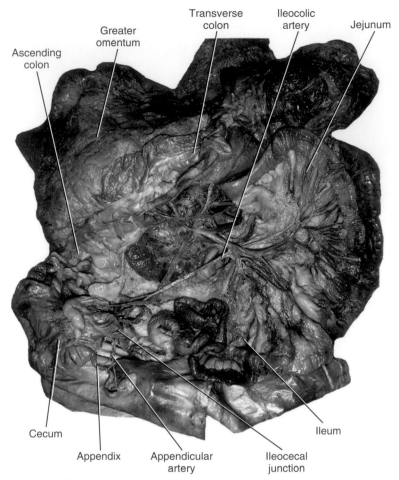

FIGURE 12-53. Lift the transverse colon and review all structures dissected out.

Retract the small intestine to the right and expose the transverse, descending, and sigmoid colon (Fig. 12-54). With scissors, continue the exposure of the inferior mesenteric vein (Fig. 12-55) toward the margins of the colon. To the right or medial to the inferior mesenteric vein, identify the *inferior mesenteric artery*. Both the inferior mesenteric artery and the inferior mesenteric vein will require additional effort to expose because of the dense nerve plexuses covering them.

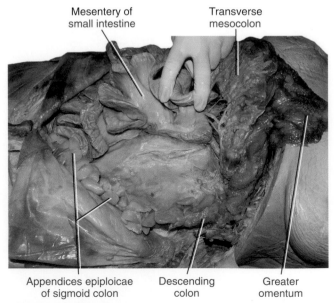

FIGURE 12-54. Retract the small intestine to the right and expose the transverse, descending, and sigmoid colon.

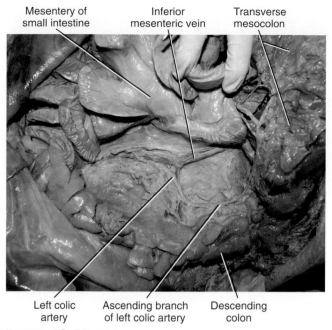

Mesentery of small intestine   Inferior mesenteric vein   Transverse mesocolon

Left colic artery   Ascending branch of left colic artery   Descending colon

FIGURE 12-55. With scissors, continue the exposure of the inferior mesenteric vein.

Mesentery of small intestine   Gallbladder   Transverse mesocolon

Sigmoid colon   Left colic artery   Marginal artery   Spleen

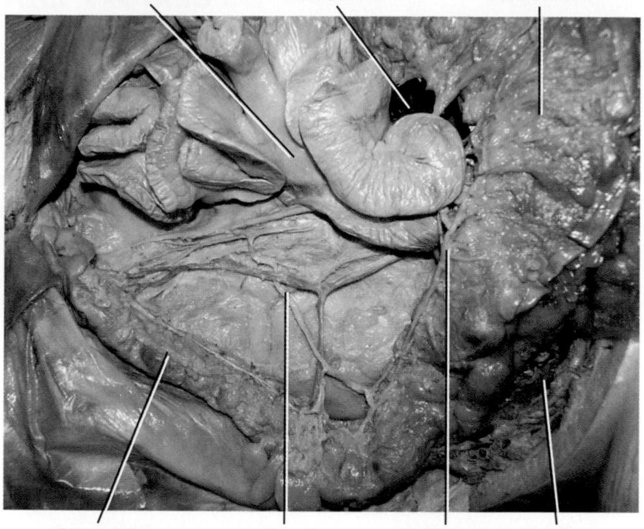

FIGURE 12-56. Identify and fully expose the branches of inferior mesenteric artery, left colic artery, and sigmoid arteries.

👆 *DISSECTION TIP:* To facilitate the dissection of the branches of the inferior mesenteric artery, make a shallow incision between the lateral wall of the descending colon and the body at the white line of Toldt (left paracolic gutter), and release the descending colon from the peritoneum. In addition, do *not* remove the nerve plexus when you expose the inferior mesenteric vessels. This nerve tissue will be examined in a later dissection of the posterior abdominal wall.

Identify the branches of the inferior mesenteric artery, the left colic artery and the sigmoid arteries and fully expose them (Fig. 12-56).

If Time Permits

Tie two strings close together around the proximal segment of the jejunum, and cut between the tied strings. Perform the same technique at a distal portion of the ileum. Clean the two segments and observe their internal morphology. Note the increased number of plicae circulares and villi, as well as increased wall thickness in the jejunum compared to the ileum.

Similarly, place a ligature at the ileocecal junction and another ligature at the midportion of the ascending colon. Remove this segment and examine its internal morphology. Identify the ileocecal valve and the plicae semilunares coli.

LABORATORY IDENTIFICATION CHECKLIST

Arteries
- ❏ Abdominal aorta
- ❏ Celiac trunk
  - ❏ Common hepatic
    - ❏ Proper hepatic
    - ❏ Gastroduodenal
      - ❏ Right gastroepiploic
    - ❏ Right gastric
  - ❏ Splenic
    - ❏ Short gastrics
  - ❏ Left gastric
    - ❏ Left gastroepiploic
- ❏ Superior mesenteric artery
  - ❏ Ileocolic
    - ❏ Appendicular
  - ❏ Right colic
  - ❏ Middle colic
- ❏ Inferior mesenteric
  - ❏ Left colic
  - ❏ Sigmoid
  - ❏ Inferior rectal
- ❏ Marginal (formed between ileocolic [right, middle] and left colic arteries)
- ❏ Jejunal and ileal arteries (arcades) and recti branches

Veins
- ❏ Inferior vena cava
  - ❏ Hepatic
- ❏ Portal
  - ❏ Superior mesenteric
  - ❏ Splenic
    - ❏ Inferior mesenteric

Lymph Nodes
- ❏ Greater omentum

Muscles
- ❏ External oblique
- ❏ Internal oblique
  - ❏ Cremaster
- ❏ Transversus abdominis
- ❏ Rectus abdominis
- ❏ Pyramidalis
- ❏ Crus (right and left) of diaphragm
- ❏ Psoas major
- ❏ Quadratus lumborum

Connective Tissue
- ❏ External oblique aponeurosis
- ❏ Greater omentum
- ❏ Lesser omentum
- ❏ Transverse mesocolon
- ❏ Sigmoid mesentery
- ❏ Appendicular mesentery
- ❏ Dorsal root mesentery
- ❏ *Liver*
  - ❏ Falciform ligament
  - ❏ Ligamentum teres

Viscera/Organs
- ❏ *Esophagus*
  - ❏ Distal esophagus
- ❏ *Stomach*
  - ❏ Fundus
  - ❏ Body
  - ❏ Cardia
  - ❏ Pylorus
  - ❏ Greater curvature
  - ❏ Lesser curvature

Viscera/Organs—cont'd
- ❏ *Small intestine*
  - ❏ Duodenum
  - ❏ Duodenal cap
  - ❏ Jejunum
  - ❏ Ileum
- ❏ *Large intestine*
  - ❏ Cecum
  - ❏ Appendix
  - ❏ Ascending colon
  - ❏ Transverse colon
  - ❏ Descending colon
  - ❏ Sigmoid colon
  - ❏ Appendices epiploicae
  - ❏ Teniae coli
- ❏ *Liver*
  - ❏ Left lobe
  - ❏ Right lobe
  - ❏ Caudate
  - ❏ Quadrate
- ❏ *Gallbladder*
  - ❏ Fundus
  - ❏ Body
  - ❏ Neck
- ❏ *Pancreas*
  - ❏ Head
  - ❏ Neck
  - ❏ Body
  - ❏ Tail
  - ❏ Uncinate process
- ❏ *Spleen*
  - ❏ Splenic notch
  - ❏ Hilum

CHAPTER 13

POSTERIOR ABDOMINAL WALL

Netter: 288, 291, 297–302, 308–322, 484–487

McMinn: 240, 242–243, 254–263

Gray's Atlas: 172–190

Cut the white lines of Toldt (paracolic gutters) along the edges of the ascending and the descending colon, and reflect the large and small intestines to the left of the abdominal cavity (Fig. 13-1). With your fingers, retract the duodenum and pancreas to the left, without disrupting their vascular supply (Fig. 13-2).

Palpate the abdominal aorta on the left and the *inferior vena cava* (IVC) on the right. With scissors, cut the peritoneum of the posterior abdominal wall and expose the IVC (Fig. 13-3). To the right of the IVC, dissect out the perirenal (renal) fascia (of Gerota), which is predominantly filled with abundant perirenal fat (Figs. 13-4 and 13-5). Trace the right ureter; expose its course from the kidney to the pelvic brim and as it cross over the iliac arteries. Remove the fat posterior to the kidney, known as *pararenal* fat (Fig. 13-6). Remove enough fascia and adipose tissue to

clearly expose the kidneys and suprarenal glands. Free up the margins of the suprarenal glands, taking care to preserve their blood vessels, especially along their medial borders.

> **✋ DISSECTION TIP:** For the removal of the perirenal and pararenal fat, use scissors or a probe and scrape it from the kidney capsule. Scrape all the fat from the posterior part of the kidney capsule. At this point, you will reflect the liver medially and expose the entire posterior abdominal wall.

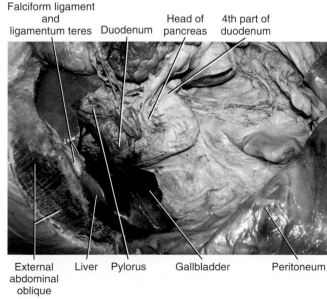

FIGURE 13-1. Lines of Toldt cut along edges of ascending and descending colon with large and small intestines reflected to left of abdominal cavity.

Labels: Falciform ligament and ligamentum teres; Duodenum; Head of pancreas; 4th part of duodenum; External abdominal oblique; Liver; Pylorus; Gallbladder; Peritoneum

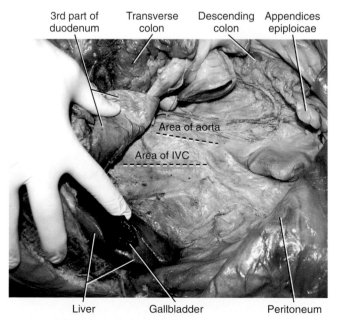

FIGURE 13-2. Left duodenum and pancreas retracted; *IVC*, inferior vena cava.

Labels: 3rd part of duodenum; Transverse colon; Descending colon; Appendices epiploicae; Area of aorta; Area of IVC; Liver; Gallbladder; Peritoneum

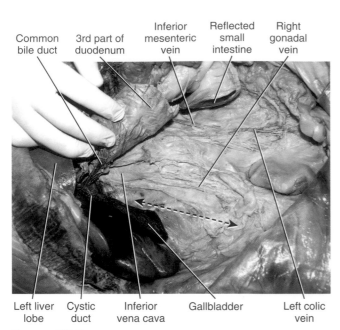

Common bile duct · 3rd part of duodenum · Inferior mesenteric vein · Reflected small intestine · Right gonadal vein

Left liver lobe · Cystic duct · Inferior vena cava · Gallbladder · Left colic vein

FIGURE 13-3. Peritoneum of posterior abdominal wall incised to expose the inferior vena cava (IVC).

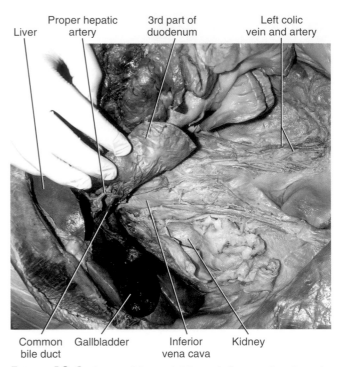

Liver · Proper hepatic artery · 3rd part of duodenum · Left colic vein and artery

Common bile duct · Gallbladder · Inferior vena cava · Kidney

FIGURE 13-4. Perirenal fascia (of Gerota) dissected to the right of the IVC.

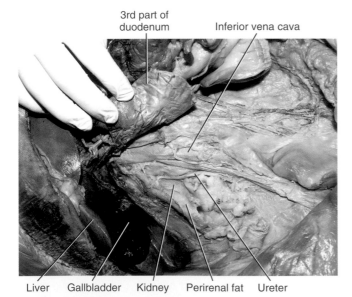

3rd part of duodenum · Inferior vena cava

Liver · Gallbladder · Kidney · Perirenal fat · Ureter

FIGURE 13-5. Appreciate the abundant perirenal fat.

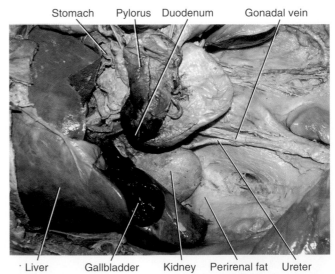

Stomach · Pylorus · Duodenum · Gonadal vein

Liver · Gallbladder · Kidney · Perirenal fat · Ureter

FIGURE 13-6. Right ureter exposed as it leaves the right kidney, toward the pelvic brim and over the iliac arteries. Pararenal fat has been removed posterior to the kidney.

Cut the falciform, left triangular, and coronary ligaments. Place your fingertips underneath the lateral side of the liver, lift it up slightly, and cut the right triangular ligament (Fig. 13-7). Pull the liver inferiorly, and in the space between the diaphragm and the

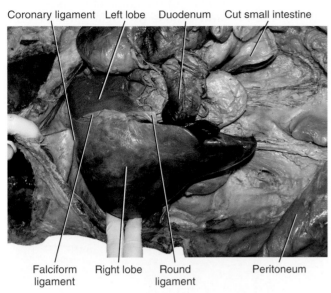

Coronary ligament   Left lobe   Duodenum   Cut small intestine

Falciform ligament   Right lobe   Round ligament   Peritoneum

FIGURE 13-7. Falciform, left triangular, and coronary ligaments cut and right triangular ligament incised on lifting liver.

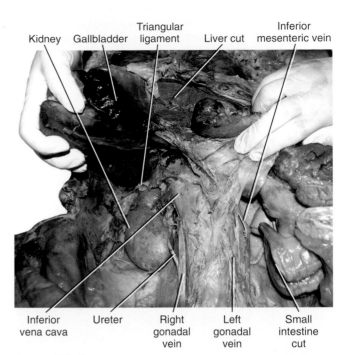

Kidney   Gallbladder   Triangular ligament   Liver cut   Inferior mesenteric vein

Inferior vena cava   Ureter   Right gonadal vein   Left gonadal vein   Small intestine cut

FIGURE 13-9. Liver lifted upward and to the left exposing infrahepatic portion of IVC.

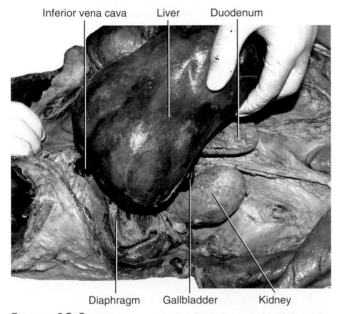

Inferior vena cava   Liver   Duodenum

Diaphragm   Gallbladder   Kidney

FIGURE 13-8. With liver pulled inferiorly, cut the IVC in the space between superior aspect of the liver and the undersurface of the diaphragm.

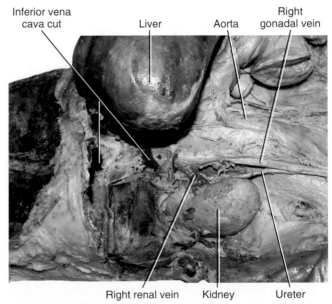

Inferior vena cava cut   Liver   Aorta   Right gonadal vein

Right renal vein   Kidney   Ureter

FIGURE 13-10. Incision through IVC superior to level of renal veins, with liver reflected.

liver, cut the IVC (Fig. 13-8). Lift the liver upward and to the left; expose the infrahepatic portion of IVC away from the body wall (Fig. 13-9). Gently pull the liver to the left; otherwise, you will damage the right adrenal vein as it enters the IVC. With a scalpel, make

an incision through the IVC superior to the level of the renal veins and reflect the liver to the left (Fig. 13-10). The liver is attached to the abdominal cavity only by the portal vein, hepatic artery, and common bile duct.

On the reflected liver, identify the right and left lobes (divided by the falciform ligament), as well as the quadrate and caudate lobes of the right lobe. Identify the fissure for the ligamentum venosum and the ligamentum teres (round ligament). Identify the round ligament, ligamentum venosum, right and left triangular ligaments, and coronary ligament (Fig. 13-11). To identify the ligamentum venosum, reflect the caudate lobe and clean the fissure for the ligament (Fig. 13-12).

Reflect the inferior vena cava slightly inferiorly and expose the suprarenal gland and the bare area of the liver (Fig. 13-13). Clean out the connective tissue and fat over the IVC and expose the right gonadal vein and right renal vein (Figs. 13-14 and 13-15). Continue the exposure of the left renal vein to the left and

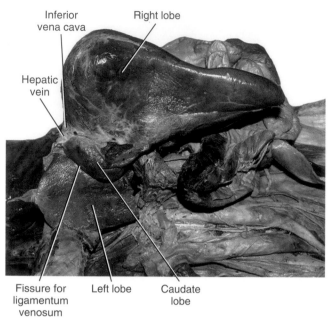

FIGURE 13-11. Identify the right and left lobes of the liver. Trace the inferior vena cava and the haptic vein. Identify the fissure for the ligamentum venosum between the left lobe of the liver and the caudate lobe.

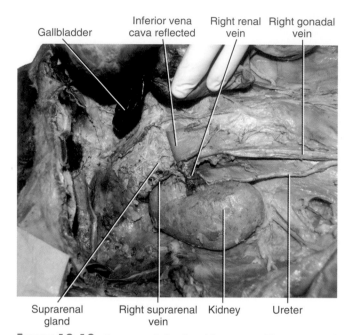

FIGURE 13-13. Suprarenal gland and bare area of liver exposed by reflecting the IVC slightly inferiorly.

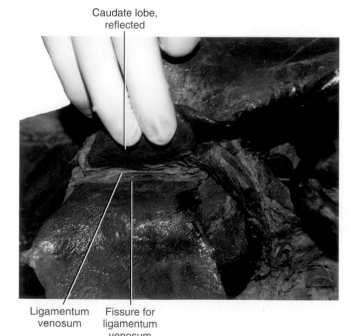

FIGURE 13-12. Caudate lobe reflected and fissure cleaned to locate the ligamentum venosum.

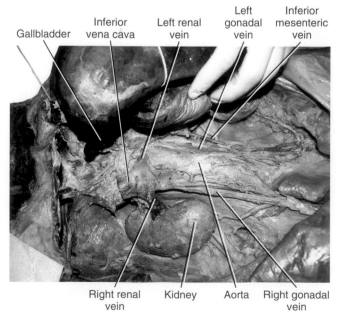

FIGURE 13-14. Fat and connective tissue cleaned over IVC, exposing right gonadal vein and right renal vein.

clean the fat and connective tissue over the abdominal aorta (Fig. 13-16). Pay special attention identifying the gonadal artery arising from the aorta just inferior to the level of the right renal vein. In the space between the IVC and aorta, identify the right lymphatic trunk and the sympathetic fibers ascending from the superior hypogastric plexus. This plexus is located just anterior to the promontory of the

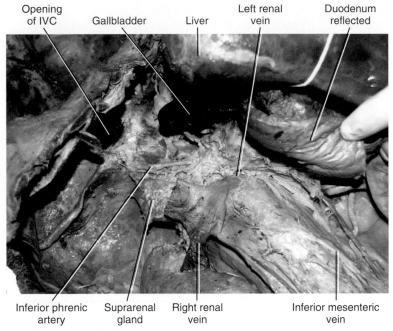

FIGURE 13-15. Left renal vein exposed; *IVC*, inferior vena cava.

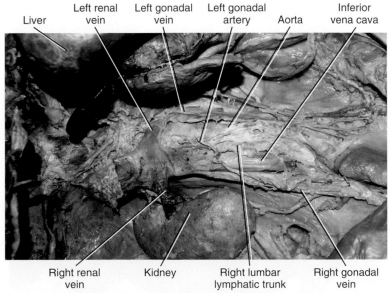

FIGURE 13-16. Left renal vein exposed, showing left gonadal vein, with gonadal artery from aorta just inferior to right renal vein.

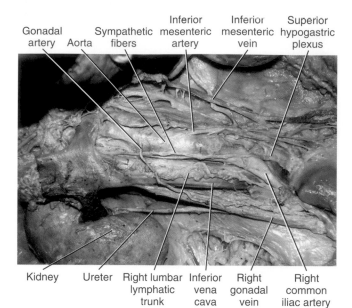

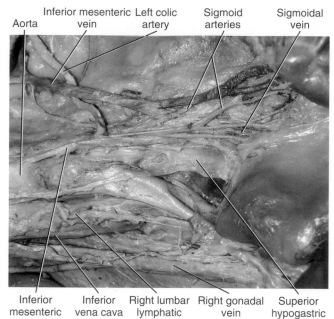

FIGURE 13-17. Right lymphatic trunk and sympathetic fibers ascending from superior hypogastric plexus.

FIGURE 13-18. Dissection completed by exposing inferior mesenteric artery.

sacrum (Fig. 13-17). Complete the dissection by exposing the branches of the *inferior mesenteric artery* (Figs. 13-18 and 13-19).

Identify and expose the renal arteries and veins. The left renal vein crosses over the aorta, inferior to

☝ *DISSECTION TIP:* Additional renal arteries are often seen arising from the aorta; these are normal variations.

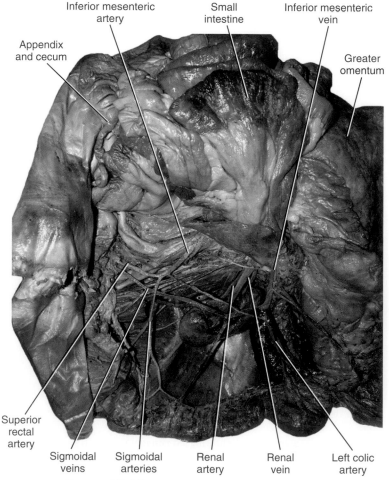

FIGURE 13-19. Structures of the abdominal wall.

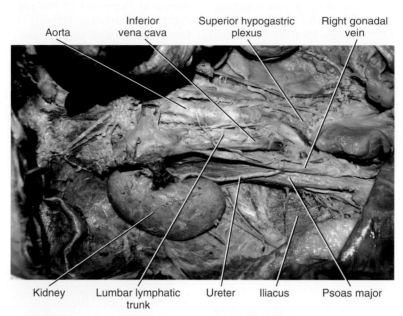

Aorta   Inferior vena cava   Superior hypogastric plexus   Right gonadal vein

Kidney   Lumbar lymphatic trunk   Ureter   Iliacus   Psoas major

FIGURE 13-20. Locate and expose the renal arteries and veins.

the origin of the superior mesenteric artery, to reach the IVC. In contrast, the right renal artery passes posterior to the IVC (Fig. 13-20).

Identify the right suprarenal gland with its connection between the right suprarenal vein and the IVC (see Fig. 13-13). This vein is very short. Dissect out the right superior, middle, and inferior suprarenal arteries, typically arising from the inferior

phrenic artery, aorta, and renal artery, respectively (Fig. 13-21). Notice the drainage of the right gonadal vein directly into the IVC. Identify the left suprarenal gland, and expose the left suprarenal vein and left gonadal vein draining into the left renal vein. With a scalpel, make a coronal incision and expose the outer cortex, as well as the inner medulla, of the adrenal gland.

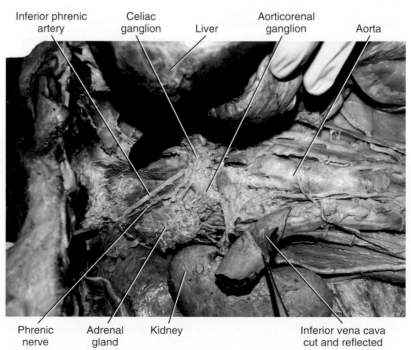

Inferior phrenic artery   Celiac ganglion   Liver   Aorticorenal ganglion   Aorta

Phrenic nerve   Adrenal gland   Kidney   Inferior vena cava cut and reflected

FIGURE 13-21. Dissect the right superior, middle, and inferior suprarenal arteries typically arising from the inferior phrenic artery, aorta, and renal artery, respectively.

Hold one of the two kidneys in your hand. Make a vertical incision along its lateral border, and transect the kidney into two parts (Fig. 13-22). Open and inspect the inner part of the kidney. Identify the outer layer, the renal cortex, and the inner layer, the *renal medulla.* Realize that the cortex sends extensions into the medulla, the *renal columns.* The renal medulla is composed of *pyramids,* projections of the renal *papillae,* which contain collecting ducts that drain urine into the minor *calyces.* About 10 minor calyces combine to form three major calyces; all major calyces combine to form the *renal pelvis,* located at the hilum of the kidney (Fig. 13-23).

Between the inferior vena cava and the abdominal aorta, at the level of the right renal vein, locate the right sympathetic trunk (Fig. 13-24). You can also trace the sympathetic chain just underneath the IVC, between the psoas major muscle and the vertebral column (Figs. 13-25 and 13-26). The sympathetic chain will contribute lumbar splanchnic nerves to the superior hypogastric plexus (Fig. 13-25).

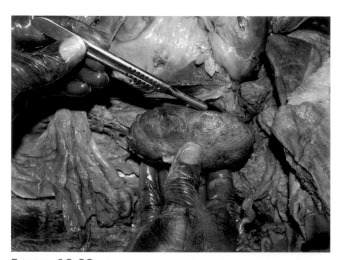

FIGURE 13-22. An incision into the kidney along its border allows access to its internal structures.

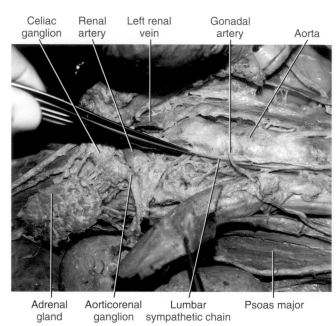

FIGURE 13-24. Right sympathetic chain between the IVC and abdominal aorta.

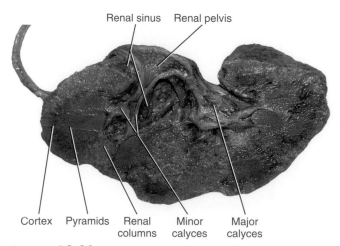

FIGURE 13-23. Inside the kidney, note the cortex, medulla, calyces, pyramids, and columns.

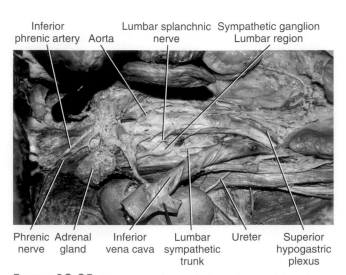

FIGURE 13-25. The sympathetic chain is shown giving rise to lumbar splanchnic nerves that contribute to the pancreatic and superior hypogastric plexuses.

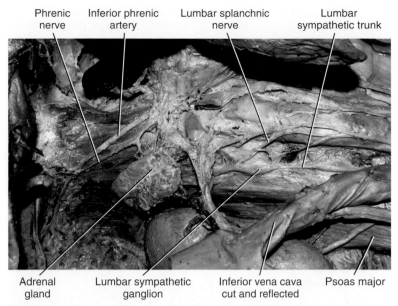

Phrenic nerve   Inferior phrenic artery   Lumbar splanchnic nerve   Lumbar sympathetic trunk

Adrenal gland   Lumbar sympathetic ganglion   Inferior vena cava cut and reflected   Psoas major

FIGURE 13-26. Sympathetic chain courses underneath the IVC between psoas major muscle and vertebral column.

The right and left renal arteries are surrounded by a dense network of neural fibers (Fig. 13-24). Identify the *aorticorenal ganglion*. This ganglion further connects with the celiac ganglion, occupying the area over the celiac trunk (Fig. 13-24). Preganglionic sympathetic fibers reach the celiac, aorticorenal, and superior mesenteric ganglia by way of the greater, lesser, and least splanchnic nerves, respectively. These fibers synapse in the ganglia, and postganglionic fibers travel along the arteries of the abdomen.

Lift the kidney upward, and clean out the posterior surface of the renal hilum (Fig 13-27). Identify the

psoas major muscle, and remove the fascia over the right crus of the diaphragm and psoas major muscle (Fig. 13-28). At the opening of the IVC, look for the inferior phrenic artery, and trace it to its origin from the aorta.

☞ *DISSECTION TIP:* In some cases, the inferior phrenic artery originates from the celiac trunk.

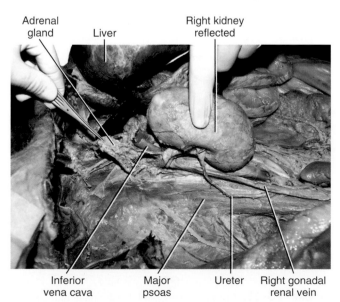

Adrenal gland   Liver   Right kidney reflected

Inferior vena cava   Major psoas   Ureter   Right gonadal renal vein

FIGURE 13-27. Right kidney lifted upward in order to clean out posterior surface of renal hilum.

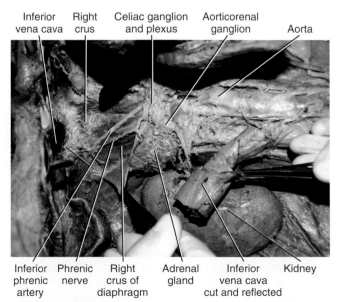

Inferior vena cava   Right crus   Celiac ganglion and plexus   Aorticorenal ganglion   Aorta

Inferior phrenic artery   Phrenic nerve   Right crus of diaphragm   Adrenal gland   Inferior vena cava cut and reflected   Kidney

FIGURE 13-28. Fascia removed over right crus of diaphragm and psoas major muscle.

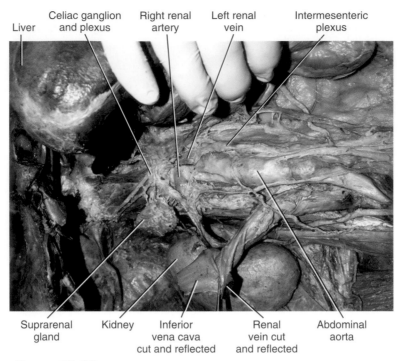

Liver   Celiac ganglion   Right renal   Left renal   Intermesenteric
        and plexus   artery   vein   plexus

Suprarenal   Kidney   Inferior   Renal   Abdominal
gland   vena cava   vein cut   aorta
                      cut and reflected   and reflected

FIGURE 13-29. Continuation of splanchnic nerves into abdominal cavity.

Next to the inferior phrenic artery, dissect out the continuation of the phrenic nerve into the abdominal cavity (Fig. 13-29). The phrenic nerve accompanies the inferior phrenic artery and is related to the phrenic ganglion.

Lift the kidney upward, and look between the superomedial border of the psoas major and the right crus of the diaphragm for the greater, lesser, and least splanchnic nerves (Figs. 13-30 and 13-31). You may also pull the celiac ganglion upward and look for the greater splanchnic nerve underneath. Trace these nerves to their terminations at the celiac ganglion (for the greater), aorticorenal ganglion (for the lesser), and superior mesenteric ganglion (for the least).

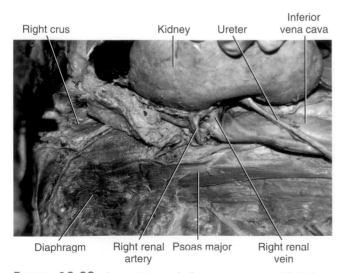

Right crus   Kidney   Ureter   Inferior
                                    vena cava

Diaphragm   Right renal   Psoas major   Right renal
            artery   vein

FIGURE 13-30. Appreciate underlying structures with kidney lifted.

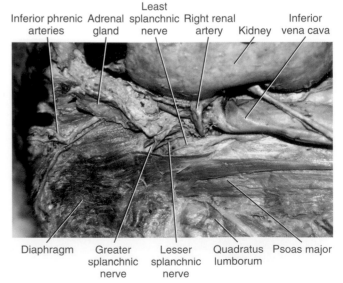

                        Least
Inferior phrenic Adrenal splanchnic Right renal   Inferior
arteries   gland   nerve   artery   Kidney   vena cava

Diaphragm   Greater   Lesser   Quadratus   Psoas major
            splanchnic   splanchnic lumborum
            nerve   nerve

FIGURE 13-31. Greater, lesser, and least splanchnic nerves coursing between the superomedial border of the psoas major muscle and the right crus of diaphragm.

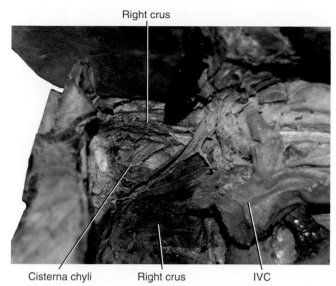

FIGURE 13-32. Vertical incision at right crus of diaphragm exposes cisterna chyli; *IVC,* inferior vena cava.

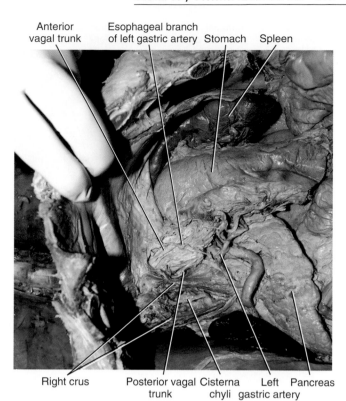

FIGURE 13-33. Thoracic cavity opened and anterior and posterior vagal trunks around lower esophagus used to locate anterior and posterior trunks in the abdominal cavity.

Between the abdominal aorta and the IVC and at the left side of the aorta, identify the right and left lumbar lymph trunks, respectively. These lymph trunks will eventually join the intestinal lymph trunk and form the *cisterna chyli.* Make a vertical incision at the right crus of the diaphragm, and expose the cisterna chyli (Fig. 13-32).

Open up the thoracic cavity and identify the anterior and posterior vagal trunks around the lower part of the esophagus. Place slight traction on the anterior vagal trunk, which primarily originates from the left vagus nerve, and look anterior to the cardio-esophageal junction for a mobile structure. Locate the anterior vagal trunk and expose its branches. Similarly, place slight traction on the posterior vagal trunk in the thorax (primarily right vagus nerve) and find the medial side of the *esophageal hiatus,* or the right side of the esophagus, for identification of the posterior vagal trunk (Fig. 13-33).

Inspection of Posterior Abdominal Structures

Observe the thoracic and abdominal surfaces of the diaphragm. Note the central tendinous portion of the diaphragm, the *central tendon.* Lateral to the esophagus, identify the *right and left crura,* the two muscular extensions of the diaphragm arising from the central tendon to insert onto the 2nd or 3rd lumbar (L2 or L3) vertebra. Fibers from the right and left crura intermix to encircle the esophagus as it passes through the diaphragm. Just superior to the celiac trunk, the right and left crura are united by a midline tendon, the *median arcuate ligament.*

Laterally, the diaphragm attaches to the ribs and inferolaterally it attaches to the psoas major forming a thickened connective tissue band, the *medial arcuate ligament.* More laterally, the diaphragm arches over the quadratus lumborum to attach to the 12th rib, forming another thickened connective tissue band over the quadratus lumborum, the *lateral arcuate ligament* (see Fig. 13-31).

Remove any remaining fat inferior to the right and left kidneys to expose the lumbar plexus and the underlying muscles (Fig. 13-34). Identify the psoas major muscle and, lateral to it, the quadratus lumborum muscle. Inferior to the quadratus lumborum, identify the iliacus muscle, which lies in the iliac fossa. Palpate the 12th rib and at its inferior border, expose the *subcostal nerve.*

On the lateral side of the psoas major muscle, identify the *genitofemoral nerve* as it travels on its anterior surface. A few centimeters below the origin of the *iliohypogastric nerve,* identify the *ilioinguinal nerve,* which travels from the lateral side of the psoas major muscle toward the anterior superior iliac spine. At the lateral side of the distal end of the psoas major muscle in the abdominal cavity, identify the *femoral nerve* and, lateral to it, the much smaller, *lateral femoral cutaneous nerve.*

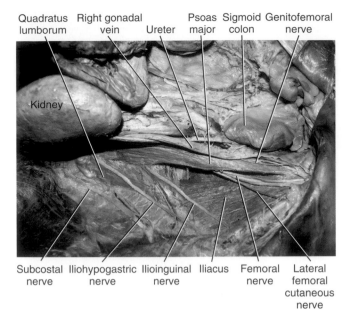

Quadratus lumborum · Right gonadal vein · Ureter · Psoas major · Sigmoid colon · Genitofemoral nerve

Kidney

Subcostal nerve · Iliohypogastric nerve · Ilioinguinal nerve · Iliacus · Femoral nerve · Lateral femoral cutaneous nerve

FIGURE 13-34. Removal of fat inferior to right and left kidneys exposes branches of the lumbar plexus and underlying muscles.

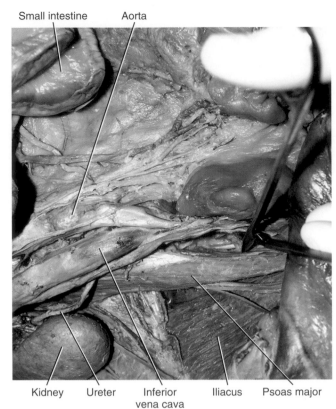

Small intestine · Aorta

Kidney · Ureter · Inferior vena cava · Iliacus · Psoas major

FIGURE 13-35. Psoas major muscle separated from adjacent external iliac artery and vein.

Medial to the psoas major muscle, place a probe or a pair of scissors and separate the psoas major from the adjacent external iliac artery and vein (Fig. 13-35). Deep and medial to the psoas major muscle, identify the *obturator nerve* (Fig. 13-36).

Once all branches of the lumbar plexus are identified, on one side of the cadaver, carefully remove the psoas major muscle in a piecemeal fashion, and expose the origin of the nerves of the lumbar plexus (Fig. 13-37).

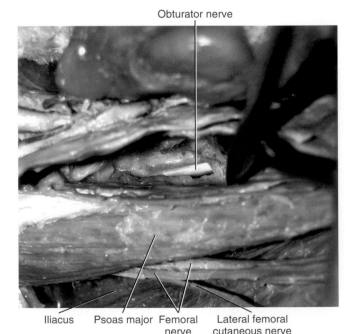

Obturator nerve

Iliacus · Psoas major · Femoral nerve · Lateral femoral cutaneous nerve

FIGURE 13-36. Obturator nerve lies deep and medial to the psoas major muscle.

> ☞ *DISSECTION TIPS*
> - In about 50% of cadaveric donors, the psoas minor muscle will be evident on the anterior surface of the psoas major.
> - In most cadavers, the lumbar plexus will exhibit great variation.
>   1. The most common variation is that the ilioinguinal and iliohypogastric nerves fuse and split into their terminal branches just proximal to the *anterior superior iliac spine*.
>   2. Similarly, the subcostal and iliohypogastric nerves can be fused and split more distally.

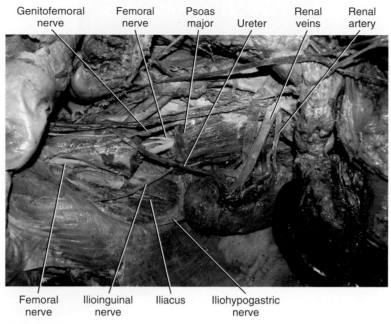

FIGURE 13-37. Psoas major muscle removed exposing origin of lumbar plexus nerves.

LABORATORY IDENTIFICATION CHECKLIST

Nerves/Connective Tissue
❒ Iliohypogastric
❒ Ilioinguinal
❒ Genitofemoral
❒ Lateral femoral cutaneous
❒ Femoral
❒ Obturator
❒ Accessory obturator
   (variation)
❒ Lumbosacral trunk
❒ Sympathetic trunk
   ❒ Gray/white rami
      communicantes
   ❒ Sympathetic ganglion
   ❒ Lumbar splanchnic
❒ Celiac ganglia
❒ Celiac plexus
❒ Suprarenal plexus
❒ Aorticorenal ganglion
❒ Superior mesenteric plexus
❒ Intermesenteric (aortic)
   plexus

Arteries
❒ Right and left inferior phrenic
❒ Superior suprarenal
❒ Middle suprarenal
❒ Inferior suprarenal
❒ Renal
❒ Gonadal
❒ Lumbar 1-4
❒ Subcostal
❒ Iliolumbar

Veins
❒ Inferior vena cava (IVC)
❒ Inferior phrenic
❒ Suprarenal
❒ Renal
❒ Gonadal
❒ Lumbar 1-4
❒ Iliolumbar

Lymph
❒ Cisterna chyli

Muscles/Connective Tissue
❒ Right crus
   ❒ Ligament of Treitz
❒ Left crus
❒ Psoas major
❒ Psoas minor
❒ Quadratus lumborum
❒ Transversus abdominis
❒ Median arcuate ligament
❒ Medial arcuate ligament
❒ Lateral arcuate ligament

Organs
❒ Kidney
❒ Ureter
❒ Adrenal or suprarenal gland

Bones
❒ Coxal, right and left
❒ Sacrum
❒ Vertebrae
   ❒ 12th thoracic (T12)
   ❒ 1st to 5th lumbar: (L1-L5)

PERITONEAL ASPIRATION/LAVAGE

Gray's Anatomy for Students: 279

Netter: 247, 255

Clinical Application

Procedure introducing a trocar to withdraw fluid or to introduce saline into the peritoneal cavity for irrigation.

Anatomic Landmarks (Figs V-1 and V-2)

- Infraumbilical region
- Skin
- Subcutaneous tissue
- Linea alba/rectus abdominis muscle
- Transversalis fascia
- Extraperitoneal fat
- Parietal peritoneum
- Umbilicus
- Anterior superior iliac spine (ASIS)

PARACENTESIS

Gray's Anatomy for Students: 279

Netter: 247, 255

Clinical Application

Withdraw fluid (e.g., ascites) from the peritoneal cavity.

Anatomic Landmarks

Infraumbilical Region

- Skin
- Subcutaneous tissue
- Linea alba
- Median umbilical fold/ligament
- Medial umbilical fold/ligament
- Transversalis fascia
- Extraperitoneal fat/space
- Peritoneal sac

About 5 cm superior to ASIS

Layers traversed
- Skin (lateral to rectus)
- Subcutaneous tissue
- External oblique aponeurosis
- Internal oblique muscle

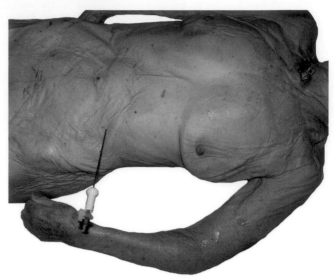

FIGURE V-1.

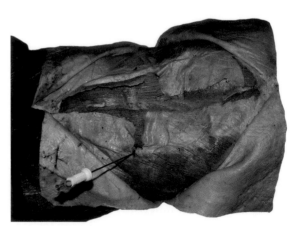

FIGURE V-2.

- Transversus abdominis muscle
- Transversalis fascia
- Extraperitoneal fat/space
- Peritoneum

PUDENDAL NERVE BLOCK

Gray's Anatomy for Students: 446

Netter: 385, 391, 393

Clinical Application

Procedure to place a bolus of local anesthetic into the pudendal canal, anesthetizing the pudendal nerve and its branches.

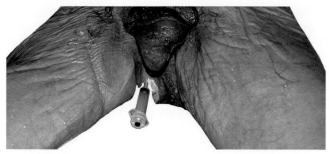

Figure V-3.

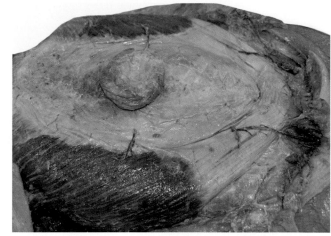

Figure V-5.

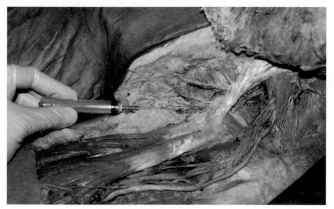

Figure V-4.

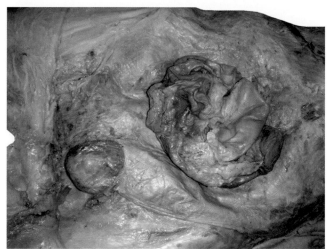

Figure V-6.

Anatomic Landmarks (Figs. V-3 and V-4)

- Vagina introitus
- Lateral vagina wall and mucosa
- Vaginal mucosa
- Ischial spine
- Coccygeus
- Sacrospinous ligament (resistance)
- Pudendal canal (Alcock's canal)
- Pudendal nerve
- Internal pudendal artery
- Internal pudendal vein

HERNIATIONS AND OTHER PATHOLOGIES

The following cadavers exhibited marked herniations and other examples of abdominal and vascular abnormalities, including life-threatening aortic aneurysm.
- Umbilical hernia (Fig. V-5)
- Umbilical hernia and an indirect inguinal hernia (Figs. V-6 and V-7)

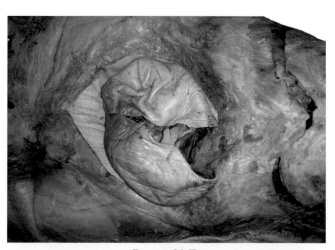

Figure V-7.

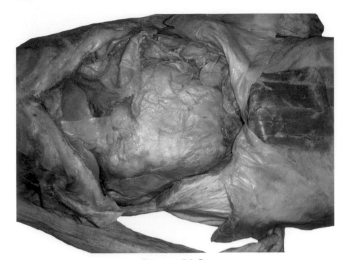

FIGURE V-8.

- Massive malignancies in the abdominal cavity and the liver (Fig V-8).
- Multiple malignant nodules in a sagittal section of the liver (Fig. V-9).
- Example of hepatomegaly (Fig. V-10).
- Dissected liver with evident hepatic arteries and veins (Fig. V-11).
- Example of splenomegaly (Fig. V-12).

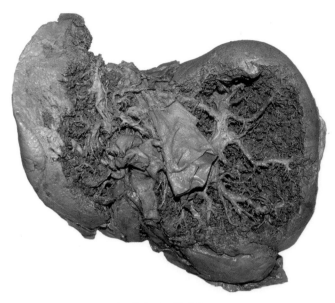

FIGURE V-11.

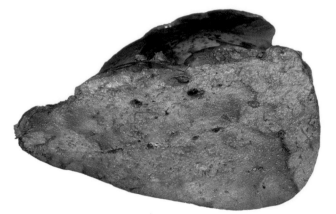

FIGURE V-9.

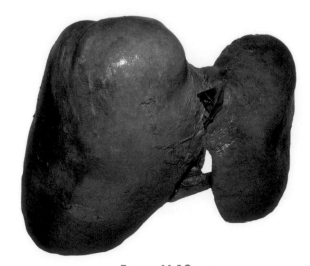

FIGURE V-10.

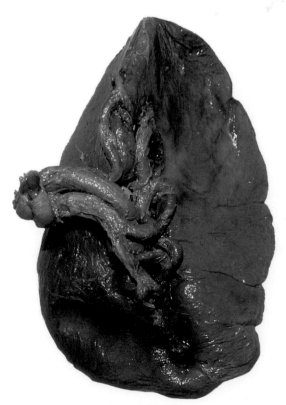

FIGURE V-12.

- Examples of kidneys with cysts (Figs. V-13, V-14, and V-15).
- Abdominal aortic aneurysm; large Gortex tube placed at site is visible (Fig. V-16).
- Large abdominal aortic aneurysm (Fig. V-17).

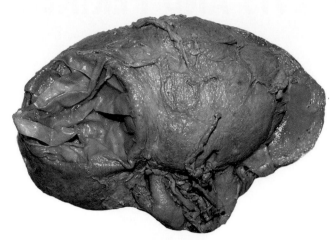

FIGURE V-13.

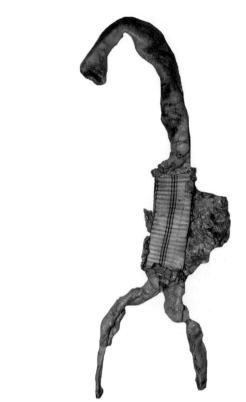

FIGURE V-16.

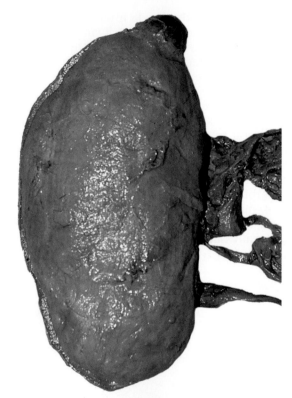

FIGURE V-14.

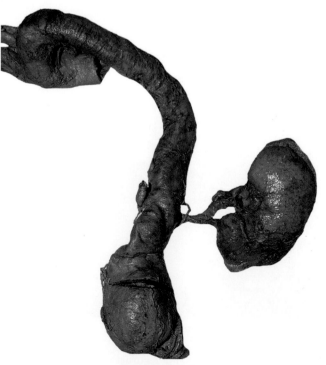

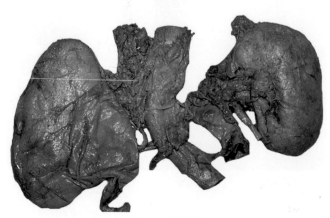

FIGURE V-15.

FIGURE V-17.

CHAPTER 14

PELVIS

Netter: 332–355, 371–374, 378–383, 388–390, 392, 394, 484–487

McMinn: 262–287

Gray's Atlas: 198–223, 227–240, 254–256

MIDLINE HEMIPELVECTOMY (MALE)

Several techniques are available for dissection of the pelvis. This chapter describes the traditional midline hemipelvectomy.

Identify the rectosigmoid junction and expose the rectum (Fig. 14-1). Posterior to the pubic symphysis, palpate the urinary bladder and note its peritoneal covering. With a probe or scissors, dissect out and reflect the peritoneum from the posterior surface of the urinary bladder (Figs. 14-2 and 14-3). Notice the median umbilical ligament connecting to the urinary bladder (urachus).

The adipose tissue between the posterior surface of the urinary bladder and the peritoneum is termed *preperitoneal fat.* Place your fingertips, using blunt dissection, between the urinary bladder and the pubic symphysis into the retropubic space of Retzius

(Fig. 14-4). Pull on the fascia attached to the lateral sides of the median umbilical ligament and at the superior part of the urinary bladder, the *vesicoumbilical fascia,* and reflect it posteriorly. With this maneuver, observe the expansion of the retropubic space of Retzius.

Mobilize the rectum and the bladder. With a saw, cut the pubic symphysis vertically 2 to 3 cm (~1 inch) lateral to the midline (Fig. 14-5). Mobilize the rectum laterally, and with a scalpel, extend the incision from the pubic symphysis backward toward the sacrum and pelvis (Fig. 14-6). Cut the peritoneum, urinary bladder, aorta, and all soft tissues. With a scalpel, make a second horizontal incision starting from the aorta, at the level of the kidneys, and extending laterally along the borders of the iliac crest (Fig. 14-7).

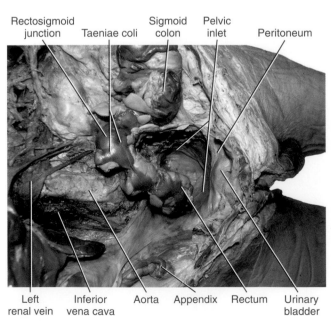

FIGURE 14-1. Identification of rectosigmoid junction and exposure of rectum.

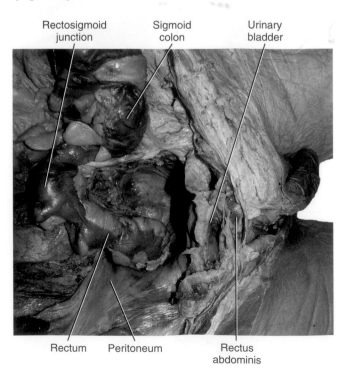

FIGURE 14-2. Urinary bladder posterior to pubic symphysis.

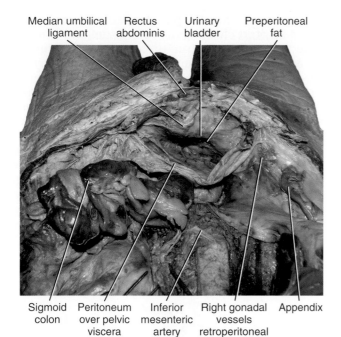

Median umbilical ligament | Rectus abdominis | Urinary bladder | Preperitoneal fat

Sigmoid colon | Peritoneum over pelvic viscera | Inferior mesenteric artery | Right gonadal vessels retroperitoneal | Appendix

FIGURE 14-3. Peritoneum reflected from posterior surface of urinary bladder.

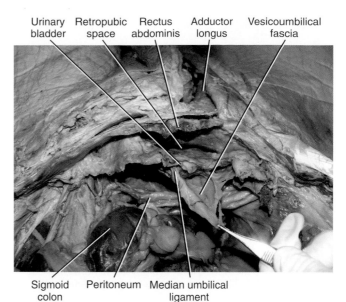

Urinary bladder | Retropubic space | Rectus abdominis | Adductor longus | Vesicoumbilical fascia

Sigmoid colon | Peritoneum | Median umbilical ligament

FIGURE 14-4. Blunt dissection between urinary bladder and pubic symphysis into retropubic space.

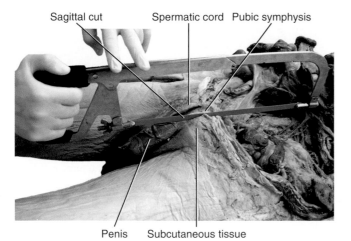

Sagittal cut | Spermatic cord | Pubic symphysis

Penis | Subcutaneous tissue

FIGURE 14-5. Pubic symphysis cut vertically about 1 inch lateral to midline.

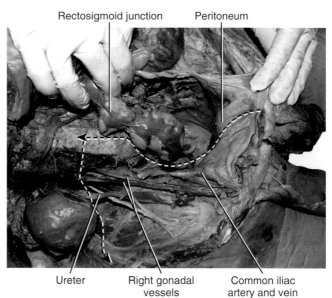

Rectosigmoid junction | Peritoneum

Ureter | Right gonadal vessels | Common iliac artery and vein

FIGURE 14-6. Incision extended from pubic symphysis back toward sacrum and pelvis *(dashed line with arrowheads).*

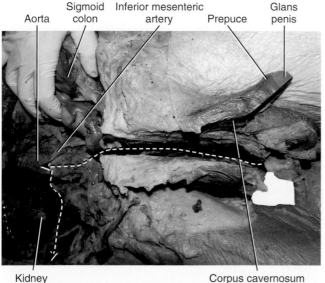

Aorta | Sigmoid colon | Inferior mesenteric artery | Prepuce | Glans penis

Kidney | Corpus cavernosum

FIGURE 14-7. Second horizontal incision from aorta extends laterally along iliac crest.

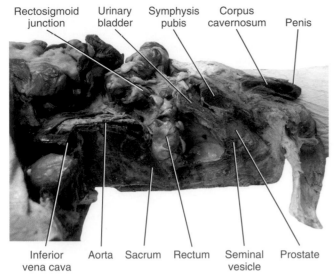

Rectosigmoid junction   Urinary bladder   Symphysis pubis   Corpus cavernosum   Penis

Inferior vena cava   Aorta   Sacrum   Rectum   Seminal vesicle   Prostate

FIGURE 14-8. After the cadaver is turned on its side, the saw is passed through the open pubic symphysis. A horizontal cut is made alongside the iliac crest and this portion is detached.

With the cadaver on its side, and using a saw, cut the sacrum through its promontory, up through the 4th lumbar vertebra. Saw through the pubic symphysis and make a horizontal incision alongside the iliac crest (as previously described) and detach this portion of the body (Fig. 14-8).

> ✋ *DISSECTION TIP:* For the hemipelvectomy, you will need the help of your colleagues to lift and turn the cadaver on its side.

With scissors, reflect the parietal peritoneum upward (Fig. 14-9). Start cleaning the soft tissues and adipose tissue around larger structures (Fig. 14-10). Identify the aorta and expose the external iliac artery (Fig. 14-11). Trace the vas deferens and expose it toward the prostate. On top of the external iliac artery, identify the ureter. Trace and expose the ureter to its entrance to the urinary bladder (Fig. 14-12).

Inferior to the external iliac artery, expose the external iliac vein. Retract the external iliac vein inferiorly and clean the adipose tissue superior to it (Fig. 14-13). Just inferior to the course of the external iliac vein, identify the obturator nerve and trace it to the obturator foramen. Identify the internal iliac artery and expose its anterior and posterior divisions.

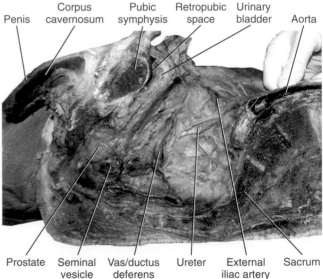

Penis   Corpus cavernosum   Pubic symphysis   Retropubic space   Urinary bladder   Aorta

Prostate   Seminal vesicle   Vas/ductus deferens   Ureter   External iliac artery   Sacrum

FIGURE 14-10. Soft tissue and adipose tissue cleaned around large structures.

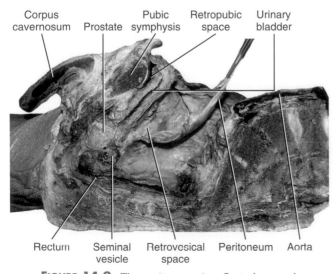

Corpus cavernosum   Prostate   Pubic symphysis   Retropubic space   Urinary bladder

Rectum   Seminal vesicle   Retrovesical space   Peritoneum   Aorta

FIGURE 14-9. The peritoneum is reflected upward.

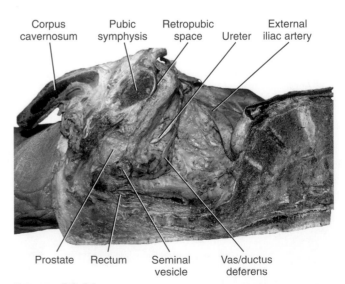

Corpus cavernosum   Pubic symphysis   Retropubic space   Ureter   External iliac artery

Prostate   Rectum   Seminal vesicle   Vas/ductus deferens

FIGURE 14-11. Exposure of external iliac artery, with vas/ductus deferens exposed toward prostate and ureter to its entrance.

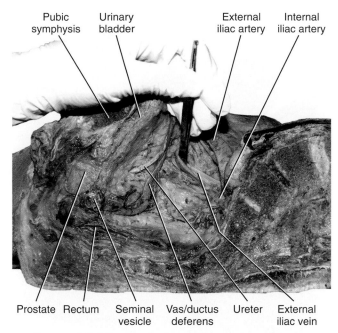

FIGURE 14-12. External iliac vein retracted inferiorly.

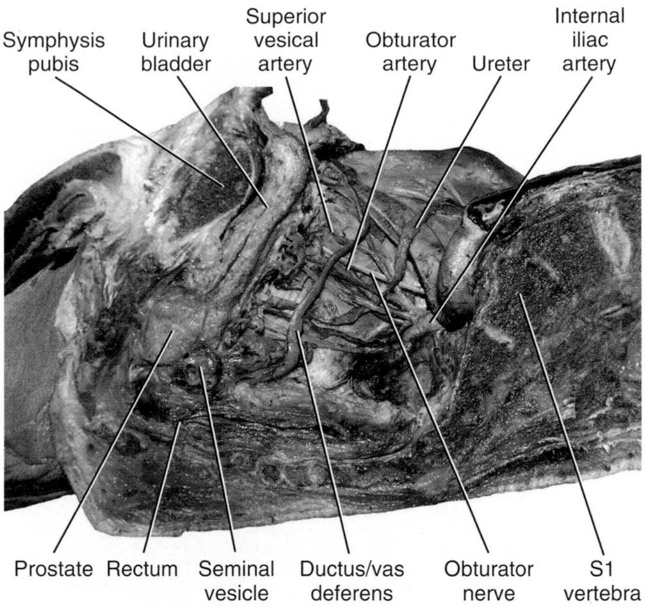

Pubic symphysis · Urinary bladder · External iliac artery · Internal iliac artery

Prostate · Rectum · Seminal vesicle · Vas/ductus deferens · Ureter · External iliac vein

FIGURE 14-14. Internal iliac artery with anterior and posterior divisions.

Symphysis pubis · Urinary bladder · Superior vesical artery · Obturator artery · Ureter · Internal iliac artery

Prostate · Rectum · Seminal vesicle · Ductus/vas deferens · Obturator nerve · S1 vertebra

> **✋ DISSECTION TIP:** The branches of the internal iliac artery are very variable. An easy way to avoid confusion is to rely on landmarks (see Dissection Tips), and always name the artery based on its distribution, not its origin.

Expose the branches of the anterior division of the internal iliac artery. These branches are the umbilical, obturator, inferior gluteal, internal pudendal, middle rectal, inferior vesical, and uterine arteries (Figs. 14-14 to 14-23).

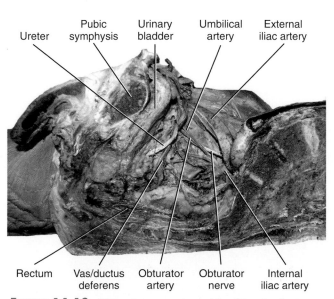

Ureter · Pubic symphysis · Urinary bladder · Umbilical artery · External iliac artery

Rectum · Vas/ductus deferens · Obturator artery · Obturator nerve · Internal iliac artery

FIGURE 14-13. Obturator nerve traced to obturator foramen.

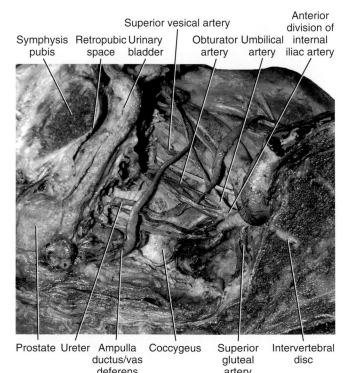

Symphysis pubis · Retropubic space · Urinary bladder · Superior vesical artery · Obturator artery · Umbilical artery · Anterior division of internal iliac artery

Prostate · Ureter · Ampulla ductus/vas deferens · Coccygeus · Superior gluteal artery · Intervertebral disc

FIGURE 14-15. Branches of anterior division of internal iliac artery.

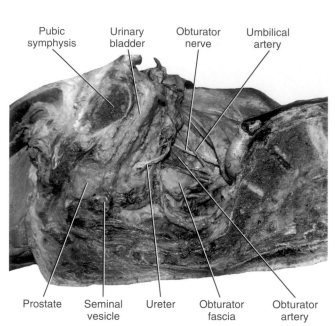

FIGURE 14-16. Appreciate major landmarks of pelvis in relation to branches of the internal iliac artery.

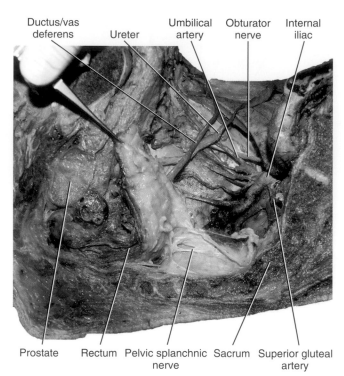

FIGURE 14-18. Sympathetic trunk exposed in pelvis with gray communicating rami passing lateral to nerves of sacral plexus.

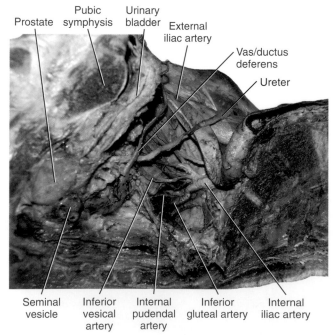

FIGURE 14-17. Appreciate branches of the anterior division of the internal iliac artery.

DISSECTION TIPS

Branches of Internal Iliac Artery: Anterior Division

Umbilical artery: Usually the first branch of the anterior division. The umbilical artery courses upward and superior to the urinary bladder to become the median umbilical ligament (Fig. 14-20). The umbilical artery often gives off the superior vesical branches that supply the superior portion of the urinary bladder; in 75% of cases, there are two or three superior vesical arteries.

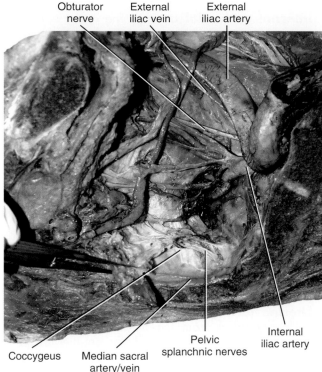

Obturator
nerve   External
iliac vein   External
iliac artery

Coccygeus   Median sacral
artery/vein   Pelvic
splanchnic nerves   Internal
iliac artery

FIGURE 14-19. To expose pelvic splanchnic nerves fully, lift the rectum and anal canal superiorly.

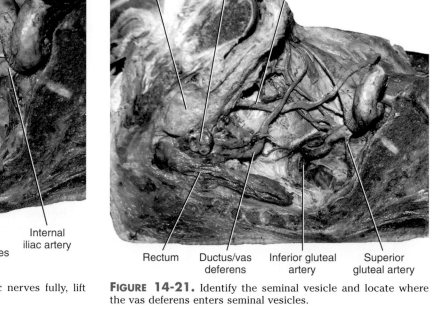

Prostate   Seminal
vesicle   Ureter

Rectum   Ductus/vas
deferens   Inferior gluteal
artery   Superior
gluteal artery

FIGURE 14-21. Identify the seminal vesicle and locate where the vas deferens enters seminal vesicles.

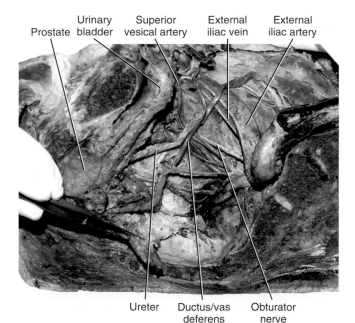

Prostate   Urinary
bladder   Superior
vesical artery   External
iliac vein   External
iliac artery

Ureter   Ductus/vas
deferens   Obturator
nerve

FIGURE 14-20. To expose pubococcygeus and iliococcygeus muscles, you need to clean all the pelvic fascia and adipose tissue over the levator ani inferior to the prostate gland.

Obturator artery: Usually arises parallel to the origin of the umbilical artery; travels with the obturator nerve to split into anterior and posterior branches in the obturator foramen (Figs. 14-19 to 14-21). The obturator artery travels anterior to the obturator internus and its fascia and is crossed medially by the ureter and the vas deferens. It gives rise to small branches: iliac, vesical, and pubic.

The main variation of the obturator artery is that in 30% of cases, it arises from the inferior epigastric artery.

Inferior gluteal artery: Arises at the posterior side of the anterior division and is mainly distributed to the buttocks. The landmark for identifying the inferior gluteal artery is to look for the artery passing between the 1st and 2nd sacral nerves and between the piriformis and coccygeus muscles (Figs. 14-22 and 14-23).

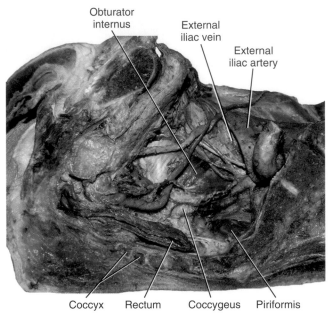

Obturator internus
External iliac vein
External iliac artery
Coccyx   Rectum   Coccygeus   Piriformis

FIGURE 14-22. Locate coccygeus muscle that arises from ischial spine and sacrospinous ligament and attaches to the coccyx and lower part of the sacrum.

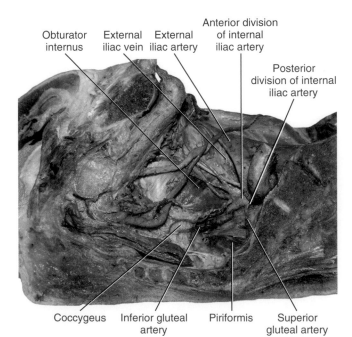

Obturator internus
External iliac vein
External iliac artery
Anterior division of internal iliac artery
Posterior division of internal iliac artery
Coccygeus   Inferior gluteal artery   Piriformis   Superior gluteal artery

FIGURE 14-23. Obturator internus fascia cleaned the exposing obturator internus muscle.

Internal pudendal artery: The artery is more anterior in position than the inferior gluteal artery as these arteries leave the pelvis. The internal pudendal artery does not pass between S1 and S2 nerves but typically courses lower between the piriformis and coccygeus muscles (Figs. 14-22 and 14-23). It will also accompany the pudendal nerve to the Alcock's canal. Several small branches arise from the internal pudendal artery: inferior rectal, perineal, artery of the bulb, urethral artery, deep artery of the penis or clitoris, and dorsal artery of the penis or clitoris.

Middle rectal: It arises with or from the internal pudendal, inferior vesical, or inferior gluteal arteries; mainly supplies the rectum.

Inferior vesical (vaginal in females): Usually arises from the internal pudendal artery. The inferior vesical artery supplies the fundus of the urinary bladder, the prostate, and the seminal vesicles.

Uterine (artery to vas deferens in males): Usually arises from the medial surface of the anterior trunk. It runs medially on the levator ani and the broad ligament and at about 2 cm at the cervix of the uterus it crosses in front of the ureter, to anastomose with the ovarian artery. The uterine artery typically gives off a *superior* branch supplying the body and fundus of the uterus and a *vaginal* branch supplying the cervix and vagina.

Expose the branches of the posterior division of the internal iliac artery: These branches are the iliolumbar, lateral sacral, and the superior gluteal arteries.

☞ *DISSECTION TIPS*

Branches of Internal Iliac Artery: Posterior Division

Iliolumbar: This artery is typically found between the lumbosacral trunk and the obturator nerve. It then ascends superolaterally to the iliac fossa, finally to reach the psoas muscle. The iliolumbar artery gives off an iliac and a lumbar branch.

Lateral sacral: Usually, two lateral sacral arteries are present, superior and inferior. The *superior* lateral sacral artery usually enters the 1st or 2nd sacral foramina. The *inferior* lateral sacral artery runs obliquely across the piriformis muscle to the medial side of the sacral foramina. It anastomoses with the middle sacral artery.

Superior gluteal: Largest branch of the posterior trunk and a direct continuation of its posterior trunk. The superior gluteal artery runs backward between the lumbosacral trunk and the 1st sacral nerve (see Fig. 14-30). It divides into superficial and deep branches in the buttock.

Behind the internal and external iliac arteries, identify the obturator internus muscle covered with the obturator fascia (a part of the endopelvic fascia). Expose the inferior part of the obturator fascia and note its white, thickened band of fibers, the *tendinous arch of the levator ani* (arcus tendineus levator ani). The tendinous arch runs from the obturator internus to the posterior part of the pubic bone and serves as an attachment site for the fibers of the levator ani muscle (see Figs. 14-16, 14-17, and 14-22). The tendinous arch is continuous with the obturator internus fascia.

The floor of the pelvis is mainly composed of the levator ani (anteriorly) and the coccygeus (posteriorly) muscles, forming the *pelvic diaphragm* (Figs. 14-22 and 14-23). The levator ani consists mainly of the pubococcygeus muscle arising from the anterior/middle portion of the tendinous arch of levator ani and the iliococcygeus. It further divides into the puborectalis and pubovaginalis (in females) muscles and the levator prostatae (in males) muscles. The iliococcygeus muscle arises mainly from the tendineus arch of the levator ani and attaches to the coccyx. The coccygeus muscle arises from the ischial spine and sacrospinous ligament and attaches to the coccyx and lower part of the sacrum (Fig. 14-22).

DISSECTION TIP: To expose the pubococcygeus and the iliococcygeus muscles, you need to clean all the pelvic fascia and adipose tissue over the levator ani muscle inferior to the prostate gland (Figs. 14-20 and 14-21). These muscles are often atrophied, and clear borders may be difficult to identify.

Clean the superior fascia of the pelvic diaphragm, which covers the levator ani. Note the continuity of the tendinous arch of the levator ani and the obturator internus fascia (Figs. 14-17 to 14-19). Clean the obturator internus fascia and expose the obturator internus muscle (Figs. 14-22 and 14-23).

Expose the sympathetic trunk in the pelvis, and observe the pelvic gray communicating rami passing lateral to nerves of the sacral plexus (there are no white communicating rami below the level of L2 or L3) and the origins of the pelvic splanchnic nerves (Figs. 14-18 to 14-20). To expose the pelvic splanchnic nerves completely, lift the rectum and anal canal superiorly. Note the pelvic splanchnic nerves penetrating the piriformis and coccygeus muscles to reach the lateral wall of the rectum. Trace the obturator nerve through the obturator foramen, and expose the lumbosacral trunk and the sacral nerves.

Expose the vas deferens to the seminal vesicles. Expose the dilatation of the vas deferens near the seminal vesicle, the *ampulla.* Expose the seminal vesicles, and identify the ejaculatory duct formed by the union of the vas deferens and the seminal vesicle.

Identify the prostate gland and expose its superior portion, the base, which is in contact with the urinary bladder. On either side of the prostate, palpate, if possible, the lateral lobes. Look for the wedge-shaped median lobe, located anterior to the ejaculatory ducts. Palpate the posterior lobe.

Dissection of the Female

Identify the broad ligament with its different portions—the mesosalpinx, mesovarium, and mesometrium. Identify the ovaries and the peritoneal fold covering the ovarian vessels, the suspensory ligament (infundibulopelvic) (Fig. 14-24). Identify the proper ligament of the ovary.

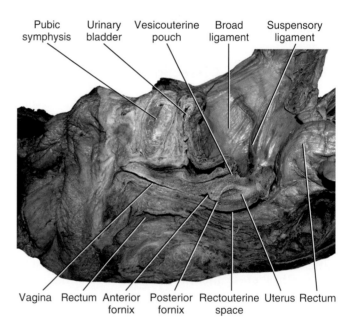

FIGURE 14-24. Broad ligament of uterus and suspensory ligament of ovary; appreciate the relationship between the rectum and uterus forming the pouch of Douglas (retrovesical space).

DISSECTION TIP: This ovarian ligament connects to the body of the uterus and the round ligament of the uterus.

At the base of the broad ligament, look for a thickening of the endopelvic fascia, the cardinal ligament (ligament of Mackenrodt). Inferiorly, identify the uterosacral ligament connecting the uterus to the sacrum.

✋ *DISSECTION TIP:* The cardinal and uterosacral ligaments may be difficult to identify in the cadaver. However, by pulling the uterus anteriorly toward the pubic symphysis and to the right, you may feel the left uterosacral ligament.

On the hemisected uterus, identify the fundus, body and cervix. Anterior to the cervix, identify the vagina. The deepest portion of the vagina behind the cervix is the posterior fornix (Fig. 14-25).

On the hemisected pelvis observe the most inferior portion of the abdomen, the pouch of Douglas (rectouterine pouch) (Fig. 14-24). A connective tissue septum extends inferiorly from the pouch of Douglas (retrovesical space) between the rectum and the vagina/uterus to attach to the perineal body, the rectovaginal septum (fascia of Denonvilliers). Its counterpart in the male is the rectoprostatic septum.

Ongoing Male Dissection

With a paper towel, clean the contents of the rectum and anal canal. Internally, identify the transverse folds of the rectum (valves of Houston), the anal columns (of Morgagni), and the pectinate line (Fig. 14-26).

Make a midsagittal incision through the prostate gland, and identify the three portions of the urethra: prostatic, membranous, and the spongy (Fig. 14-27). Within the prostatic urethra, identify an elevation, the *urethral crest,* and in the midline, the opening of the prostatic utricle. Lateral and distal to the prostatic utricle, identify the ejaculatory ducts. Lateral to the urethral crest, identify the openings of the prostatic ducts.

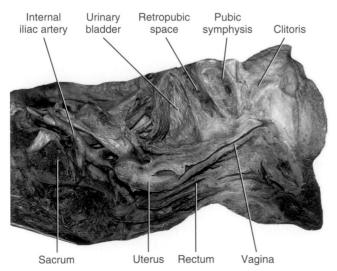

FIGURE 14-25. Vaginal canal with anterior and posterior fornices.

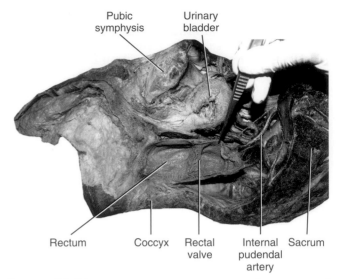

FIGURE 14-26. In this specimens, note internal structures of rectum and anal canal (transverse folds, valves of Houston).

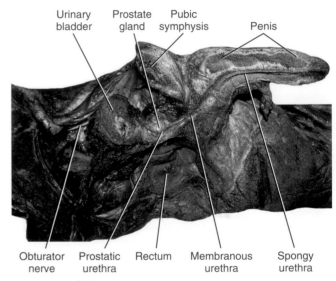

FIGURE 14-27. In this hemisected pelvis, appreciate anatomic components of urethra (prostatic, membranous, and spongy parts).

In Figure 14-28 the arteries and veins have been removed and the underlying musculature has been exposed.

Pull the hemisected urinary bladder medially and posteriorly, and identify the puboprostatic ligaments (pubovesical in females) lying laterally between the pubic symphysis and the bladder (Fig. 14-29). Identify the trigone of the urinary bladder.

✋ *DISSECTION TIP:* Trigone identification will be difficult in the hemisected specimen because the incision plane usually transects it.

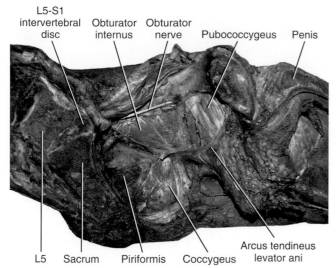

FIGURE 14-28. Arteries and veins removed and musculature exposed; *L5,* 5th lumbar; *S1,* 1st sacral.

Identify the ureteric orifice and the interureteric ridge or crest created by a muscular fold between the two ureteric orifices. The orifice of the urethra forms a muscular elevation, the *uvula.*

Lift the rectum upward, and expose the pelvic splanchnic nerves (Fig. 14-30).

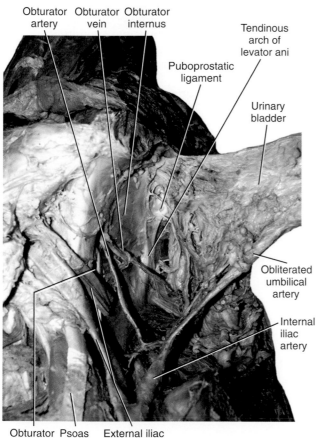

FIGURE 14-29. Urinary bladder retracted medially and puboprostatic ligaments identified in the space between the obturator internus muscle and urinary bladder, just behind the pubic symphysis.

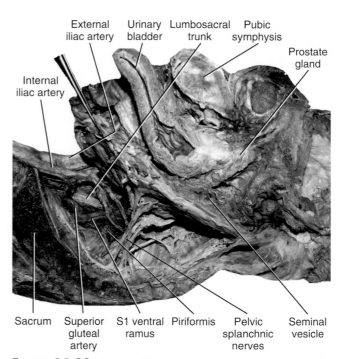

FIGURE 14-30. Rectum lifted upward to expose pelvic splanchnic nerves; *S1,* 1st sacral vertebra.

LABORATORY IDENTIFICATION CHECKLIST

Nerves
- ❏ Pudendal
- ❏ Obturator
- ❏ Lumbosacral trunk
- ❏ S1 ventral rami
- ❏ S2 ventral rami
- ❏ S3 ventral rami
- ❏ S4 ventral rami
- ❏ Pelvic splanchnic
- ❏ Sacral sympathetic chain/ ganglia
- ❏ Superior hypogastric plexus
- ❏ Inferior hypogastric plexus
- ❏ Sacral splanchnic nerves

Arteries
- ❏ Aorta
- ❏ Middle sacral
- ❏ Common iliac
  - ❏ External iliac
  - ❏ Internal iliac
    - ❏ *Anterior division*
    - ❏ Umbilical
    - ❏ Superior vesical
    - ❏ Obturator
    - ❏ Uterine
    - ❏ Vaginal
    - ❏ Inferior gluteal
    - ❏ *Posterior division*
    - ❏ Lateral sacral
    - ❏ Iliolumbar
    - ❏ Superior gluteal
- ❏ Gonadal (testicular/ovarian)
- ❏ Internal pudendal
- ❏ Superior rectal

Veins
- ❏ Inferior vena cava
- ❏ Common iliac
  - ❏ External iliac
  - ❏ Internal iliac

Muscles
- ❏ Piriformis
- ❏ Obturator internus
- ❏ Levator ani
- ❏ Coccygeus
- ❏ Pubococcygeus
- ❏ Iliococcygeus

Connective Tissue
- ❏ Pelvic fascia
- ❏ Obturator fascia

Ligaments
- ❏ Sacrotuberous
- ❏ Sacrospinous
- ❏ Iliolumbar
- ❏ Broad
- ❏ Uterosacral
- ❏ Lateral (cardinal, Mackenrodt)

Organs/Urinary/ Reproductive
- ❏ Urinary bladder
- ❏ Ureter
- ❏ Sigmoid colon
- ❏ Rectosigmoid junction
- ❏ Rectum
- ❏ Anal canal

Male
- ❏ Prostate gland
- ❏ Seminal vesicle
- ❏ Vas/ductus deferens

Female
- ❏ Uterus
- ❏ Fallopian tube
- ❏ Ovary

Spaces
- ❏ Retropubic
- ❏ Retrovesical (pouch of Douglas)
- ❏ Retrouterine

Bones
- ❏ Sacrum
- ❏ Coccyx
- ❏ Os coxae (hip bone)
  - ❏ Ilium
  - ❏ Ischium
  - ❏ Pubic

CHAPTER 15

PERINEUM

Netter: 356–365, 375–376, 384–387, 391, 393

McMinn: 278–280

Gray's Atlas: 226, 241–253, 257

DISSECTION OF THE MALE CADAVER

Dissection differences for the **female cadaver** are mentioned when appropriate.

> ✋ *DISSECTION TIP:* To best dissect the perineum, first perform the gluteal region dissection, including the ischioanal fossae and thighs. This will make it much easier to expose and dissect the structures of the perineum.

Place the cadaver in the supine position. Place a block under the sacrum and abduct the thighs as far as possible. A wooden block or rod is placed between the thighs at the level of the femoral condyles to maintain them in abduction (Fig. 15-1).

Identify the adductor longus and gracilis muscles. These muscles can be transected so that the thighs can be abducted more easily. In this specimen, it was not necessary to transect these muscles (Fig. 15-2).

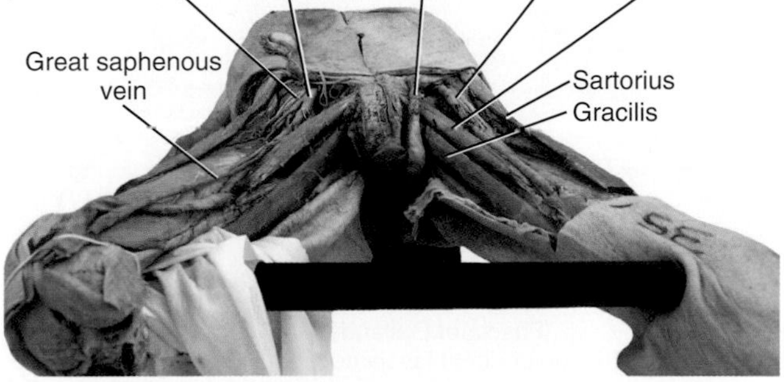

Draw imaginary lines outlining the borders of the *urogenital triangle:* a line between the ischial tuberosities and two lines along the ischiopubic rami to the pubic symphysis (Fig. 15-3). At the midpoint of a line connecting the two ischial tuberosities, palpate a fibromuscular mass of tissue, the *perineal body.* As described later, the perineal body is an important structure because the superficial and deep transverse perineus muscles, the bulbospongiosus muscle, the levator ani muscle, and the external anal sphincter muscles are attached to it.

Remove the skin of the urogenital region, including the scrotum. Reflect the testis toward the inguinal ligament, and expose the urogenital triangle. Lift the penis upward, and remove the adipose tissue and the rich venous network (Fig. 15-4). The fat that is removed here is located in the superficial perineal fascia (of Colles). This fascia is the continuation of Scarpa's fascia (membranous layer of anterior abdominal wall) into the perineum (Figs. 15-5 and 15-6). Camper's fascia (fatty layer of anterior abdominal wall) continues into the perineum.

FIGURE 15-1. Male cadaver in supine position with block under sacrum with thighs abducted.

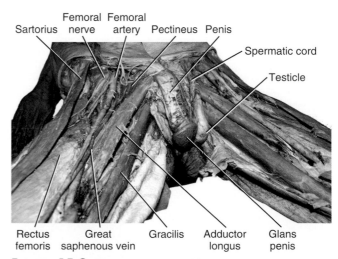

FIGURE 15-2. Transecting the adductor longus and gracilis muscles to abduct thighs more easily was not necessary in this cadaver.

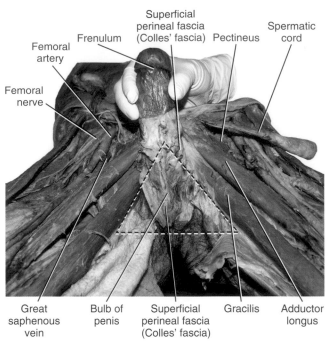

FIGURE 15-3. Urogenital triangle *(dashed outline)*, with line between ischial tuberosities and two lines along ischiopubic rami to pubic symphysis.

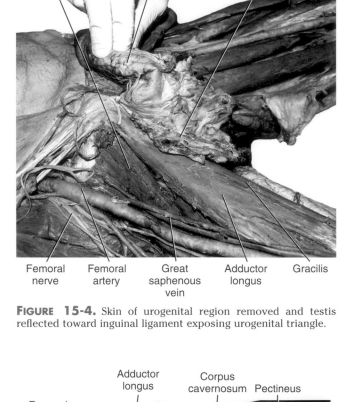

FIGURE 15-4. Skin of urogenital region removed and testis reflected toward inguinal ligament exposing urogenital triangle.

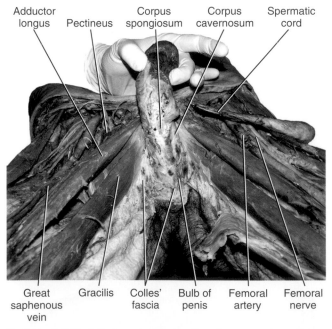

FIGURE 15-5. Lift the penis upward and remove the adipose tissue and the rich venous network.

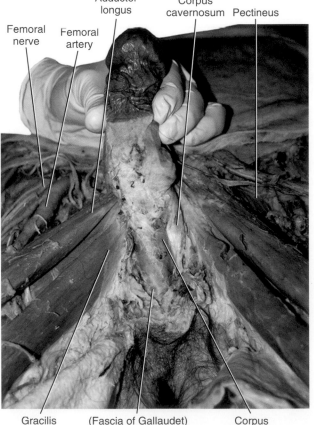

FIGURE 15-6. Colles' fascia removed to identify corpus cavernosum laterally and corpus spongiosum medially. Bulbospongiosus muscle is covered with deep perineal fascia.

If you are dissecting a **female cadaver,** make an incision into the skin around the vaginal orifice, leaving the labia minora and clitoris intact.

> **DISSECTION TIP:** The superficial perineal fascia is fairly thick and intermingled with the adipose tissue of the urogenital triangle. This fascia attaches laterally to the ischiopubic rami.

Remove Colles' fascia, and identify the corpus cavernosum laterally and the corpus spongiosum medially (Fig. 15-6). Expose the bulbospongiosus muscle covered with a fascial layer, the *deep perineal fascia* (Gallaudet's fascia). The deep perineal fascia invests the bulbospongiosus muscle, superficial transverse perineal muscles, and ischiocavernosus muscles.

Continue the exposure of the bulbospongiosus inferiorly, exposing the deep perineal fascia. The potential space between the superficial perineal fascia and deep perineal fascia is called the *superficial perineal cleft* (space between Colles' and Gallaudet's fasciae) (Figs. 15-7 and 15-8).

> **DISSECTION TIP:** During the removal of the superficial perineal cleft, you may encounter branches of the posterior femoral cutaneous nerve, as well as scrotal vessels and nerves.

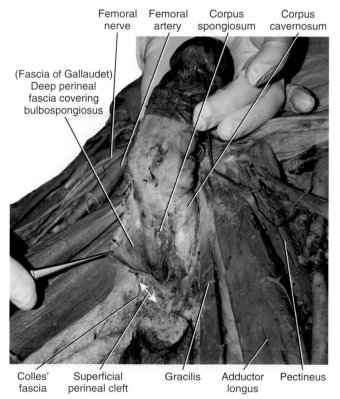

FIGURE 15-7. Exposure of bulbospongiosus muscle continued inferiorly, further revealing the deep perineal fascia.

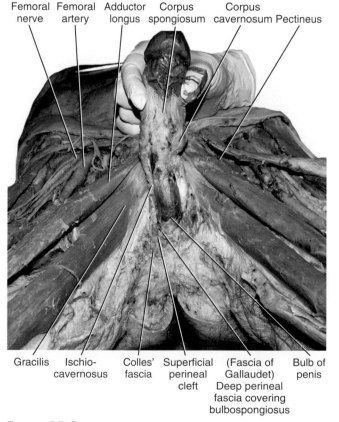

FIGURE 15-8. Ischiocavernosus muscle arises from ischiopubic rami.

Dissect lateral to the bulbospongiosus muscle and identify the ischiocavernosus muscle arising from the ischiopubic rami (Fig. 15-8). The ischiocavernosus surrounds the crus of the penis (corpora cavernosa), a bilateral collection of erectile tissue (Fig. 15-9).

The inferior portion of the corpus spongiosum becomes dilated, forming the bulb of the penis. At the level of the bulb, remove the superficial perineal fascia and identify the superficial perineal muscle laterally (Figs. 15-10 and 15-11).

☝ *DISSECTION TIP:* The superficial transverse perineal muscle is absent in some cadavers. It has also been shown that these muscles atrophy with age.

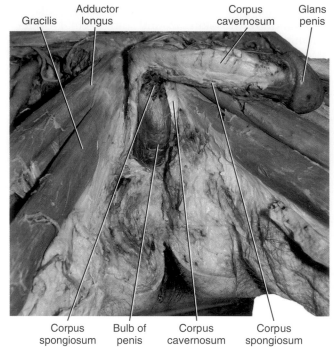

FIGURE 15-10. Dilated corpus spongiosum forms bulb of penis.

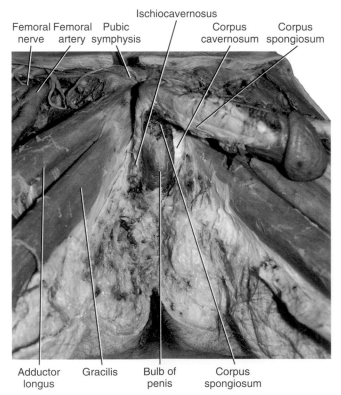

FIGURE 15-9. Crus of penis is surrounded by ischiocavernosus muscle.

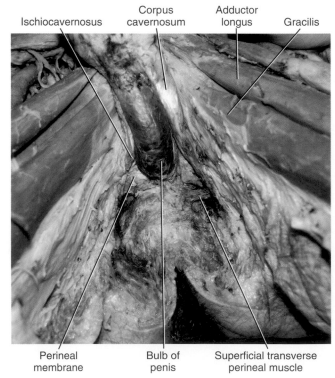

FIGURE 15-11. Superficial fascia removed at level of penile bulb to identify superficial perineal muscle laterally.

Clean the superficial transverse perineal muscles, and superior to them, expose the perineal membrane (Fig. 15-12). Inferior and lateral to the transverse perineal muscles, expose the perineal nerve and perineal artery, which are branches of the pudendal nerve and internal pudendal artery, respectively (Figs. 15-11 and 15-12).

Expose the ischiocavernosus muscle along the ischiopubic rami (Fig. 15-13).

Lift the penis and expose the crus. Make an incision into the crus and expose its spongy matrix and its *tunica albuginea,* the outer covering of the corpus (Fig. 15-14). Observe the pubic symphysis for the *suspensory ligament* of the penis, arising from deep fascia of the anterior abdominal wall, and the *fundiform ligament,* arising from the membranous layer of the superficial fascia of the abdomen.

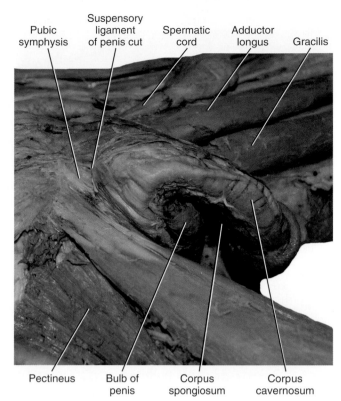

FIGURE 15-13. Ischiocavernosus muscle along ischiopubic rami.

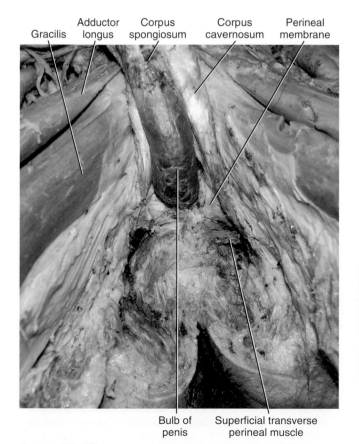

FIGURE 15-12. Superficial transverse perineal muscles cleaned, exposing perineal membrane. Perineal nerve and artery are inferior and lateral to transverse perineal muscle.

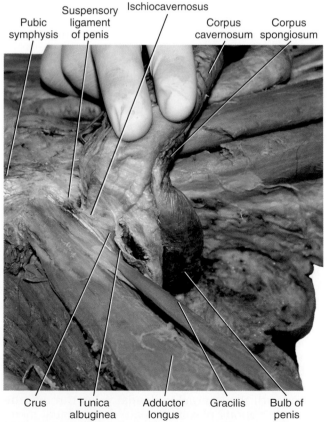

FIGURE 15-14. Penis lifted to expose crus with incision revealing spongy matrix and tunica albuginea.

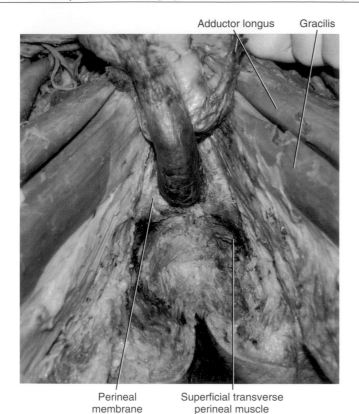

Adductor longus   Gracilis

Perineal membrane   Superficial transverse perineal muscle

FIGURE 15-15. Ischiocavernosus muscle reflected anteriorly to expose perineal membrane.

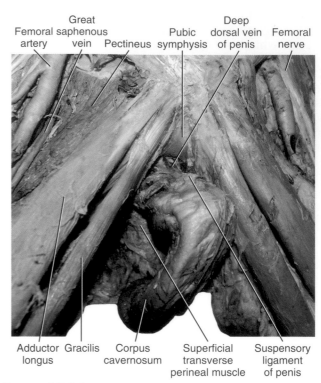

Great Femoral saphenous artery   vein   Pectineus   Pubic symphysis   Deep dorsal vein of penis   Femoral nerve

Adductor longus   Gracilis   Corpus cavernosum   Superficial transverse perineal muscle   Suspensory ligament of penis

FIGURE 15-16. Suspensory and fundiform ligaments cut and penis pushed downward.

Cut the ischiocavernosus muscle and reflect it anteriorly to expose the perineal membrane (Fig. 15-15).

In the **female cadaver,** reflect the vestibular bulb and identify the greater vestibular gland (Bartholin's gland) lateral to the vaginal opening.

> ☜ *DISSECTION TIP:* The bulbourethral gland in males may be difficult to find deep in the urogenital diaphragm.

Cut the suspensory and fundiform ligaments of the penis and push the penis downward (Fig. 15-16). With a scalpel, cut through the bulb of the penis at the perineal membrane and remove the penis (Fig. 15-17).

Identify the deep dorsal vein of the penis, the urethra, and the perineal body, and appreciate the dimensions of the perineal membrane. The deep dorsal vein of the penis is a large vein located deep to Buck's fascia (of the penis) just inferior to the arcuate pubic ligament. The deep dorsal vein anastomoses with the internal pudendal veins through the prostatic venous plexus. Palpate the perineal membrane between the deep dorsal vein of the penis and the urethra, and note its thickening, the *transverse perineal ligament* (Fig. 15-17).

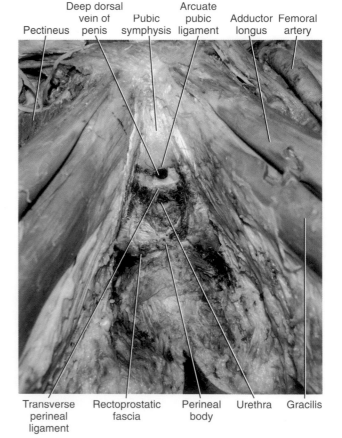

Deep dorsal vein of   Pubic   Arcuate pubic   Adductor   Femoral
Pectineus   penis   symphysis   ligament   longus   artery

Transverse perineal ligament   Rectoprostatic fascia   Perineal body   Urethra   Gracilis

FIGURE 15-17. Bulb cut from perineal membrane and penis removed revealing deep dorsal vein, urethra, and perineal body.

✍ DISSECTION TIP: Inferior and lateral to the superficial transverse perineal muscle, locate the perineal nerve and the perineal artery, tracing these toward the ischioanal fossa if time permits.

Reflect the deep perineal membrane, and expose the underlying musculature, the deep transverse perineal muscle and sphincter urethrae (Fig. 15-18).

✍ DISSECTION TIP: If time permits, cut the external urethral orifice of the penis and open the corpus spongiosum to expose the urethra. Extend the incision throughout the entire course of the urethra.

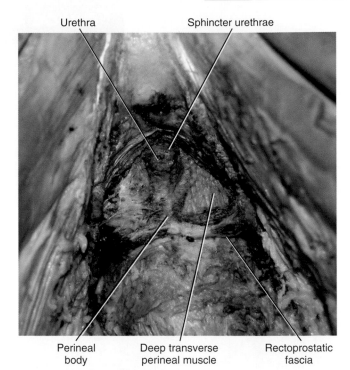

FIGURE 15-18. Deep perineal membrane reflected, exposing underlying musculature, deep transverse perineal muscle, and sphincter urethrae.

LABORATORY IDENTIFICATION CHECKLIST

Nerves
❐ Femoral
  ❐ Motor branches
  ❐ Cutaneous branches
❐ Obturator
  ❐ Anterior branch
  ❐ Posterior branch
❐ Ilioinguinal
❐ Pudendal

Arteries
❐ Femoral
❐ Obturator
❐ Deferential
❐ Perineal

Veins
❐ Great saphenous
❐ Femoral
❐ Deep dorsal of penis

Muscles
❐ Sartorius
❐ Gracilis
❐ Adductor longus
❐ Pectineus
❐ Iliopsoas
❐ Bulbospongiosus
❐ Ischiocavernosus
❐ Superficial transverse perineus
❐ Deep transverse perineus
❐ Sphincter urethrae

Connective Tissue
❐ Superficial perineal fascia
❐ Corpora cavernosa
❐ Bulb of penis
❐ Bulb of vestibule
❐ Corpus spongiosum
❐ Crus of penis/clitoris

Connective Tissue—cont'd
❐ Perineal membrane
❐ Perineal body
❐ Suspensory ligament of penis/clitoris
❐ Prepuce of penis/clitoris
❐ Glans of penis/clitoris
❐ Spermatic cord
❐ Scrotum
❐ Testicles
❐ Labia majora
❐ Labia minora
❐ Urethra
❐ Rectoprostatic fascia
❐ Pubic symphysis

Bones
❐ Right/left pubic bone
❐ Ischial spine

Clinical Application

Figures VI-1 and VI-2 depict the pelvic cavity with viscera removed. Note the superior and inferior hypogastric plexuses.

Figures VI-3 and VI-4 show large tumors in the uterus.

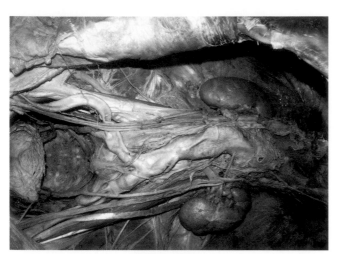

FIGURE VI-1.

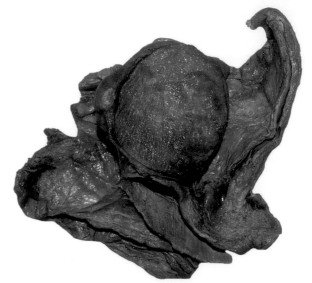

FIGURE VI-3.

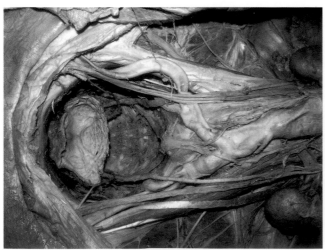

FIGURE VI-2.

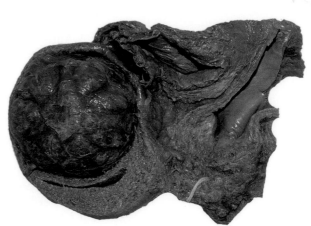

FIGURE VI-4.

CHAPTER 16

GLUTEAL REGION

Netter: 482–483, 490–491

McMinn: 278, 316–319

Gray's Atlas: 280–283, 287, 293–295

Typically, you will not need to make additional skin incisions if you continue the dissection on the same cadaver that you performed the dissection of the back (Fig. 16-1). If not, place the cadaver in the prone position, and incise the skin and subcutaneous tissues along the iliac crest to the posterior superior iliac spine (Figs. 16-2 and 16-3). Extend this incision medially to the intergluteal cleft, anterior to the area covering the perineum. Reflect the skin and superficial fascia from the gluteal region and posterior thigh by making a longitudinal midline skin incision distally to the knee. Make a circumferential incision through the skin of the leg, just distal to the knee (Fig. 16-3). There is typically a large amount of adipose tissue over the gluteus maximus muscle. Remove the adipose tissue and deep fascia in the gluteal region, exposing the gluteus maximus muscle (Figs. 16-4 to 16-6).

> ☝ *DISSECTION TIP:* In many atlases, you will find the gluteus maximus muscle shown with no fat. To create a clean specimen, remove the fat between the longitudinal fibers of the gluteus maximus muscle (Fig. 16-6).

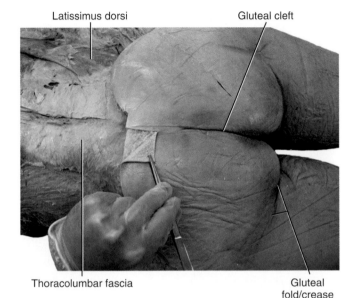

FIGURE 16-2. Gluteal region with reflected skin, demonstrating dissection from the midline.

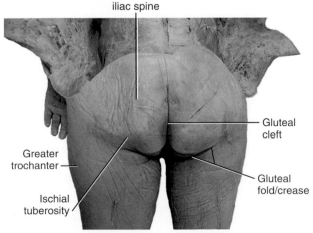

FIGURE 16-1. Surface anatomy landmarks of the gluteal region.

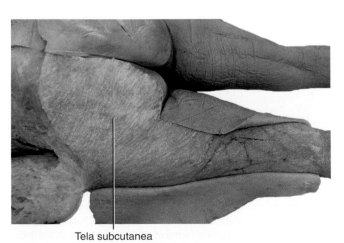

FIGURE 16-3. Gluteal and posterior thigh regions with dermis reflected, revealing membranous layer of subcutaneous tissue (tela subcutanea).

241

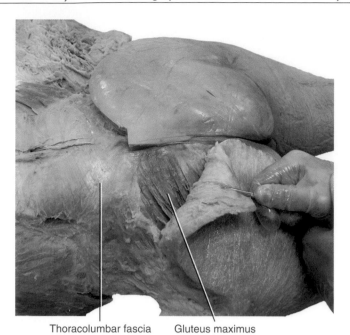

Thoracolumbar fascia   Gluteus maximus

FIGURE 16-4. Gluteal region with thoracolumbar fascia superiorly and reflected subcutaneous tissue, revealing gluteus maximus muscle inferiorly.

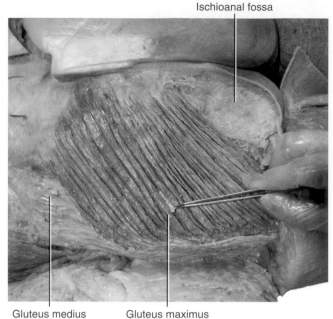

Ischioanal fossa

Gluteus medius   Gluteus maximus

FIGURE 16-6. Closer view highlighting the gluteus medius (covered with fascia) muscle superiorly, the gluteus maximus muscle inferiorly, and the ischioanal fossa medially.

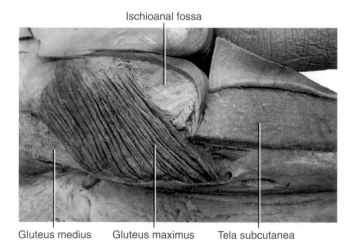

Ischioanal fossa

Gluteus medius   Gluteus maximus   Tela subcutanea

FIGURE 16-5. Further gluteal region dissection, revealing the gluteus medius (covered with fascia) muscle superiorly, the gluteus maximus muscle inferiorly, and the ischioanal fossa and tela subcutanea medially.

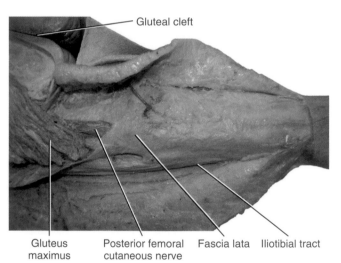

Gluteal cleft

Gluteus   Posterior femoral   Fascia lata   Iliotibial tract
maximus   cutaneous nerve

FIGURE 16-7. Posterior thigh region with skin and subcutaneous tissue reflected, revealing the posterior cutaneous nerve, fascia lata, and iliotibial tract.

Reflect the skin over the posterior portion of the thigh. The adipose tissue and deep fascia will be removed later during the dissection (Fig. 16-7). As you delineate the superior and inferior borders of the gluteus maximus muscle, protect the posterior femoral cutaneous nerve from damage by being cautious along the inferior border of the gluteus maximus muscle.

Palpate the sacrotuberous ligament at the medial border of the gluteus maximus muscle by placing your fingertips into the ischioanal fossa (Fig. 16-8). Palpate the superior border of the gluteus maximus and insert your fingertips into the space between the gluteus maximus muscle and fascia over the gluteus medius muscle (Fig. 16-9).

In most cadavers, the deep fascia and aponeurotic tissues along the superior border of the gluteus maximus muscle blend with those of the gluteus medius muscle. However, the muscular fibers of the gluteus medius muscle run almost perpendicular to

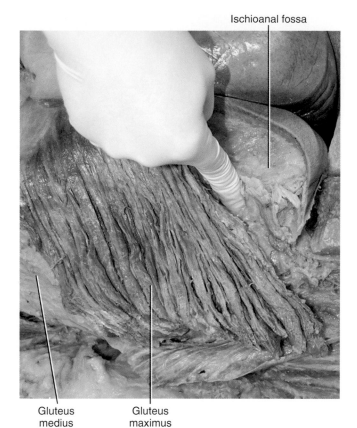

Ischioanal fossa

Gluteus
medius

Gluteus
maximus

FIGURE 16-8. Fingertips in gluteal region highlight gluteus medius superiorly, gluteus maximus inferiorly, and ischioanal fossa medially (palpation of lateral wall of fossa–obturator internus).

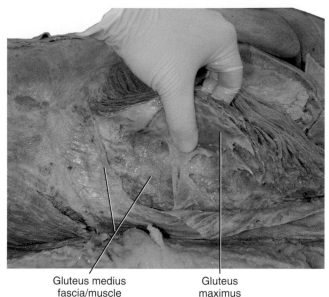

Gluteus medius
fascia/muscle

Gluteus
maximus

FIGURE 16-10. Reflecting the gluteus maximus muscle demonstrates the deeper lying muscle fibers of the gluteus medius muscle.

the orientation of the gluteus maximus muscle, and the two muscles can be readily separated once you have clearly exposed their fibers.

Using your fingertips, lift the upper portion of the gluteus maximus muscle from the underlying gluteus medius muscle.

Make an incision at the lateral border of the gluteus maximus muscle, separating it from its connection to the iliotibial tract (Fig. 16-10). Lift the gluteus maximus medially toward the sacrum, and identify the greater trochanter and trochanteric bursa (Figs. 16-11 and 16-12).

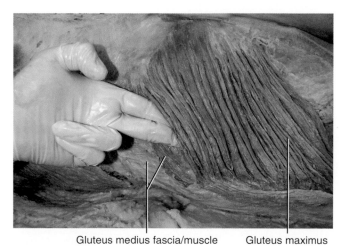

Gluteus medius fascia/muscle   Gluteus maximus

FIGURE 16-9. Gluteal region after dissecting superior border of gluteus maximus muscle superficially, revealing deeper gluteus medius fascia and muscle.

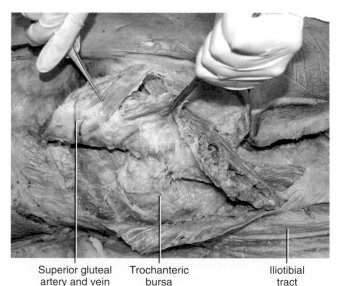

Superior gluteal
artery and vein

Trochanteric
bursa

Iliotibial
tract

FIGURE 16-11. Reflection of superolateral border of gluteus maximus muscle, revealing superior gluteal artery and vein and trochanteric bursa.

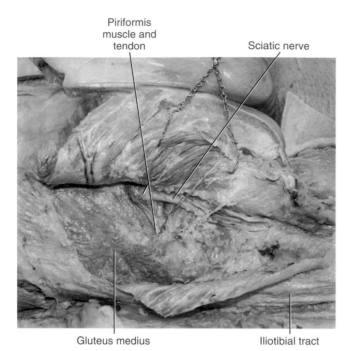

FIGURE 16-12. Gluteal region with reflected gluteus maximus muscle, revealing gluteus medius and piriformis muscles and sciatic nerve.

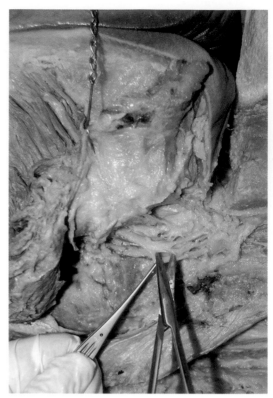

FIGURE 16-13. Connective tissue cleaned around posterior femoral cutaneous and sciatic nerves.

> **DISSECTION TIP:** The trochanteric bursa appears as loose connective tissue over the greater trochanter, intermingled with adipose tissue. It is often cleaned away during routine dissection.

Reflect the gluteus maximus muscle medially from the gluteal tuberosity of the femur; remove the deep fascia and adipose tissue along its inferior border (Fig. 16-13). Clean the sciatic and the posterior femoral cutaneous nerves from the adipose tissue, and trace them proximally from under the piriformis muscle (Fig. 16-14). Once you identify the posterior femoral cutaneous nerve, identify its perineal branch traveling medially.

> **DISSECTION TIP:** To identify the posterior femoral cutaneous nerve, make a small opening through the fascia lata on the posterior aspect of the thigh, and identify the sciatic nerve. Medial to the sciatic nerve, you will be able to identify the posterior femoral cutaneous nerve. In some specimens, the sciatic nerve may split in the gluteal region, with one part traveling above or through and the other part below the piriformis muscle.

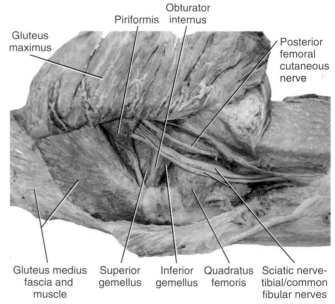

FIGURE 16-14. Reflected gluteus maximus muscle, revealing gluteus medius, rotator muscles (piriformis, superior/inferior gemelli, obturator internus, quadratus femoris), sciatic nerve, and posterior femoral cutaneous nerve.

The gluteus maximus muscle is partially attached to the sacrotuberous ligament. Palpate the sacrotuberous ligament as you did earlier (see Fig. 16-8); reflect the gluteus maximus muscle medially toward the sacrum, and expose the sacrotuberous ligament. Use a scalpel to cut the attachment of the gluteus maximus muscle from the sacrotuberous ligament. With scissors, cut the lateral portion of the sacrotuberous ligament, and free the gluteus maximus muscle (Fig. 16-15). Clean and expose the inferior gluteal vessels and nerve from the deep surface of the gluteus maximus muscle (Figs. 16-16 and 16-17).

> ☛ *DISSECTION TIP:* The obturator internus, superior gemellus, and inferior gemellus muscles are often seen as a combined tripartite tendon with indistinguishable borders. With scissors or a probe, separate these three muscles at the margin of the lesser sciatic foramen.

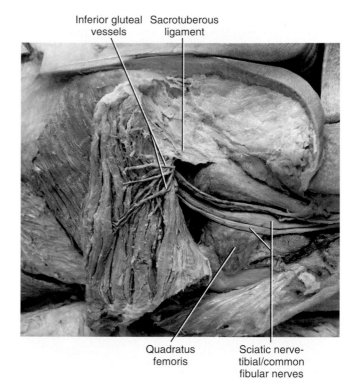

FIGURE 16-16. Gluteus maximus muscle reflected superiorly, revealing inferior gluteal vessels, quadratus femoris muscle, and tibial and common fibular nerves.

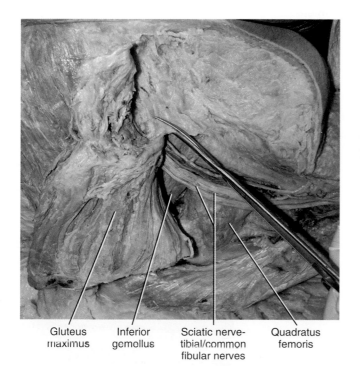

FIGURE 16-15. Reflected gluteus maximus muscle revealing quadratus femoris muscle and tibial and common fibular nerves.

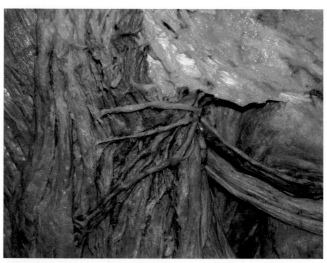

FIGURE 16-17. Closer view of Figure 16-16 showing gluteal region with gluteus maximus reflected, revealing inferior gluteal artery and vein and sacrotuberous ligament.

Lift the posterior femoral cutaneous and sciatic nerves, and clean the adipose and connective tissues from the structures that lie deep to the gluteus maximus muscle, such as the piriformis, obturator internus, and superior and inferior gemellus muscles (Figs. 16-18 and 16-19). Inferior to the obturator internus and gemelli muscles, identify the quadratus femoris muscle.

Identify the borders of the gluteus medius and tensor fasciae latae muscles. The tensor fasciae latae muscle arises from the anterior portion of the iliac crest. Its tendon is covered by fascia lata and continues distally as the iliotibial tract. Place your fingertips at the inferior border of the gluteus medius muscle and lift it upward (Fig. 16-20).

At the superior space between the gluteus maximus and gluteus medius muscles, identify the superficial branch of the superior gluteal artery (Figs. 16-21 and 16-22). Cut the attachment of the gluteus medius from the greater trochanter and reflect it superiorly. On its deep surface, identify the deep branch of the superior gluteal artery (Fig. 16-22). The muscle exposed underneath the reflected gluteus medius is the gluteus minimus muscle. Deep and inferior to the sacrotuberous ligament, identify the nerve to the obturator internus, internal pudendal artery, its venae comitantes, and the pudendal nerve (Fig. 16-23). The venae comitantes are the pair of veins that accompany the internal pudendal artery.

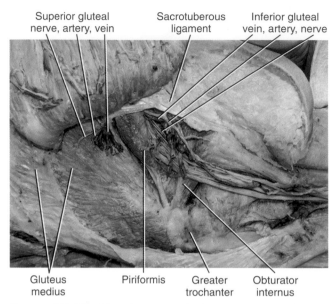

FIGURE 16-18. Gluteal region with gluteus maximus reflected, revealing superior and inferior gluteal artery and vein oriented around piriformis muscle.

> ☞ *DISSECTION TIP:* The nerve to the quadratus femoris and inferior gemellus muscles is a small branch that may be found by retracting the sciatic nerve posteromedially; observe this small nerve traveling deep to the gemelli and obturator internus.

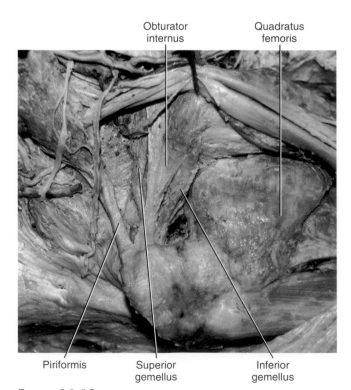

FIGURE 16-19. Gluteal region close-up view highlighting rotator muscles (piriformis, superior/inferior gemelli, obturator internus, quadratus femoris) with sciatic nerve reflected medially.

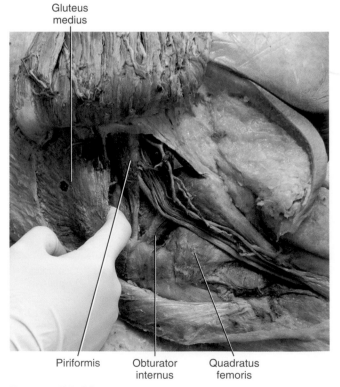

FIGURE 16-20. Reflected gluteus maximus muscle reveals gluteus medius muscle, "rotators" (piriformis, obturator internus, quadratus femoris muscles), and the sciatic nerve.

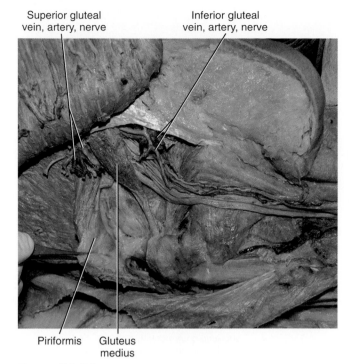

Superior gluteal vein, artery, nerve

Inferior gluteal vein, artery, nerve

Piriformis   Gluteus medius

FIGURE 16-21. Gluteus maximus reflected, revealing piriformis muscle and superior and inferior gluteal neurovascular bundles.

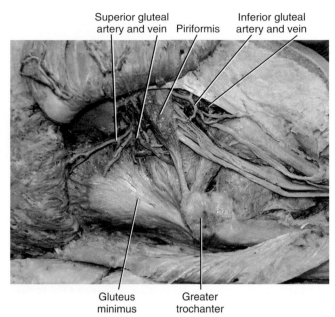

Superior gluteal artery and vein   Piriformis   Inferior gluteal artery and vein

Gluteus minimus   Greater trochanter

FIGURE 16-23. Gluteal region with reflection of the gluteus maximus muscle medially and the gluteus medius muscle superiorly, revealing the gluteus minimus muscle and the superior gluteal neurovascular bundle lying superficial to the gluteus minimus muscle.

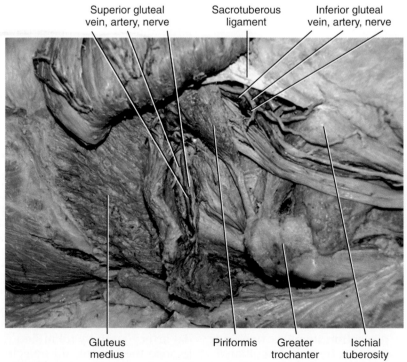

Superior gluteal vein, artery, nerve

Sacrotuberous ligament

Inferior gluteal vein, artery, nerve

Gluteus medius   Piriformis   Greater trochanter   Ischial tuberosity

FIGURE 16-22 Gluteus maximus muscle reflected, highlighting piriformis muscle and superior and inferior gluteal neurovascular bundles.

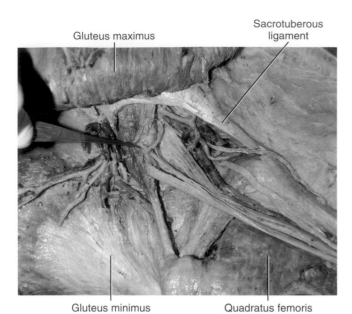

Gluteus maximus | Sacrotuberous ligament

Gluteus minimus | Quadratus femoris

FIGURE 16-24. Gluteal region with reflection of the gluteus maximus muscle medially and gluteus medius muscle superiorly, revealing the gluteus minimus muscle and the superior gluteal neurovascular bundle lying superficial to the gluteus minimus muscle.

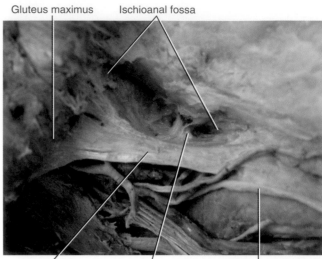

Gluteus maximus | Ischioanal fossa

Sacrotuberous ligament | Neurovascular bundle of pudendal nerve, artery, and vein covered with lunate fascia | Posterior femoral cutaneous nerve

FIGURE 16-26. Gluteus maximus reflected, revealing ischioanal fossa, sacrotuberous ligament, pudendal neurovascular bundle, and posterior femoral cutaneous nerve.

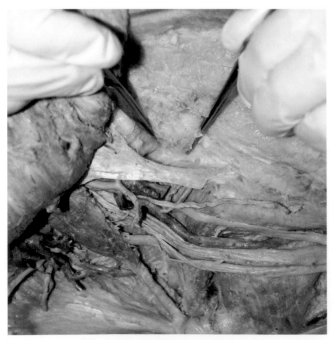

FIGURE 16-25. Gluteal region with reflection of gluteus maximus, highlighting piriformis muscle, sacrotuberous ligament, and superior/inferior gluteal neurovascular bundles.

NOTE: This part of the dissection involves opening the pudendal canal and dissecting the ischioanal fossa; it may also be performed separately with the dissection of the perineum.

Dissect and clean away the adipose tissue of the structures inferior to the sacrotuberous ligament, and identify the internal pudendal artery, its venae comitantes and the pudendal nerve (Fig. 16-24). Identify the continuation of the obturator fascia at the ischioanal fossa, the *lunate fascia*. This fascia encircles the internal pudendal artery and vein and pudendal nerve branches (Figs. 16-25 and 16-26).

> ☝ *DISSECTION TIP:* Identifying the lunate fascia and the point of entrance of the internal pudendal artery and vein and the pudendal nerve into the gluteal region is useful for exposing these structures when a large amount of adipose tissue is present.

Separate the inferior border of the sacrotuberous ligament with scissors, and cut its inferior attachment from the ischial tuberosity (Fig. 16-27). Reflect the sacrotuberous ligament upward toward the reflected gluteus maximus muscle, and expose the contents of the pudendal canal (Alcock's canal) (Figs. 16-28 and 16-29).

Expose the pudendal, inferior rectal, and perineal nerves (Fig. 16-30). Remove all the adipose tissue from the ischioanal fossa thoroughly so that the branches of the pudendal nerve and internal pudendal artery are fully identified (Figs. 16-31 and 16-32). Expose the levator ani muscle and the fascia of the obturator internus muscle as well as the external anal sphincter (Figs. 16-33 and 16-34).

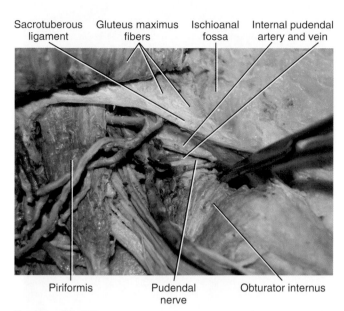

Sacrotuberous ligament   Gluteus maximus fibers   Ischioanal fossa   Internal pudendal artery and vein

Piriformis   Pudendal nerve   Obturator internus

FIGURE 16-27. Gluteus maximus muscle reflected, revealing sacrotuberous ligament, gluteus maximus fibers, ischioanal fossa border, obturator internus muscle, and pudendal neurovascular bundle.

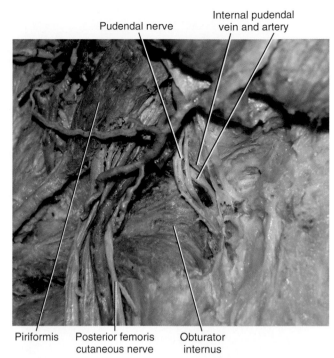

Pudendal nerve   Internal pudendal vein and artery

Piriformis   Posterior femoris cutaneous nerve   Obturator internus

FIGURE 16-29. Gluteus maximus muscle reflected, revealing piriformis muscle, posterior femoral cutaneous nerve, obturator internus muscle, ischioanal fossa, pudendal nerve, and internal pudendal artery and vein.

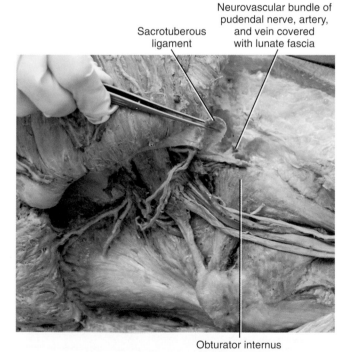

Sacrotuberous ligament   Neurovascular bundle of pudendal nerve, artery, and vein covered with lunate fascia

Obturator internus

FIGURE 16-28. Sacrotuberous ligament held between forceps with gluteus maximus muscle reflected, revealing ischioanal fossa border, obturator internus muscle, and pudendal neurovascular bundle within lunate fascia.

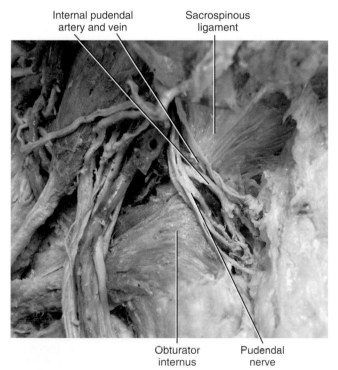

Internal pudendal artery and vein   Sacrospinous ligament

Obturator internus   Pudendal nerve

FIGURE 16-30. Sacrotuberous ligament reflected, revealing obturator internus muscle, pudendal nerve, internal pudendal artery and vein, and sacrospinous ligament.

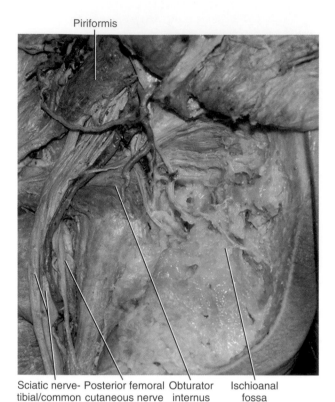

Piriformis

Sciatic nerve- Posterior femoral Obturator Ischioanal
tibial/common cutaneous nerve internus fossa
fibular nerves

FIGURE 16-31. Reflected gluteus maximus muscle reveals piriformis and obturator internus muscles, tibial and common fibular nerves of sciatic nerve, posterior femoral cutaneous nerve, and ischioanal fossa.

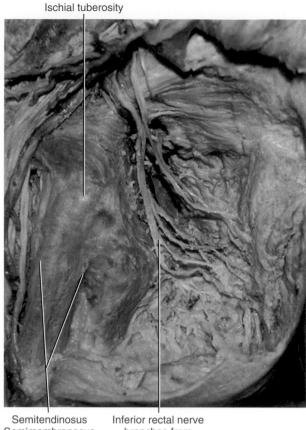

Ischial tuberosity

Semitendinosus Inferior rectal nerve
Semimembranosus branches from
Long head of pudendal nerve
biceps femorias

FIGURE 16-33. Superior aspect of posterior thigh and ischioanal fossa, highlighting ischial tuberosity, "hamstring" muscles (semitendinosus, semimembranosus, long head of biceps femoris), and inferior rectal nerve branches.

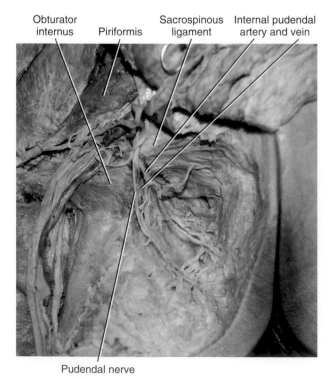

Obturator Piriformis Sacrospinous Internal pudendal
internus ligament artery and vein

Pudendal nerve

FIGURE 16-32. Sacrotuberous ligament reflected, revealing obturator internus, pudendal nerve, internal pudendal artery and vein, and sacrospinous ligament.

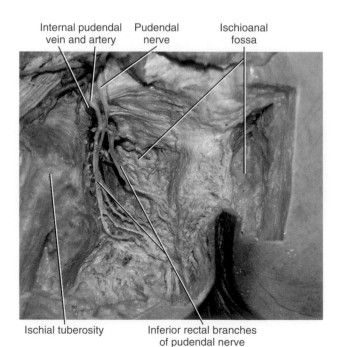

Internal pudendal Pudendal Ischioanal
vein and artery nerve fossa

Ischial tuberosity Inferior rectal branches
of pudendal nerve

FIGURE 16-34. Bilateral ischioanal fossae highlighting subcutaneous fat, pudendal nerve, internal pudendal artery and vein, and inferior rectal nerve branches.

Palpate the iliotibial tract, the band into which the tensor fasciae latae and the gluteus maximus muscles (partially) insert. Note the lateral intermuscular septum, which begins from the deep surface of the fascia lata and attaches to the *linea aspera* (rough line). Identify the space between the quadratus femoris and adductor magnus (adductor minimus) muscles, and find the medial femoral circumflex artery (Fig. 16-35).

With blunt dissection, separate the muscles of the posterior thigh ("hamstrings"), and identify the long and short heads of the biceps femoris muscle as well as the semitendinosus and semimembranous muscles (Fig. 16-36). Dissect out their origins from the ischial tuberosity. Retract the long head of the biceps femoris laterally to expose the sciatic nerve. Note the division of the sciatic nerve into the tibial and common fibular (peroneal) nerves as it approaches the popliteal fossa (Fig. 16-37).

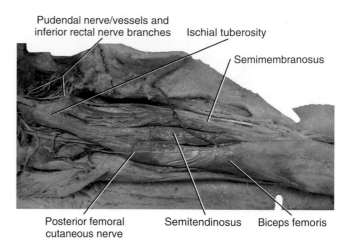

FIGURE 16-36. Reflected skin and subcutaneous tissue of posterior thigh and ischioanal fossa, revealing pudendal nerve superiorly and inferior rectal nerve inferiorly, internal pudendal artery and vein, ischial tuberosity, and biceps femoris, semitendinosus, and semimembranosus muscles.

👆 *DISSECTION TIP:* Typically, the division of the sciatic nerve into the tibial and common fibular nerves occurs near the popliteal fossa. However, some cadavers may have a high split of the sciatic nerve, or two nerves may exit from the inferior border of the piriformis muscle, with a lateral nerve (common fibular) and a medial nerve (tibial).

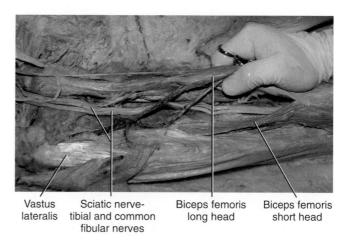

FIGURE 16-37. Posterior thigh, highlighting sciatic nerve (tibial/common fibular nerves) and biceps femoris muscle (long and short heads).

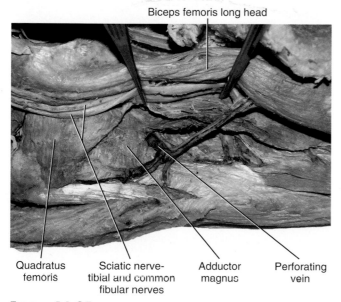

FIGURE 16-35. Superior posterior thigh with retracted tibial and common fibular nerves and long head of biceps femoris muscle, highlighting quadratus femoris and adductor longus muscles and perforating vein.

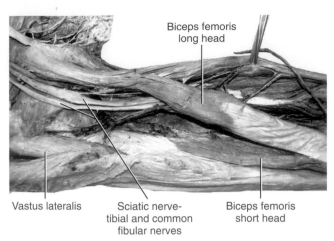

FIGURE 16-38. Posterior thigh, showing tibial and common fibular nerves of sciatic nerve long and short heads of biceps femoris muscle.

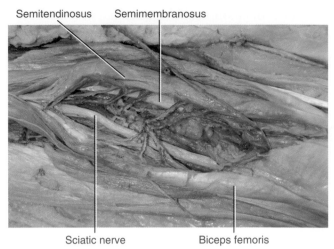

FIGURE 16-39. Posterior thigh, highlighting sciatic nerve between "hamstrings": biceps femoris lateral, semitendinosus medial and superficial, and semimembranosus muscle medial and deep.

Look at the lateral aspect of the sciatic nerve. The only branches to arise from its lateral surface innervate the short head of the biceps femoris muscle (Fig. 16-38). Clean the perforating arteries and veins, which provide the arterial supply and venous drainage of the posterior thigh (Figs. 16-39 to 16-41).

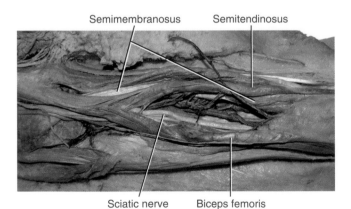

FIGURE 16-40. Posterior thigh, showing sciatic nerve between hamstring muscles' (biceps femoris, semitendinosus, semimembranosus).

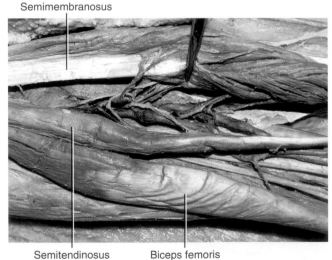

FIGURE 16-41. Posterior thigh revealing musculature: biceps femoris laterally, semitendinosus reflected laterally, and semimembranosus medially.

LABORATORY IDENTIFICATION CHECKLIST

Nerves
❏ Superior gluteal
❏ Inferior gluteal
❏ Pudendal
  ❏ Inferior rectal
❏ Posterior femoral cutaneous
❏ Sciatic
❏ Tibial (medial)
❏ Common fibular (lateral)

Arteries
❏ Superior gluteal
❏ Inferior gluteal
❏ Internal pudendal
  ❏ Inferior rectal
❏ Medial femoral circumflex
❏ Perforating arteries

Veins
❏ Superior gluteal
❏ Inferior gluteal
❏ Internal pudendal
❏ Perforating veins

Muscles
❏ Gluteus maximus
❏ Gluteus medius
❏ Gluteus minimus
❏ Piriformis
❏ Superior gemellus
❏ Obturator internus
❏ Inferior gemellus
❏ Quadratus femoris
❏ Semimembranosus
❏ Semitendinosus
❏ Biceps femoris
  ❏ Long head
  ❏ Short head
❏ Adductor minimus
❏ Tensor fasciae latae
❏ Levator ani
❏ External anal sphincter

Ligaments
❏ Sacrotuberous
❏ Sacrospinous

Fossa/Canal
❏ Ischioanal fossa
❏ Alcock's canal

Fascia
❏ Gluteal
❏ Obturator internus
❏ Lunate
❏ Fascia lata
❏ Iliotibial tract

Bursa
❏ Trochanteric bursa

CHAPTER 17

THIGH AND LEG

Netter: 471–481, 488–489

McMinn: 320–323

Gray's Atlas: 272–279, 284–292

BEFORE DISSECTION

Palpate the following bony landmarks on the cadaver or on yourself:

- Anterior superior iliac spine
- Pubic tubercle
- Pubic symphysis
- Greater trochanter of femur
- Medial and lateral femoral condyles

- Patella
- Tibial tuberosity
- Head and neck of fibula
- Medial and lateral malleoli of tibia and fibula, respectively

Make a horizontal skin incision 2 to 3 cm (~1 inch) on the thigh inferior and parallel to the inguinal ligament. Leave the skin intact over the external genitalia. At the midpoint of this horizontal incision, make a vertical incision to the anterior portion of the patella. Make an encircling incision around the knee (Fig. 17-1). Reflect the skin medially over the thigh, and identify the superficial veins (Fig. 17-2).

Continue the dissection by making a vertical incision from the knee toward the ankle (Fig. 17-3). Make a transverse incision between the malleoli. Reflect the skin of the leg laterally (Fig. 17-4). Start exposing the superficial veins of the leg and thigh (Figs. 17-5 and 17-6). Identify the great saphenous vein and saphenous nerve.

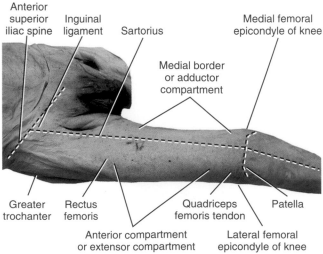

FIGURE 17-1. Three thigh dissection incisions: horizontal cut inferior and parallel to inguinal ligament, vertical cut to anterior patella at midpoint of horizontal incision, and encircling cut around knee.

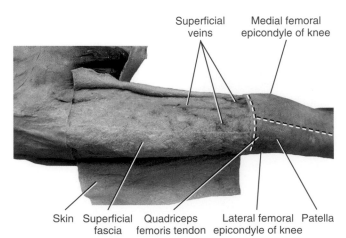

FIGURE 17-2. Skin reflected medially over thigh, revealing superficial veins.

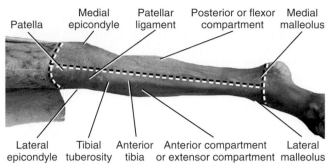

Patella • Medial epicondyle • Patellar ligament • Posterior or flexor compartment • Medial malleolus • Lateral epicondyle • Tibial tuberosity • Anterior tibia • Anterior compartment or extensor compartment • Lateral malleolus

FIGURE 17-3. Vertical incision from knee toward ankle.

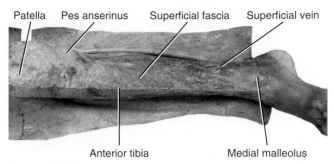

Patella • Pes anserinus • Superficial fascia • Superficial vein • Anterior tibia • Medial malleolus

FIGURE 17-4. Transverse cut between malleoli, with skin of leg reflected laterally.

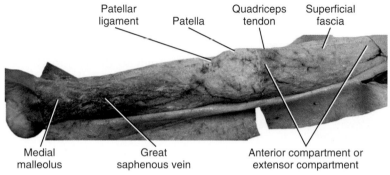

Patellar ligament • Patella • Quadriceps tendon • Superficial fascia • Medial malleolus • Great saphenous vein • Anterior compartment or extensor compartment

FIGURE 17-5. Exposure of superficial veins of the leg and thigh.

Clean the superficial fascia over the *great saphenous vein,* starting from the ankle toward the knee (Fig. 17-7). Around the knee, the saphenous nerve is located deep to the great saphenous vein. In the leg medial to the tibia, however, the great saphenous vein runs parallel with the saphenous nerve (Fig. 17-8).

The great saphenous vein arises from the medial side of the dorsal venous arch of the foot and ascends anterior to the medial malleolus, along the medial side of the leg and thigh, finally draining into the femoral vein.

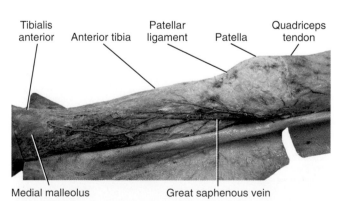

Tibialis anterior • Anterior tibia • Patellar ligament • Patella • Quadriceps tendon • Medial malleolus • Great saphenous vein

FIGURE 17-6. Skin of leg reflected, showing great saphenous vein and tibialis anterior muscle.

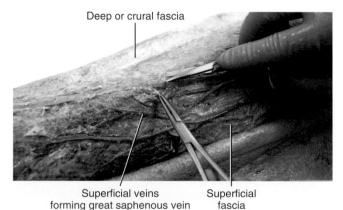

Deep or crural fascia • Superficial veins forming great saphenous vein • Superficial fascia

FIGURE 17-7. Superficial fascia cleaned over great saphenous vein.

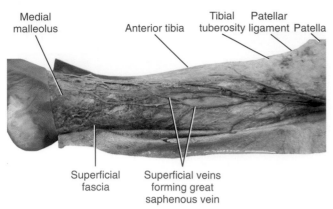

Medial malleolus — Anterior tibia — Tibial tuberosity — Patellar ligament — Patella — Superficial fascia — Superficial veins forming great saphenous vein

FIGURE 17-8. In the leg medial to the tibia, note how the great saphenous vein runs parallel with the saphenous nerve.

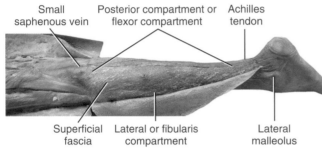

Small saphenous vein — Posterior compartment or flexor compartment — Achilles tendon — Superficial fascia — Lateral or fibularis compartment — Lateral malleolus

FIGURE 17-9. Skin of leg reflected to the ankle.

Remove the skin from the posterior aspect of the leg to the ankle (Fig. 17-9). Leave the superficial and deep fasciae (crural fascia) intact. Identify the *small (lesser) saphenous vein,* which begins from the lateral aspect of the dorsal venous arch of the foot. The small saphenous vein ascends just inferior to the lateral malleolus, accompanying the sural nerve, and finally drains into the popliteal vein (Fig. 17-10). Observe the sural nerve and the small saphenous vein as they penetrate the deep crural fascia to travel to the popliteal fossa (Fig. 17-11). On the anterior part of the leg, on its medial side over the patellar ligament, expose the infrapatellar branch of the saphenous nerve (Fig. 17-12).

Follow the great saphenous vein toward the thigh, and clean the fat of the superficial fascia around the vein (Fig. 17-13). Expose the great saphenous vein toward the *fossa ovalis* (saphenous hiatus), the opening in the deep fascia, where the vein travels through to drain into the femoral vein. Expose the superficial and deep perforating tributaries of the great saphenous vein (Fig. 17-14).

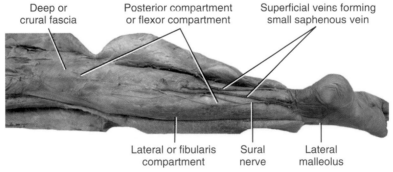

Deep or crural fascia — Posterior compartment or flexor compartment — Superficial veins forming small saphenous vein — Lateral or fibularis compartment — Sural nerve — Lateral malleolus

FIGURE 17-10. Skin of leg reflected, revealing posterior and lateral compartments, deep fascia, and small saphenous vein.

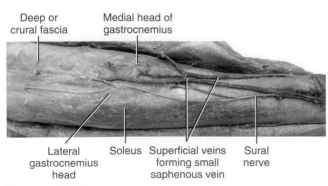

Deep or crural fascia — Medial head of gastrocnemius — Lateral gastrocnemius head — Soleus — Superficial veins forming small saphenous vein — Sural nerve

FIGURE 17-11. Reflected view shows sural nerve and small saphenous vein penetrating deep (crural) fascia to travel to popliteal fossa.

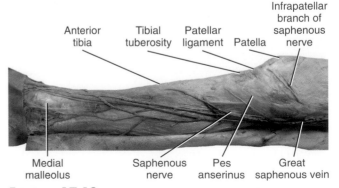

Anterior tibia — Tibial tuberosity — Patellar ligament — Patella — Infrapatellar branch of saphenous nerve — Medial malleolus — Saphenous nerve — Pes anserinus — Great saphenous vein

FIGURE 17-12. Infrapatellar branch of saphenous nerve exposed on medial side of anterior leg over patellar ligament.

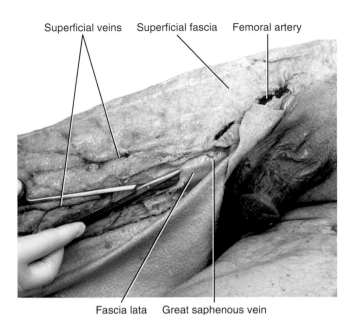

Superficial veins   Superficial fascia   Femoral artery

Fascia lata   Great saphenous vein

FIGURE 17-13. Fat of superficial fascia cleaned around great saphenous vein.

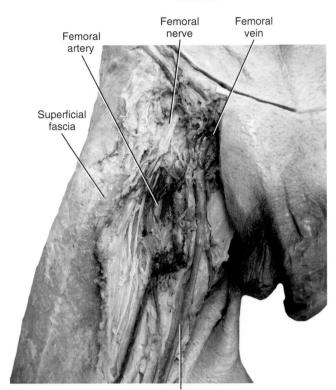

Femoral artery   Femoral nerve   Femoral vein

Superficial fascia

Great saphenous vein

FIGURE 17-15. Fat cleaned around saphenous vein, with dissection extended medially and laterally.

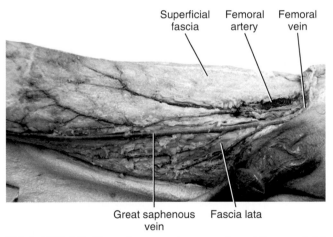

Superficial fascia   Femoral artery   Femoral vein

Great saphenous vein   Fascia lata

FIGURE 17-14. View of great saphenous vein and its superficial and deep perforating tributaries.

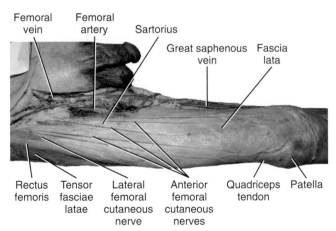

Femoral vein   Femoral artery   Sartorius   Great saphenous vein   Fascia lata

Rectus femoris   Tensor fasciae latae   Lateral femoral cutaneous nerve   Anterior femoral cutaneous nerves   Quadriceps tendon   Patella

FIGURE 17-16. Appreciate anterior cutaneous branches of femoral nerve intermingled with tributaries of great saphenous vein and rectus femoris muscle with lateral femoral cutaneous nerve.

Start cleaning fat from around the great saphenous vein, extending the dissection medially and laterally (Fig. 17-15). Do not cut through the deep fascia of the thigh, but identify the anterior cutaneous branches of the femoral nerve intermingled with the tributaries of the great saphenous vein. Lateral to the vein, identify the rectus femoris muscle. On top of and lateral to the muscle, identify the lateral femoral cutaneous nerves (Fig. 17-16).

> ⚓ *DISSECTION TIP:* Observe the lymphatics in the area of the fossa ovalis, but do not spend time exposing all of them. Realize that the inguinal lymph nodes are so named based on their position relative to the deep fascia. The deep inguinal lymph nodes are located deep to it, whereas the superficial nodes are superficial to the deep fascia.

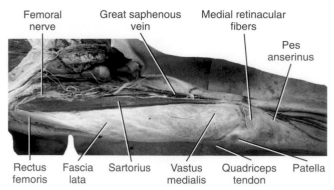

Femoral nerve — Great saphenous vein — Medial retinacular fibers — Pes anserinus

Rectus femoris — Fascia lata — Sartorius — Vastus medialis — Quadriceps tendon — Patella

FIGURE 17-17. Distal ends of dissected cutaneous nerve reflected, with deep fascia (fascia lata) cut, exposing sartorius muscle.

Cut the distal ends of the cutaneous nerves you previously dissected; reflect the nerves medially and preserve them. Cut the deep fascia of the thigh, *fascia lata,* and expose the sartorius muscle (Fig. 17-17).

Continue reflecting the fascia lata over the vastus medialis muscle (Fig. 17-18). Expose the quadriceps femoris muscles of the extensor compartment of the thigh; the vastus medialis, lateralis, and intermedius muscles; and the rectus femoris muscle and their tendons attaching to the patella. Continue the exposure by noting the fascia lata laterally and its thickened distal part, the *iliotibial tract,* attaching to the lateral condyle of the tibia (Fig. 17-19).

Reflect the rectus femoris muscle medially, and expose the vastus intermedius muscle underneath (Fig. 17-20). Place the cutaneous nerves back in their original position over the dissected muscles, and appreciate their location (Fig. 17-21).

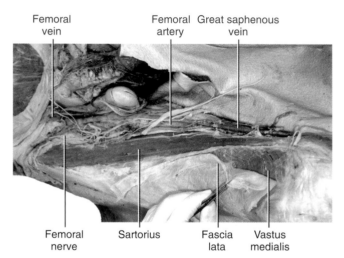

Femoral vein — Femoral artery — Great saphenous vein

Femoral nerve — Sartorius — Fascia lata — Vastus medialis

FIGURE 17-18. View of fascia lata reflected over vastus medialis muscle.

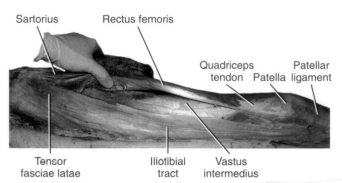

Sartorius — Rectus femoris — Quadriceps tendon — Patella — Patellar ligament

Tensor fasciae latae — Iliotibial tract — Vastus intermedius

FIGURE 17-20. Rectus femoris muscle reflected medially, exposing vastus intermedius muscle.

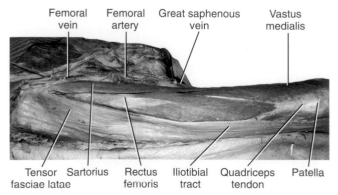

Femoral vein — Femoral artery — Great saphenous vein — Vastus medialis

Tensor fasciae latae — Sartorius — Rectus femoris — Iliotibial tract — Quadriceps tendon — Patella

FIGURE 17-19. Exposed quadriceps femoris muscles of extensor compartment of thigh with tendon attaching to patella.

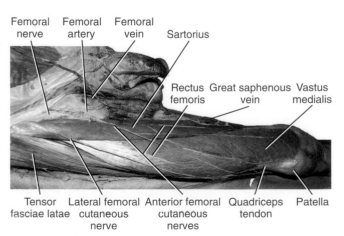

Femoral nerve — Femoral artery — Femoral vein — Sartorius

Rectus femoris — Great saphenous vein — Vastus medialis

Tensor fasciae latae — Lateral femoral cutaneous nerve — Anterior femoral cutaneous nerves — Quadriceps tendon — Patella

FIGURE 17-21. Appreciate the position of the cutaneous nerves of the anterior thigh.

Expose the femoral vein, and dissect out the *cribriform fascia*, which fills the saphenous hiatus (Fig. 17-22). Cut the femoral sheath around the femoral artery and vein. Note the relationship between the femoral artery and vein; the femoral artery is located lateral to the femoral vein. The femoral nerve lies lateral to the femoral artery (Fig. 17-23). Clean the fascia covering the femoral artery and vein, and trace these vessels underneath the inguinal ligament to the femoral canal.

Continue removing fat, and expose the adductor longus and gracilis muscles medially (Fig. 17-24). Retract the femoral artery laterally from the femoral vein and deep between these vessels note the iliopsoas muscle lying over the anterior aspect of the hip joint (Fig. 17-25).

> ☝ **DISSECTION TIP:** The area you just dissected is called the *femoral triangle*, formed by the inguinal ligament superiorly, the sartorius muscle laterally, and the adductor longus muscle medially. The pectineus and iliopsoas muscles form the floor of the triangle.

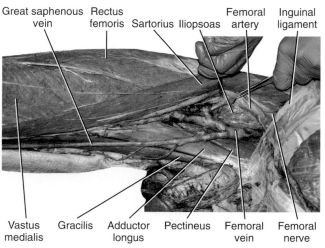

FIGURE 17-24. View of femoral artery and vein underneath inguinal ligament showing adductor longus and gracilis muscles.

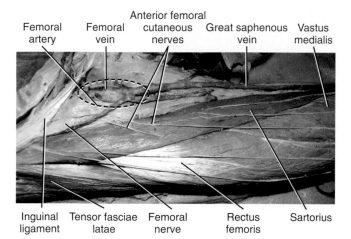

FIGURE 17-22. Femoral vein exposed, and the cribriform fascia that fills saphenous hiatus *(outlined oval)* is dissected.

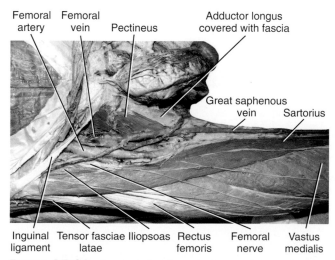

FIGURE 17-23. Femoral sheath incised around femoral artery and vein to appreciate their relationship.

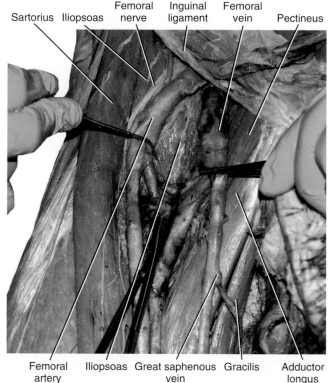

FIGURE 17-25. Femoral artery retracted laterally from femoral vein, highlighting deep-lying iliopsoas muscle over anterior aspect of capsule of hip joint.

Cut the smaller venous tributaries draining to the femoral vein for better exposure of the femoral triangle. Medial to the iliopsoas muscle, note the pectineus muscle, and more medially, the adductor longus muscle. Clean the femoral artery and vein proximal to the femoral canal, and trace the lateral femoral cutaneous nerve underneath the inguinal ligament, just medial to the anterior superior iliac spine (Fig. 17-26).

Cut the sartorius muscle at its distal quarter, and expose the adductor canal (Figs. 17-27 and 17-28).

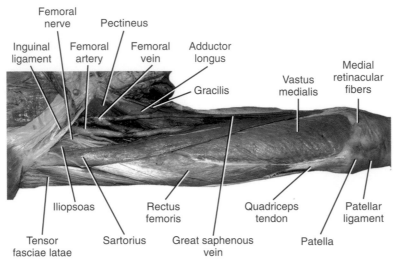

FIGURE 17-26. Femoral artery and vein cleaned proximal to femoral canal, showing lateral femoral cutaneous nerve.

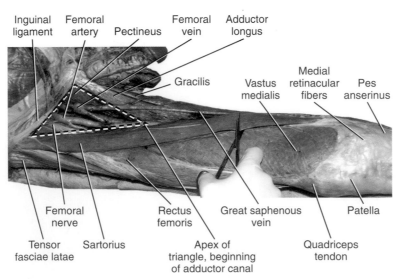

FIGURE 17-27. Smaller tributaries draining the femoral vein cut to expose femoral triangle *(outline)* and appreciate the pectineus and adductor longus muscles.

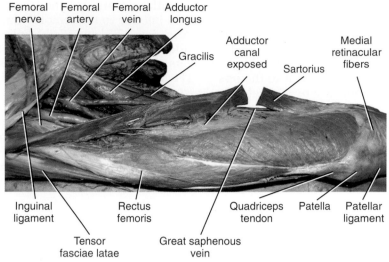

Femoral nerve   Femoral artery   Femoral vein   Adductor longus

Gracilis   Adductor canal exposed   Sartorius   Medial retinacular fibers

Inguinal ligament   Rectus femoris   Quadriceps tendon   Patella   Patellar ligament

Tensor fasciae latae   Great saphenous vein

FIGURE 17-28. View of cut sartorius muscle, exposing adductor canal.

The adductor canal is formed by the adductor magnus, adductor longus, and vastus medialis muscles. The canal begins at the apex of the femoral triangle and ends at the adductor hiatus, which is the canal formed by the adductor magnus tendon at the posterior knee. After passing through the adductor hiatus and reaching the posterior part of the knee, the femoral artery and femoral vein are termed the *popliteal artery* and *popliteal vein*. Within the adductor canal, expose and identify the femoral artery, femoral vein, saphenous nerve, nerve to the vastus medialis muscle, and descending genicular artery (Fig. 17-29).

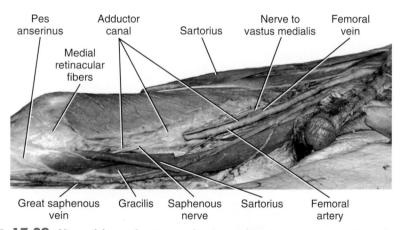

Pes anserinus   Adductor canal   Sartorius   Nerve to vastus medialis   Femoral vein

Medial retinacular fibers

Great saphenous vein   Gracilis   Saphenous nerve   Sartorius   Femoral artery

FIGURE 17-29. View of femoral artery and vein, saphenous nerve, nerve to vastus medialis muscle, and descending genicular artery within adductor canal.

Expose the aperture in the tendon of insertion of the adductor magnus, the adductor hiatus (Fig. 17-30). Identify the nerve to the vastus medialis muscle, and trace the nerve to its termination on the muscle. Distal to the level of the adductor hiatus, trace the saphenous nerve and expose it to the posteromedial aspect of the knee where it meets the great saphenous vein.

With scissors, cut the femoral vein a few centimeters inferior to the femoral canal and reflect it inferiorly (Figs. 17-31 and 17-32). Fully expose the pectineus, adductor longus, and gracilis muscles. Pull the femoral artery medially, and dissect out its branches (Figs. 17-33 and 17-34). Identify the lateral femoral circumflex artery, and expose its descending branch supplying the vastus lateralis, which travels in the muscle between the vastus lateralis and vastus intermedius (this is a fairly constant dissection landmark). The lateral femoral artery also gives off several perforating branches to the vastus intermedius.

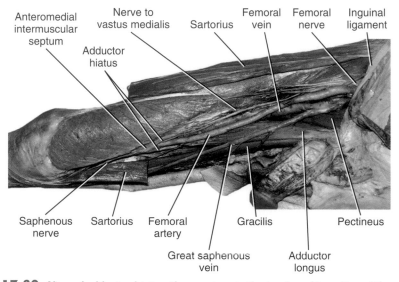

FIGURE 17-30. View of adductor hiatus, the aperture in the tendon of insertion of the adductor magnus muscle.

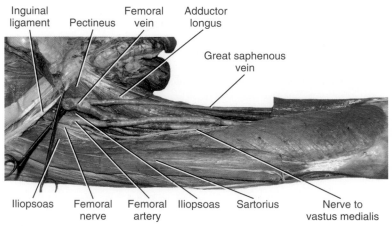

FIGURE 17-31. View of musculature with femoral vein incised inferior to the femoral canal.

Continue the dissection by exposing the deep femoral artery *(profunda femoris)* deep to the adductor longus muscle (Figs. 17-33 and 17-34). Expose several of the perforating branches mainly supplying the posterior compartment of the thigh. Identify the medial femoral circumflex artery, and expose it between the iliopsoas and pectineus muscles.

> ✍ *DISSECTION TIP:* If large enough, dissect out the transverse branch of the lateral femoral circumflex artery running to the posterior surface of the femur below the greater trochanter and contributing to the so-called cruciate anastomosis. Look for an ascending branch from the lateral circumflex artery that runs upward to anastomose with the deep circumflex iliac and superior gluteal arteries. In some specimens, a retractor is useful to retract the tissues between the adductor longus and vastus intermedius muscles.

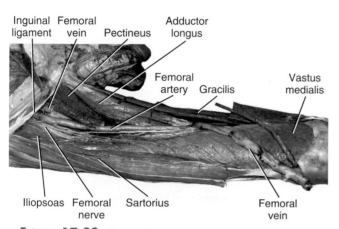

FIGURE 17-32. View with femoral vein reflected inferiorly.

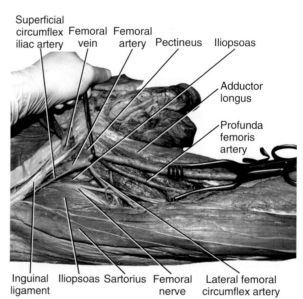

FIGURE 17-33. Femoral artery pulled medially and its branches dissected.

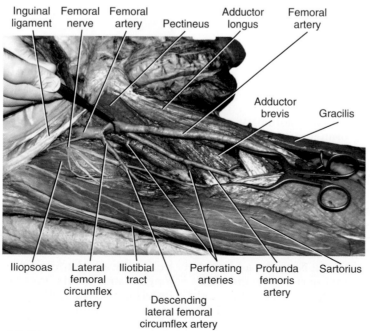

FIGURE 17-34. Appreciate lateral femoral circumflex artery and its descending branch.

DISSECTION TIP: Remember that an artery's name is based on its distribution, not its origin. The lateral circumflex femoral, medial circumflex femoral, and deep femoral arteries typically originate from a common trunk.

If time permits, from the exposed femoral artery, look for the following arteries:
- Superficial circumflex iliac artery, which travels toward the anterior superior iliac spine.
- Superficial epigastric artery, which travels upward toward the anterior abdominal wall, crossing over the inguinal canal.
- Superficial and deep external pudendal vessels typically are small arteries that anastomose with branches of the internal pudendal artery. Do not attempt to identify these two vessels.

The so-called cruciate anastomosis classically involves the confluence of four arteries posterior to the upper part of the femur: (1) the transverse branch of the lateral femoral circumflex artery, (2) the medial femoral circumflex artery, (3) the descending branch of the inferior gluteal artery, and (4) the ascending branch of the first perforating artery.

DISSECTION TIP: From personal observations, the *transverse* branch of the lateral femoral circumflex artery is only rarely significant in this anastomosis, although the *ascending* branch does participate.

In actuality, the transverse branch of the lateral femoral circumflex may be very small or absent. Anastomoses around the hip also involve other vessels like the superior gluteal, iliolumbar, deep circumflex iliac, ascending branch of the lateral circumflex, and the obturator arteries. Therefore, with occlusion of the femoral artery, many possible routes can form collateral circulation from the iliac arteries to the lower extremity.

In the space between the adductor longus and vastus intermedius muscles, identify the adductor brevis muscle (Fig. 17-35). With scissors, cut the pectineus muscle just inferior to the inguinal ligament, and reflect it laterally (Fig. 17-36). Note the adductor brevis fascia over the proximal part of the adductor brevis muscle. Remove the fascia carefully, and expose the obturator artery and nerve (Figs. 17-37 and 17-38).

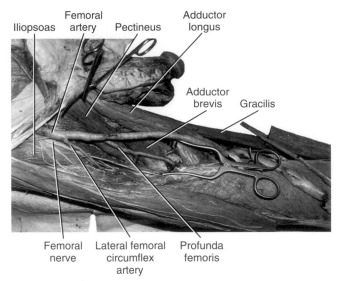

FIGURE 17-35. Appreciate adductor brevis muscle in space between adductor longus and vastus intermedius muscles.

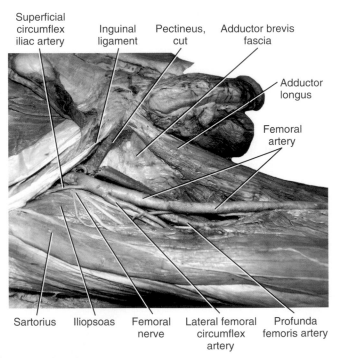

FIGURE 17-36. View with pectineus muscle incised inferior to the inguinal ligament and reflected laterally.

The *obturator nerve* splits into two divisions: anterior and posterior. The *anterior division* courses anterior to the adductor brevis to innervate the adductor longus and brevis muscles. Reflect the adductor brevis muscle laterally, and identify the *posterior division* of the obturator nerve innervating the adductor magnus.

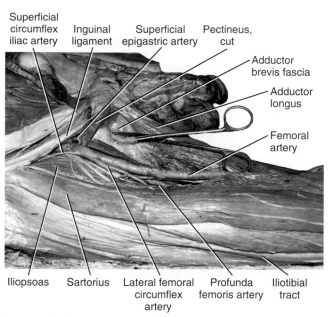

Superficial circumflex iliac artery   Inguinal ligament   Superficial epigastric artery   Pectineus, cut

Adductor brevis fascia

Adductor longus

Femoral artery

Iliopsoas   Sartorius   Lateral femoral circumflex artery   Profunda femoris artery   Iliotibial tract

FIGURE 17-37. Adductor brevis fascia removed, exposing obturator artery and nerve.

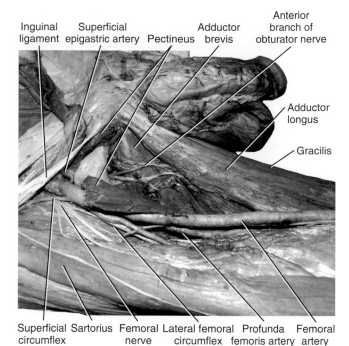

Inguinal ligament   Superficial epigastric artery   Pectineus   Adductor brevis   Anterior branch of obturator nerve

Adductor longus

Gracilis

Superficial circumflex iliac artery   Sartorius   Femoral nerve   Lateral femoral circumflex artery   Profunda femoris artery   Femoral artery

FIGURE 17-38. Adductor brevis muscle reflected laterally, revealing posterior division of obturator nerve.

LABORATORY IDENTIFICATION CHECKLIST

Nerves
❑ Femoral
   ❑ Nerve to vastus medialis
   ❑ Nerve to rectus femoris
   ❑ Nerve to vastus lateralis
   ❑ Nerve to vastus intermedius
❑ Saphenous
❑ Lateral femoral cutaneous
❑ Obturator
   ❑ Anterior division
   ❑ Posterior division
❑ Sciatic
   ❑ Tibial
   ❑ Common fibular
   ❑ Posterior cutaneous, of thigh

Arteries
❑ Femoral
❑ Superficial epigastric
❑ Superficial circumflex iliac
❑ Superficial external pudendal
❑ Deep external pudendal
❑ Profunda femoris
❑ Medial femoral circumflex
❑ Lateral femoral circumflex
❑ Perforating arteries

Arteries—cont'd
❑ Descending genicular
❑ Popliteal
❑ Superior genicular arteries
❑ Middle genicular
❑ Inferior genicular arteries
❑ Obturator
   ❑ Acetabular branch

Veins
❑ Great saphenous
❑ Small (lesser) saphenous
❑ Superficial epigastric
❑ Superficial circumflex iliac
❑ External pudendal
❑ Lateral femoral cutaneous
❑ Popliteal
❑ Profunda femoris
❑ Femoral

Connective Tissue
❑ Femoral fascia (fascia lata)
❑ Anteromedial intermuscular septum
❑ Medial intermuscular septum
❑ Lateral intermuscular septum
❑ Posterior intermuscular septum
❑ Vastoadductor membrane

Ligaments
❑ *Hip*
   ❑ Iliofemoral
   ❑ Pubofemoral
   ❑ Ischiofemoral
   ❑ Ligamentum teres
   ❑ Acetabular labrum/ transverse acetabular
❑ *Knee*
   ❑ Anterior cruciate
   ❑ Posterior cruciate
   ❑ Transverse
   ❑ Tibial (medial) collateral
      ❑ Superficial component
      ❑ Deep component
   ❑ Fibular (lateral) collateral
   ❑ Oblique popliteal (actually a tendon)

Cartilage
❑ Medial meniscus
❑ Lateral meniscus

LABORATORY IDENTIFICATION CHECKLIST—CONT'D

Muscles
- ❏ *Anterior compartment (extensor compartment)*
  - ❏ Sartorius
  - ❏ Iliopsoas
  - ❏ Iliacus
  - ❏ Rectus femoris
  - ❏ Vastus medialis
  - ❏ Vastus lateralis
  - ❏ Vastus intermedius
  - ❏ Articularis genus
- ❏ *Femoral triangle*
  - ❏ Borders
    - ❏ Inguinal ligament, superior border
    - ❏ Adductor longus, medial border
    - ❏ Sartorius, lateral border
  - ❏ Floor
    - ❏ Iliacus
    - ❏ Psoas
    - ❏ Pectineus
  - ❏ Contents (medial to lateral)
    - ❏ Femoral canal with lymphatics
    - ❏ Femoral vein
    - ❏ Femoral artery
    - ❏ Femoral nerve

Muscles—cont'd
- ❏ *Adductor canal (subsartorial, or Hunter's canal)*
  - Extends from femoral triangle apex to adductor hiatus
  - ❏ Contents
    - ❏ Femoral artery
    - ❏ Femoral vein
    - ❏ Nerve to vastus medialis
    - ❏ Saphenous nerve
    - ❏ Descending genicular
- ❏ *Tendons/retinacula*
  - ❏ Quadriceps tendon
  - ❏ Patellar ligament
  - ❏ Medial retinaculum
  - ❏ Lateral retinaculum
- ❏ *Medial compartment (adductor compartment)*
  - ❏ Gracilis
  - ❏ Pectineus
  - ❏ Obturator externus
  - ❏ Adductor longus
  - ❏ Adductor brevis
  - ❏ Adductor magnus
  - ❏ Femoral head
  - ❏ Ischial or hamstring head
  - ❏ Adductor minimus

Muscles—cont'd
- ❏ *Posterior compartment (flexor compartment)*
  - ❏ Biceps femoris
    - ❏ Long head
    - ❏ Short head
  - ❏ Semitendinosus muscle
  - ❏ Semimembranosus muscle
- ❏ *Pes anserinus*
  - ❏ Sartorius
  - ❏ Gracilis
  - ❏ Semitendinosus

Bursae
- ❏ Suprapatellar
- ❏ Prepatellar
- ❏ Infrapatellar

Bones
- ❏ Coxal (hip bone)
- ❏ Femur
- ❏ Patella
- ❏ Proximal tibia
- ❏ Proximal fibula

CHAPTER 18

LEG AND ANKLE

Netter: 494–510

McMinn: 330–347

Gray's Atlas: 298–309, 319–328

Identify the great and small (lesser) saphenous veins and the saphenous and sural nerves, from the previous dissection of the thigh and leg in Chapter 17.

Insert scissors or a probe between the semitendinosus and biceps femoris muscles into the popliteal fossa, and remove the superficial adipose tissue (Fig. 18-1). Insert scissors or a probe underneath the crural fascia (Fig. 18-2), and divide the fascia into two parts (Fig. 18-3). Reflect the semitendinosus and biceps femoris muscles laterally, and expose the contents of the popliteal fossa (Fig. 18-4). Note the sciatic nerve dividing into the tibial and common fibular nerves.

Clean the fat and the lymphatics within the popliteal fossa and identify the following structures:
- Posterior femoral cutaneous nerve
- Small saphenous vein
- Tibial nerve
- Common fibular nerve
- Popliteal vein
- Popliteal artery

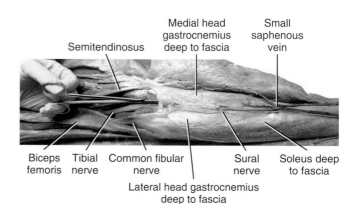

FIGURE 18-2. Scissors are placed deep to the crural fascia, highlighting the lateral and medial heads of the gastrocnemius muscle and small saphenous vein.

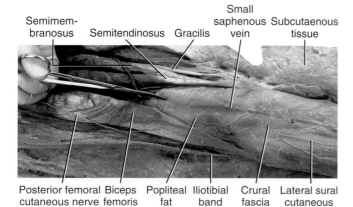

FIGURE 18-1. Scissors inserted between semitendinosus and biceps femoris muscles, into popliteal fossa, with superficial adipose tissue removed.

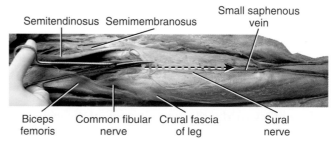

FIGURE 18-3. Broken arrow indicates crural fascia cut into two parts.

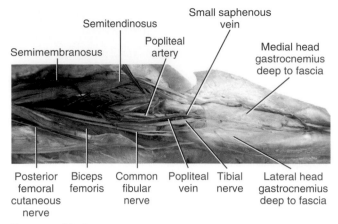

FIGURE 18-4. Semitendinosus and biceps femoris muscles reflected laterally, exposing contents of the popliteal fossa.

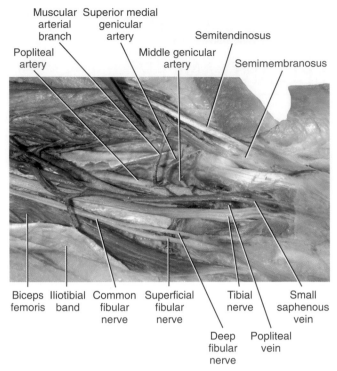

FIGURE 18-5. Appreciate the divisions of the popliteal artery into anterior and posterior tibial arteries.

👆 *DISSECTION TIP:* Identify the following landmarks (see also Chapter 17):

The *great saphenous vein* and the saphenous nerve accompany each other along the medial aspect of the leg and thigh.

The *small saphenous vein* and the sural nerve accompany each other along the posterior aspect of the leg. The small saphenous vein usually drains into the popliteal vein and often exhibits anastomoses with the great saphenous vein.

The *sural nerve* is formed by the union of the medial sural cutaneous nerve, a branch of the tibial nerve, and a communicating branch of the lateral sural cutaneous nerve arising from the common fibular nerve. The sural nerve terminates as the *lateral dorsal cutaneous nerve* on the lateral foot.

Clean the popliteal artery, and identify its division into anterior and posterior tibial arteries. Look for the popliteal artery's genicular branches, the superolateral, superomedial, inferolateral, inferomedial, and middle genicular arteries (Fig. 18-5).

Do not try to identify every branch of the genicular arteries; some are often too small. Similarly, exposing the anastomoses around the knee requires special preparation of the specimen (e.g., filling arteries with red latex).

👆 *DISSECTION TIP:*

Superolateral and superomedial genicular arteries; remove the fat just superior to the lateral and medial condyles of the femur, at the origin of the medial and lateral heads of the gastrocnemius muscle, respectively.

Middle genicular artery, usually found arising from the anterior surface of the popliteal artery (deep from your view) just posterior to the knee joint.

Inferolateral genicular artery, usually found underneath the lateral head of the gastrocnemius muscle.

Inferomedial genicular artery, usually found underneath the medial head of the gastrocnemius muscle.

Completely remove the crural fascia from the underlying muscles of the posterior compartment of the leg, without disturbing the superficial veins and cutaneous nerves (Figs. 18-6 and 18-7). Identify the medial and lateral heads of the gastrocnemius muscle, and retract them laterally (Fig. 18-8). Trace the tibial nerve and identify its medial sural cutaneous branch. Expose all the muscles of the posterior and lateral compartments (Figs. 18-9 and 18-10). Identify the common fibular nerve and trace its course from the thigh to the neck of the fibula (Fig. 18-11).

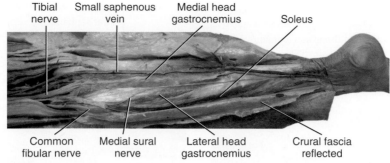

Tibial nerve · Small saphenous vein · Medial head gastrocnemius · Soleus

Common fibular nerve · Medial sural nerve · Lateral head gastrocnemius · Crural fascia reflected

FIGURE 18-6. View with crural fascia removed from underlying musculature of posterior compartment.

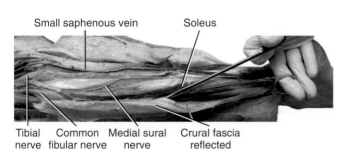

Small saphenous vein · Soleus

Tibial nerve · Common fibular nerve · Medial sural nerve · Crural fascia reflected

FIGURE 18-7. Removing fascia, being careful not to disturb superficial veins and cutaneous nerves.

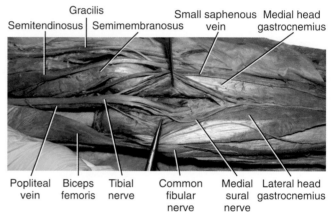

Gracilis · Semitendinosus · Semimembranosus · Small saphenous vein · Medial head gastrocnemius

Popliteal vein · Biceps femoris · Tibial nerve · Common fibular nerve · Medial sural nerve · Lateral head gastrocnemius

FIGURE 18-8. Close-up view with medial and lateral heads of gastrocnemius muscle retracted laterally.

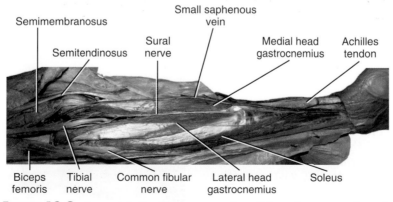

Semimembranosus · Semitendinosus · Sural nerve · Small saphenous vein · Medial head gastrocnemius · Achilles tendon

Biceps femoris · Tibial nerve · Common fibular nerve · Lateral head gastrocnemius · Soleus

FIGURE 18-9. Appreciate the tibial nerve and medial sural cutaneous branch.

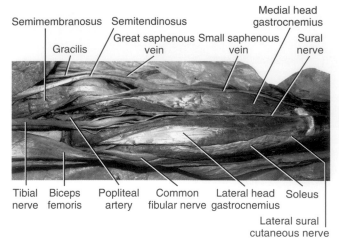

Semimembranosus Semitendinosus
Gracilis Great saphenous Small saphenous Medial head gastrocnemius
vein vein Sural nerve
Tibial Biceps Popliteal Common Lateral head Soleus
nerve femoris artery fibular nerve gastrocnemius
Lateral sural cutaneous nerve

FIGURE 18-10. Exposure of muscles of posterior and lateral compartments.

Semimembranosus Semitendinosus
Gracilis Great saphenous Popliteal Popliteal Medial head gastrocnemius
vein artery vein
Biceps Tibial Common Neck of Medial sural Lateral head
femoris nerve fibular nerve fibula nerve gastrocnemius

FIGURE 18-11. Find common fibular nerve, coursing from thigh to neck of fibula.

Detach the lateral head of the gastrocnemius muscle from the underlying soleus muscle (Fig. 18-12). Look for the *Achilles tendon,* the common tendon of the gastrocnemius and soleus muscles inserting onto the calcaneus.

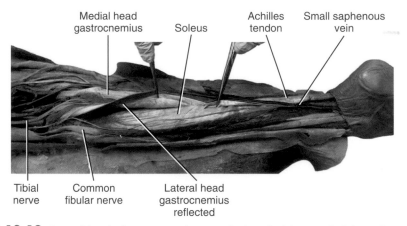

Medial head Achilles Small saphenous
gastrocnemius Soleus tendon vein
Tibial Common Lateral head
nerve fibular nerve gastrocnemius reflected

FIGURE 18-12. Lateral head of gastrocnemius muscle detached from underlying soleus muscle.

Preserve the lateral sural cutaneous nerve as you reflect the lateral head of the gastrocnemius. Similarly, preserve the medial sural cutaneous nerve and the tibial nerve as you reflect the gastrocnemius muscle.

Expose the underlying soleus muscle, and identify the tendon of the plantaris muscle on the posterior surface of the soleus (Fig. 18-13). Cut the lateral head of the gastrocnemius at the level of the femoral

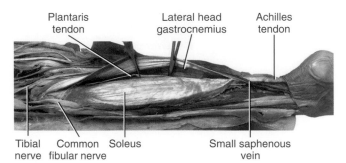

Plantaris Lateral head Achilles
tendon gastrocnemius tendon
Tibial Common Soleus Small saphenous
nerve fibular nerve vein

FIGURE 18-13. The gastrocnemius muscle reflected, preserving the lateral and medial sural cutaneous nerves and the tibial nerve, and exposing the underlying soleus muscle and the tendon of the plantaris muscle on the posterior surface of the soleus muscle.

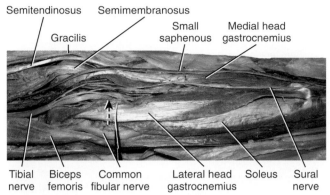

FIGURE 18-14. Lateral head of gastrocnemius muscle cut at level of femoral condyle.

condyle (Fig. 18-14). Reflect the lateral head of the gastrocnemius muscle medially, and expose the tendon of the plantaris muscle (Fig. 18-15). Identify the muscle belly of the plantaris muscle, and identify the branch from the tibial nerve, the nerve to the soleus muscle (Figs. 18-16 and 18-17).

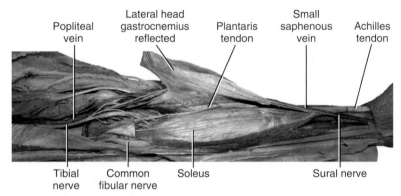

FIGURE 18-15. Lateral head of the gastrocnemius muscle reflected medially, exposing the tendon of plantaris muscle.

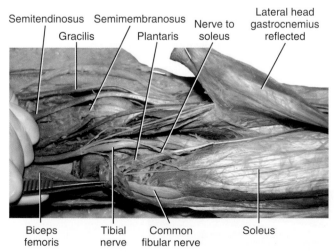

FIGURE 18-16. Close-up view highlights muscle belly of plantaris.

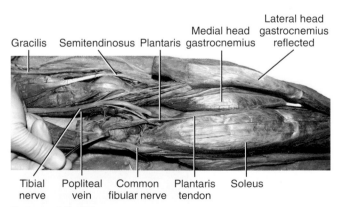

FIGURE 18-17. Further reflection, highlighting popliteal vein and tibial nerve.

With forceps, lift the lateral border of the soleus muscle and detach it from the underlying fascia over the flexor hallucis longus and flexor digitorum longus muscles (Fig. 18-18). With scissors, cut the soleus muscle close to its attachment to the tibia and fibula, and reflect it medially (Fig. 18-19). Clean the fascia and expose the flexor hallucis longus and flexor digitorum longus muscles as well as the muscles of the lateral compartment of the leg, the fibularis longus and fibularis brevis (Figs. 18-20 and 8-21).

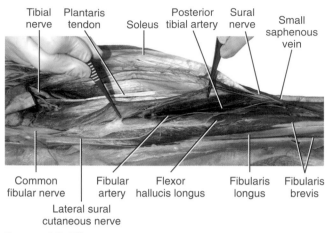

FIGURE 18-18. Lateral border of soleus muscle detached from underlying fascia over flexor hallucis longus and flexor digitorum longus muscles.

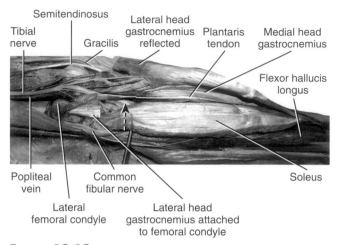

FIGURE 18-19. Soleus muscle cut (see *arrow*) proximal to tibiofibular attachment and reflected medially.

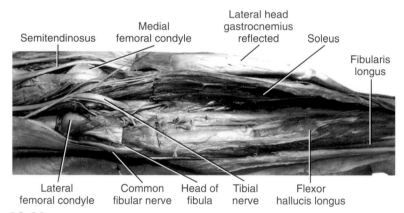

FIGURE 18-20. Fascia cleaned, exposing flexor hallucis longus, flexor digitorum longus, and lateral compartment muscles.

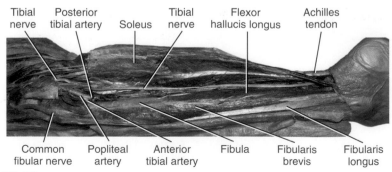

FIGURE 18-21. Fibula cleaned, exposing the division of the popliteal artery into anterior and posterior tibial arteries.

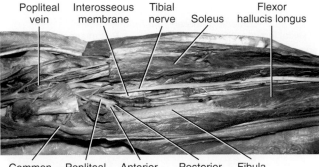

Popliteal vein   Interosseous membrane   Tibial nerve   Soleus   Flexor hallucis longus

Common fibular nerve   Popliteal artery   Anterior tibial artery   Posterior tibial artery   Fibula

FIGURE 18-22. Tibialis posterior muscle exposed along posterior surface of interosseous membrane.

Clean the fibula; lateral to it, expose the division of the popliteal artery into anterior and posterior tibial arteries (Fig. 18-22). The anterior tibial artery travels anterior to the interosseous membrane, while the posterior tibial artery gives rise to a fibular branch that travels to the lateral compartment and deep to the flexor hallucis longus muscle. Expose the tibialis posterior muscle as it travels along the posterior surface of the interosseous membrane to reach the bones of the foot (Fig. 18-22). Trace the division of the common fibular nerve into deep and superficial fibular nerves.

> **✋ DISSECTION TIP:** Soon after arriving from the common fibular nerve the superficial fibular nerve enters the lateral compartment of the leg.

Place the cadaver in the supine position, and observe the knee joint. Identify the tendon of the quadriceps femoris muscle attaching to the patella. Identify the patellar ligament and the strong, thick fascia on the medial and lateral sides of the knee joint, the *medial and lateral retinacula* of the knee (Fig. 18-23).

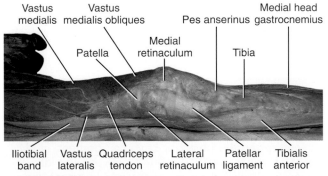

Vastus medialis   Vastus medialis obliques   Pes anserinus   Medial head gastrocnemius

Patella   Medial retinaculum   Tibia

Iliotibial band   Vastus lateralis   Quadriceps tendon   Lateral retinaculum   Patellar ligament   Tibialis anterior

FIGURE 18-23. Supine position, highlighting tendon of quadriceps femoris muscle, patellar ligament, and thick fascia on sides of knee joint (medial/lateral retinacula).

Cut the medial and lateral retinacula, and expose the patellar ligament and the tendon of the quadriceps femoris muscle (Fig. 18-24). With scissors, cut the patellar ligament close to the tibial tuberosity (Fig. 18-25). Continue the incision with a scalpel lateral and medial to the patella (Fig. 18-26).

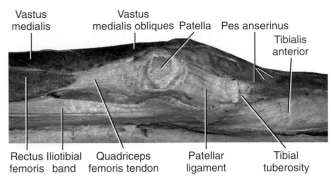

Vastus medialis   Vastus medialis obliques   Patella   Pes anserinus   Tibialis anterior

Rectus femoris   Iliotibial band   Quadriceps femoris tendon   Patellar ligament   Tibial tuberosity

FIGURE 18-24. Medial and lateral retinacula cut, exposing patellar ligament and quadriceps femoris tendon.

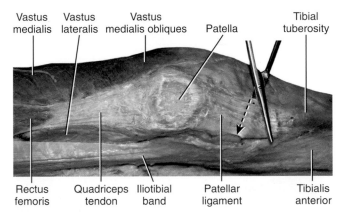

Vastus medialis   Vastus lateralis   Vastus medialis obliques   Patella   Tibial tuberosity

Rectus femoris   Quadriceps tendon   Iliotibial band   Patellar ligament   Tibialis anterior

FIGURE 18-25. Patellar ligament scissors-cut *(arrow)* close to tibial tuberosity.

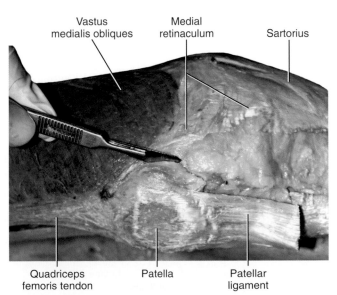

Vastus medialis obliques   Medial retinaculum   Sartorius

Quadriceps femoris tendon   Patella   Patellar ligament

FIGURE 18-26. Incision continued with scalpel lateral and medial to patella.

Detach the patella from its subcutaneous prepatellar and infrapatellar bursae and fat, and reflect it superiorly, preserving its attachment to the quadriceps femoris tendon (Fig. 18-27). Reflect the attachment of the vastus medialis muscle from the medial side of the knee, and expose this area (Figs. 18-28 and 18-29). Similarly, cut the tendon of the biceps femoris muscle from the head of the fibula. After releasing these attachments, flex the knee joint (Fig. 18-30).

On the medial side of the knee joint, inferior and medial to the tuberosity of the tibia, trace the

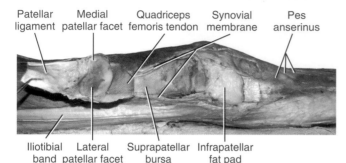

FIGURE 18-27. Patella detached from bursae and fat and reflected superiorly, retaining quadriceps femoris muscle attachment.

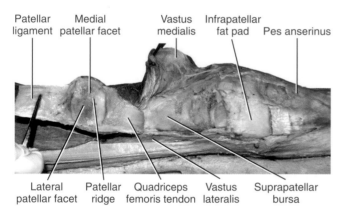

FIGURE 18-28. Vastus medialis muscle reflected from medial side of knee.

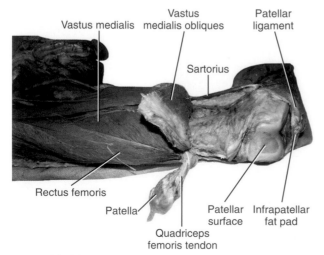

FIGURE 18-29. Tendon of biceps femoris muscle incised from the head of fibula.

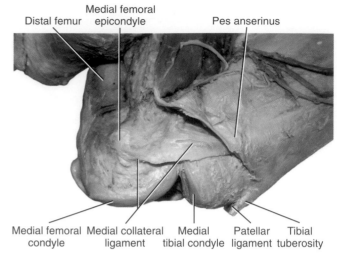

FIGURE 18-30. Knee flexed at joint to locate pes anserinus.

common insertion of the tendons of the sartorius, gracilis, and semitendinosus muscles, the *pes anserinus* (Fig. 18-30). Just superior to the pes anserinus, identify the *tibial* (medial) collateral ligament.

> ✎ *DISSECTION TIP:* The medial collateral ligament is a thick band of connective tissue that extends from the medial femoral epicondyle to the medial tibial condyle; it also attaches to the medial meniscus.

Using scissors, cut the tibial (medial) collateral ligament (Fig. 18-31). Similarly, cut the biceps femoris tendon, and identify a thick band of connective tissue extending between the lateral femoral condyle to the head of the fibula, the *fibular* (lateral) collateral ligament.

Remove the infrapatellar fat pad and infrapatellar synovial fold, to expose the anterior cruciate ligament and the medial and lateral menisci between the femur and tibia (Figs. 18-32 and 18-33). Further expose the anterior cruciate ligament (Fig. 18-34). With scissors, cut the anterior cruciate ligament and expose the posterior cruciate ligament (Figs. 18-35 and 18-36). To expose the posterior cruciate ligament clearly, flex the knee joint farther and observe the ligament as it is stretched.

> ✎ *DISSECTION TIP:* If time permits, cut the posterior part of the fibrous capsule of the knee joint. Again, identify the lateral and medial menisci and the posterior cruciate ligament. Find a thick connective tissue band between the lateral meniscus and the posterior cruciate ligament, the posterior *meniscofemoral ligament*.

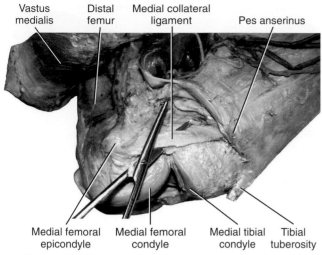

Vastus medialis — Distal femur — Medial collateral ligament — Pes anserinus

Medial femoral epicondyle — Medial femoral condyle — Medial tibial condyle — Tibial tuberosity

FIGURE 18-31. View of cut medial collateral ligament.

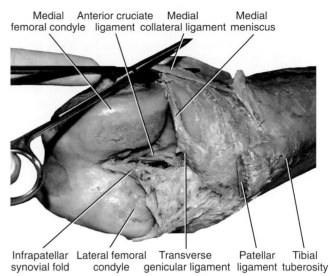

Medial femoral condyle — Anterior cruciate ligament — Medial collateral ligament — Medial meniscus

Infrapatellar synovial fold — Lateral femoral condyle — Transverse genicular ligament — Patellar ligament — Tibial tuberosity

FIGURE 18-32. Close-up view of cut lateral collateral ligament.

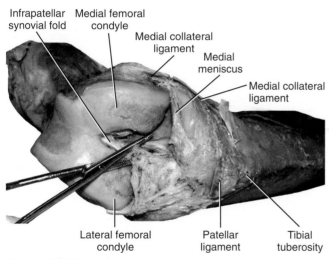

Infrapatellar synovial fold — Medial femoral condyle — Medial collateral ligament — Medial meniscus — Medial collateral ligament

Lateral femoral condyle — Patellar ligament — Tibial tuberosity

FIGURE 18-33. Infrapatellar fat pad and synovial fold removed, exposing anterior cruciate ligament and medial/lateral menisci.

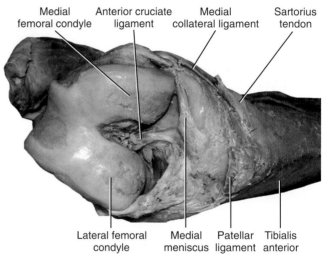

Medial femoral condyle — Anterior cruciate ligament — Medial collateral ligament — Sartorius tendon

Lateral femoral condyle — Medial meniscus — Patellar ligament — Tibialis anterior

FIGURE 18-34. View of exposed anterior cruciate ligament.

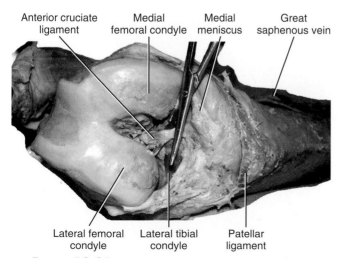

Anterior cruciate ligament — Medial femoral condyle — Medial meniscus — Great saphenous vein

Lateral femoral condyle — Lateral tibial condyle — Patellar ligament

FIGURE 18-35. View of cut anterior cruciate ligament.

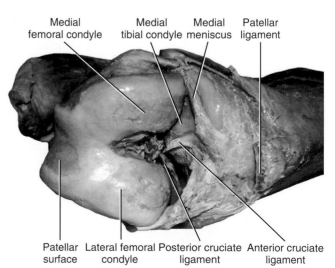

Medial femoral condyle — Medial tibial condyle — Medial meniscus — Patellar ligament

Patellar surface — Lateral femoral condyle — Posterior cruciate ligament — Anterior cruciate ligament

FIGURE 18-36. In this view, appreciate the posterior cruciate ligament.

With the cadaver supine, remove the remaining skin over the leg and expose the *crural fascia* (deep fascia) over the anterior compartment of the leg (Figs. 18-37 and 18-38). Make a midline longitudinal incision along the lateral side of the anterior border of the tibia, reflecting the crural fascia laterally (Fig. 18-39). Identify the *superior extensor retinaculum,* a flat, broad part of the deep fascia extending from the tibia to the fibula above the lateral malleolus (Fig. 18-40).

Identify the *tibialis anterior* muscle. Place your fingertip on its inferior border, and with blunt dissection, expose the extensor digitorum longus muscle. Trace its tendons onto the dorsum of the foot toward the lateral four digits (Figs. 18-41 and 18-42). Look for a tendon of the extensor digitorum longus attaching onto the base of the 5th metatarsal bone; this is the *fibularis tertius* muscle. Identify on the lateral side of the leg in the lateral compartment the fibularis longus and fibularis brevis muscles.

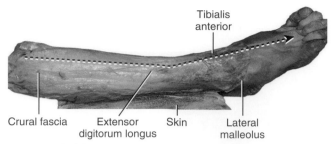

FIGURE 18-38. Broken arrow shows midline longitudinal incision along lateral side of anterior border of the tibia.

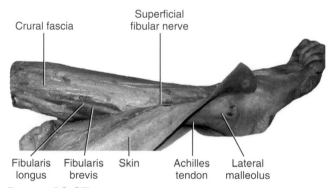

FIGURE 18-37. Remaining skin over leg removed, exposing crural fascia over anterior compartment.

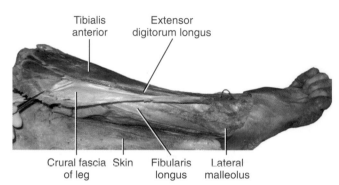

FIGURE 18-39. View of crural fascia reflected laterally.

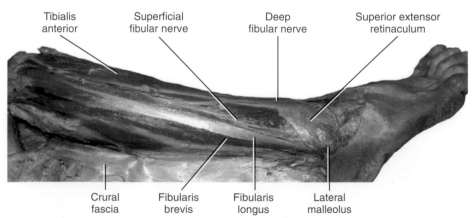

FIGURE 18-40. In this view, appreciate the superior extensor retinaculum.

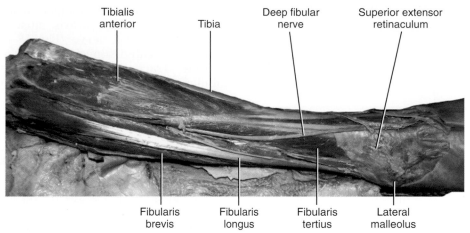

Tibialis anterior   Tibia   Deep fibular nerve   Superior extensor retinaculum

Fibularis brevis   Fibularis longus   Fibularis tertius   Lateral malleolus

FIGURE 18-41. View of tibialis anterior muscle, with exposed extensor digitorum longus muscle.

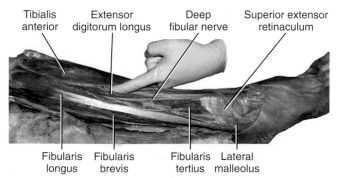

Tibialis anterior   Extensor digitorum longus   Deep fibular nerve   Superior extensor retinaculum

Fibularis longus   Fibularis brevis   Fibularis tertius   Lateral malleolus

FIGURE 18-42. Extensor digitorum longus tendons on dorsum of foot toward lateral four digits.

Identify the anterior *intermuscular septum,* which separates the anterior compartment from the lateral compartment of the leg. Appreciate the extensor hallucis longus muscle in the space between the tibialis anterior and extensor digitorum longus muscles (Fig. 18-43). Follow the tendon of the extensor hallucis longus to its insertion onto the base of the distal phalanx of the 1st digit.

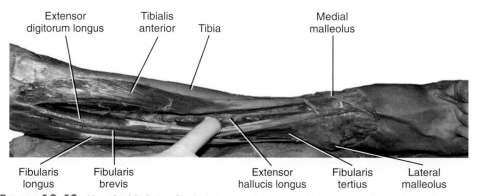

Extensor digitorum longus   Tibialis anterior   Tibia   Medial malleolus

Fibularis longus   Fibularis brevis   Extensor hallucis longus   Fibularis tertius   Lateral malleolus

FIGURE 18-43. View highlighting fibularis tertius, longus, and brevis muscles; anterior intermuscular septum; and extensor hallucis longus muscle.

DISSECTION TIP: To better visualize the deep part of the anterior compartment, place two retractors (one proximal and one distal) between the tibialis anterior and fibularis longus muscles (Fig. 18-44).

Identify the *interosseous membrane* and the area between the extensor digitorum longus and tibialis anterior muscles (Fig. 18-44). Expose the deep fibular nerve, which is accompanied by the anterior tibial artery (Fig. 18-45). Further expose the deep fibular nerve and anterior tibial artery to the dorsum of the foot (Fig. 18-46).

Reflect the fibularis longus muscle inferiorly, and expose the fibularis brevis muscle as well as the superficial fibular nerve (Fig. 18-47). The fibularis longus is located superficially to the fibularis brevis muscle. Trace the insertion of the tendon of the fibularis brevis onto the tuberosity of the 5th metatarsal bone.

DISSECTION TIP: To highlight dissection landmarks, clean the fascia over the anteromedial surface of the tibia and expose the periosteum (Fig. 18-48).

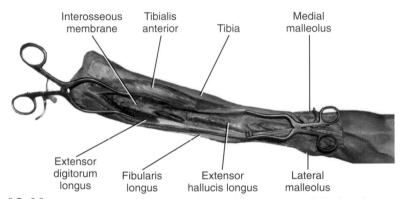

FIGURE 18-44. Retractors placed between the tibialis anterior and fibularis longus muscles, highlighting the deep part of the anterior compartment.

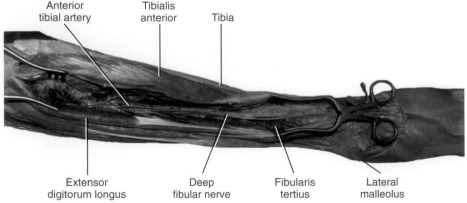

FIGURE 18-45. Appreciate the deep fibular nerve traveling anterior to the interosseous membrane.

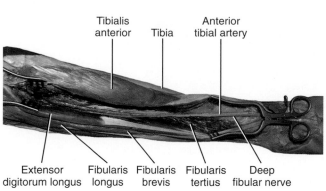

FIGURE 18-46. Deep fibular nerve and anterior tibial artery exposed to dorsum of foot.

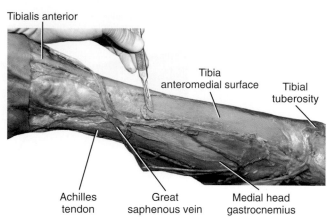

FIGURE 18-48. Cleaning fascia over anteromedial tibial surface, exposing periosteum.

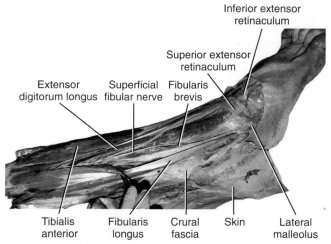

FIGURE 18-47. Fibularis longus muscle reflected inferiorly, exposing fibularis brevis muscle as well as superficial fibular nerve.

Using a scalpel, make a shallow, circumferential incision on the dorsum of the foot (Fig. 18-49). Reflect the skin over the dorsum of the foot, and expose the tendons of the extensor hallucis and extensor digitorum muscles. Identify and expose the dorsal venous arch, then trace the small saphenous vein at the lateral aspect of the arch and the great saphenous vein at the medial portion of the dorsal venous arch traveling superiorly, anterior to the medial malleolus.

✋ *DISSECTION TIP:* The skin of the dorsum of the foot is thin; therefore the incision needs to be shallow. Do not spend too much time exposing the entire dorsal venous arch.

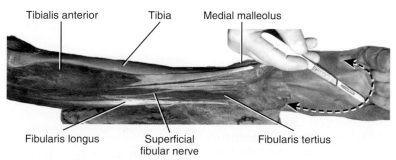

FIGURE 18-49. Shallow circumferential incision *(double-headed arrow)* on dorsum of foot.

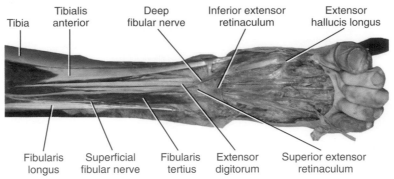

FIGURE 18-50. Appreciate superior and inferior parts of extensor retinaculum.

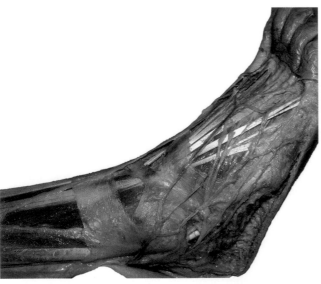

FIGURE 18-51. Note the inferior extensor retinaculum as a Y-shaped band of deep fascia forming a passage for the tendons of the extensor digitorum longus and fibularis tertius muscles.

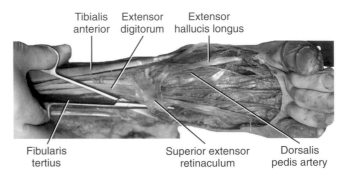

FIGURE 18-52. Superior part of extensor retinaculum cut over tendons of extensor digitorum muscle.

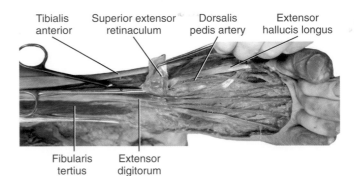

FIGURE 18-53. Inferior part of extensor retinaculum incised, showing deeper structures.

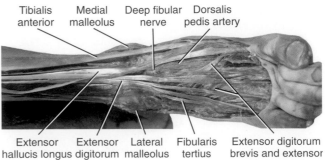

FIGURE 18-54. Tendons of extensor digitorum, extensor hallucis longus, tibialis anterior, and fibularis tertius separated from underlying bursae and soft tissue.

Identify the extensor retinaculum, divided into the superior and inferior parts. Again, the superior extensor retinaculum extends from the tibia to the fibula above the lateral malleolus as a broad, flat part of the deep fascia (Fig. 18-50). The inferior extensor retinaculum is a Y-shaped band of deep fascia forming a passage for the tendons of the extensor digitorum longus and fibularis tertius muscles. The inferior extensor retinaculum attaches to the *medial malleolus* (upper part) and to the *plantar aponeurosis* (lower band) (Figs. 18-50 and 18-51).

Cut the superior and inferior portions of the extensor retinaculum over the tendons of the extensor digitorum muscle (Figs. 18-52 and 18-53). Free the tendons of the extensor digitorum, extensor hallucis longus, tibialis anterior, and fibularis tertius muscles from the underlying bursae and soft tissues, toward their insertions (Fig. 18-54). Identify the extensor digitorum brevis and its medial part, the extensor hallucis brevis, inserting onto the base of the proximal phalanx of the first digit.

Follow the anterior tibial artery to the level of the ankle joint between the extensor hallucis and extensor digitorum longus muscles, where the anterior tibial artery becomes the dorsalis pedis artery (Fig. 18-54). The dorsalis pedis artery is absent in approximately 20% of the population.

✋ *DISSECTION TIP:* If time permits, continue the dissection as follows:
Trace out the tendon of the extensor hallucis longus muscle to the distal phalanx of the 1st digit.
Compare the extensor hallucis longus with the extensor digitorum longus muscle inserting onto the middle and distal phalanges.
Follow the terminal branches of the dorsalis pedis artery: deep plantar branch and 1st metatarsal branch.

Continue the dissection along the lateral aspect of ankle joint at the level of the *lateral malleolus* (Fig. 18-55). Expose the tendons of the fibularis brevis and fibularis longus muscles (Fig. 18-56). Clean the fat around the lateral malleolus, and expose the structures of this region (Fig. 18-57).

Cut the skin over the medial malleolus and expose the crural fascia (Figs. 18-58 and 18-59). With scissors, cut the crural fascia over the medial malleolus (Fig. 18-60). Identify the flexor retinaculum attaching between the medial malleolus and the medial surface of the calcaneus. This retinaculum forms the tarsal tunnel.

Cut the flexor retinaculum, and expose the tibial nerve, the posterior tibial artery, the tibialis posterior muscle, the flexor digitorum longus muscle, and the Achilles tendon. Clean the fascia and the soft tissues over these structures, and free them from the

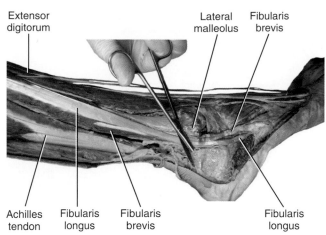

FIGURE 18-56. View of exposed tendons of fibularis brevis and fibularis longus muscles.

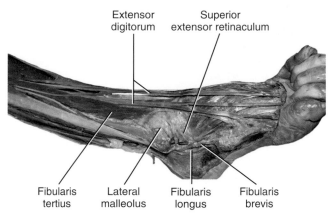

FIGURE 18-57. Fat cleaned around lateral malleolus, exposing local structures.

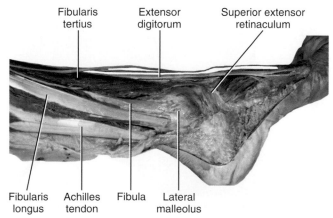

FIGURE 18-55. Dissection continued along the lateral aspect of the ankle joint at the lateral malleolus.

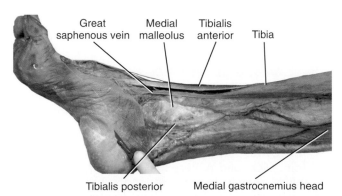

FIGURE 18-58. View of skin incision over medial malleolus.

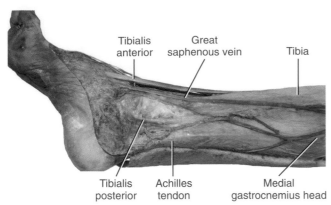

FIGURE 18-59. View with exposed crural fascia.

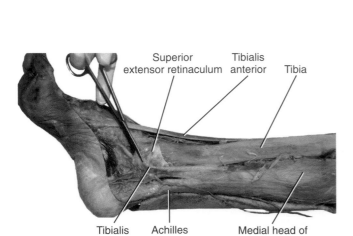

FIGURE 18-60. Crural (deep) fascia cut over medial malleolus.

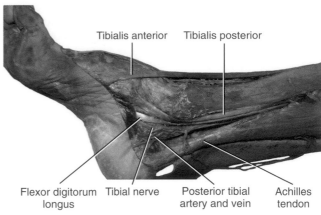

FIGURE 18-61. Flexor retinaculum cut to expose tibial nerve, posterior tibial artery, tibialis posterior and flexor digitorum longus muscles, and Achilles tendon.

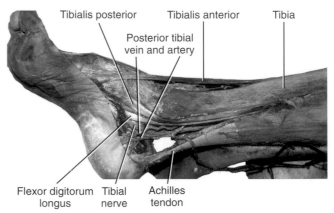

FIGURE 18-62. With fascia and soft tissue cleaned, landmarks freed from adjacent structures.

adjacent structures (Figs. 18-61 and 18-62). The relationship of these structures is important for their recognition (Figs. 18-63 and 18-64). From anterior to posterior, the structures are arranged as follows:
- Tendon of tibialis posterior muscle
- Tendon of flexor digitorum longus muscle
- Posterior tibial artery and vein
- Tibial nerve
- Flexor hallucis longus muscle

DISSECTION TIP: To remember the relationship of these structures at the medial malleolus, use one of the following mnemonics:
  Tom, Dick, And Harry
  Tom Drives A Very Nervous Horse
  Tom, Dick, and A Very Nervous Harry
If time permits, expose the tendon of the tibialis posterior muscle to the navicular (scaphoid) bone, one of its many insertion sites.

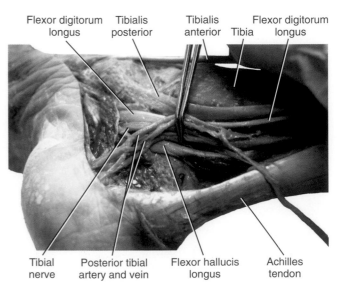

FIGURE 18-63. Note the relationship of structures passing through the tarsal tunnel.

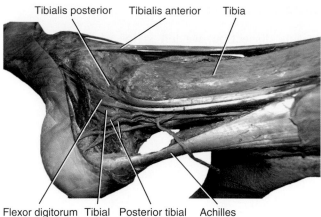

FIGURE 18-64. Appreciate the order of tendons, vessels, and nerves as they pass by the medial malleolus.

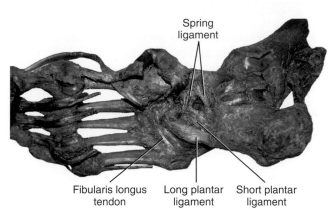

FIGURE 18-66. Optional dissection: plantar view of foot, highlighting plantar calcaneonavicular (spring) ligament and long and short plantar ligaments.

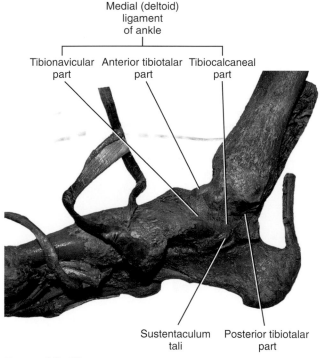

FIGURE 18-65. Optional dissection: medial view of ankle, demonstrating deltoid (medial) ligament.

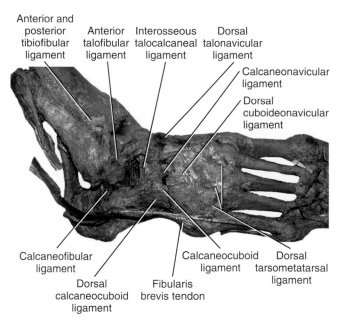

FIGURE 18-67. Optional dissection: lateral view of ankle, highlighting ligaments.

Optional Dissection of Ligaments of Foot and Ankle (Figs. 18-65 to 18-67)

Identify the lateral ligament of the ankle, formed by the anterior and posterior talofibular ligaments and the calcaneofibular ligament.

Identify the interosseous talocalcaneal ligament on the lateral side of the foot (Fig. 18-67).

Expose and cut the tendons of the tibialis anterior and tibialis posterior muscles at their insertion points. Just underneath, identify the deltoid ligament (medial side of ankle), formed of the anterior tibiotalar, tibionavicular, tibiocalcaneal, and posterior tibiotalar parts (Fig. 18-65).

Look lateral and underneath the tendon of the tibialis posterior muscle for the plantar calcaneonavicular (spring) ligament connecting the calcaneus to the navicular bones. Lateral to the calcaneonavicular ligament, expose the long and short plantar ligaments (Fig. 18-66).

See also Chapter 19.

✋ *DISSECTION TIP:* The long plantar ligament crosses over the tendon of the fibularis longus muscle. The short plantar (plantar calcaneocuboid) ligament attaches to the cuboid bone. Sometimes, the long plantar ligament may be confused with the spring ligament attached to the navicular bone (Fig. 18-66).

Creative Dissection

In this dissection, we left strips of skin intact. We dissected the intervals in between to appreciate the depth from skin to the different layers of the foot, ankle, and leg from superficial to deep (Figs. 18-68 to 18-70).

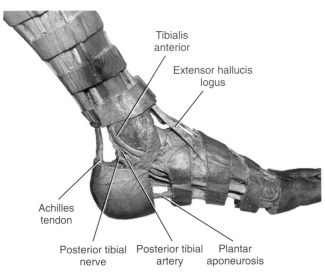

FIGURE 18-68. Special dissection: lateral view, demonstrating depth from skin to differing layers of foot, ankle, and leg, from superficial to deep.

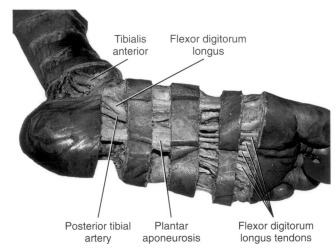

FIGURE 18-70. Special dissection: plantar view, highlighting differing layers of the foot and ankle, from superficial to deep.

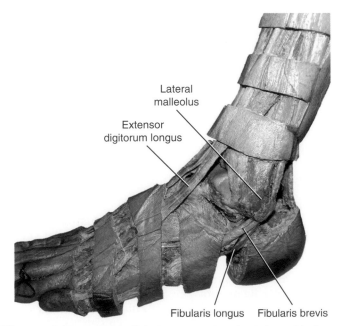

FIGURE 18-69. Special dissection: medial view; appreciate depth from skin (superficial to deep) to different layers of the foot, ankle, and leg.

LABORATORY IDENTIFICATION CHECKLIST

Nerves
- ❐ Common fibular
  - ❐ Superficial fibular
- ❐ Lateral sural cutaneous
- ❐ Sural communicating (normally formed from tibial and common fibular, but can form independently)
- ❐ Deep fibular
- ❐ Tibial nerve
  - ❐ Medial sural cutaneous
- ❐ Sural (normally formed from tibial and common fibular, but can form independently)

Arteries
- ❐ Popliteal
- ❐ Anterior tibial
- ❐ Posterior tibial
- ❐ Circumflex fibular
- ❐ Fibular

Veins
- ❐ *Superficial*
  - ❐ Great (long) saphenous
  - ❐ Small (lesser) saphenous

Veins—cont'd
- ❐ *Deep*
  - ❐ Popliteal
  - ❐ Posterior tibial
  - ❐ Fibular
  - ❐ Anterior tibial
  - ❐ Sural

Muscles
- ❐ *Anterior compartment*
  - ❐ Tibialis anterior
  - ❐ Extensor hallucis longus
  - ❐ Extensor digitorum longus
  - ❐ Fibularis tertius
- ❐ *Posterior compartment*
  - ❐ Superficial
  - ❐ Gastrocnemius
  - ❐ Soleus
  - ❐ Plantaris
- ❐ Deep
  - ❐ Popliteus
  - ❐ Flexor hallucis longus
  - ❐ Flexor digitorum longus
  - ❐ Tibialis posterior
- ❐ *Lateral compartment*
  - ❐ Fibularis longus
  - ❐ Fibularis brevis

Connective Tissue
- ❐ Anterior intermuscular septum
- ❐ Transverse intermuscular septum
- ❐ Posterior intermuscular septum
- ❐ Interosseous membrane
- ❐ Superior extensor retinaculum

Ligaments
- ❐ *Lateral ankle complex*
  - ❐ Anterior talofibular ligament (ATFL)
  - ❐ Calcaneofibular ligament (CFL)
  - ❐ Posterior talofibular ligament (PTFL)
- ❐ *Medial ankle complex*
  - ❐ Deltoid
    - ❐ Anterior tibiotalar part
    - ❐ Tibionavicular part
    - ❐ Tibiocalcaneal part
    - ❐ Posterior tibiotalar part

Bones
- ❐ Fibula
- ❐ Tibia

CHAPTER 19

FOOT

Netter: 510–525

McMinn: 350–353

Gray's Atlas: 310–318, 330–344

Before you start the dissection, identify and palpate the calcaneus, the lateral longitudinal arch, and the heads of the five metatarsal bones (Fig. 19-1).
Make a longitudinal incision starting from the lateral side of the calcaneus and following the lateral side of the lateral longitudinal arch (Fig. 19-2). Once you make the incision, reflect the skin medially (Fig. 19-3). Terminate the incision by completely reflecting the skin over the plantar portion of the foot, and maintain its attachment to the calcaneus (Fig. 19-4).

You can use the same technique for another approach: instead of starting from the calcaneus, begin the incision from the plantar surface of the base of the first digit.

> ☞ *DISSECTION TIP:* An alternate incision involves making a longitudinal cut from the calcaneus to the first digit and a second, transverse incision from the first digit to the lateral longitudinal arch, then removing the skin from the foot.

Once the skin is removed, observe the thick layer of connective tissue, the *plantar aponeurosis.* With a scalpel, make an incision from the lateral side of the calcaneus, reflecting the fat over the plantar

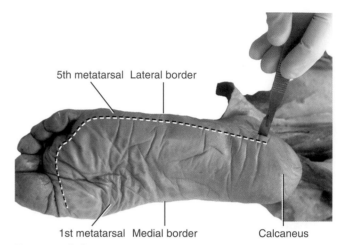

FIGURE 19-2. Longitudinal incision starts from lateral side of calcaneus and follows lateral longitudinal arch.

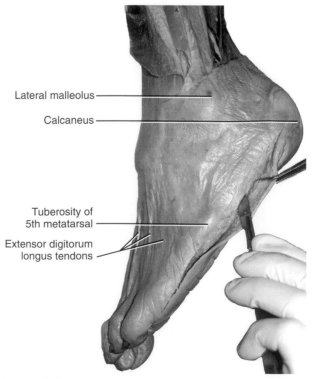

FIGURE 19-3. Skin reflected medially, highlighting key foot landmarks.

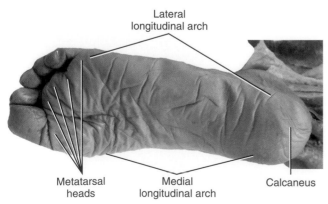

FIGURE 19-1. View of the plantar surface of the foot for identifying calcaneus, lateral longitudinal arch, and five metatarsal heads.

aponeurosis medially (Fig. 19-5). Remove the fat (plantar subcutaneous tissue) and expose the plantar aponeurosis with its fibrous slips to the digits (Fig. 19-6). On the lateral side of the foot, identify the abductor digiti minimi muscle and the underlying flexor digiti minimi muscle.

With a scalpel, cut the plantar aponeurosis at its junction with the flexor digiti minimi muscle, and reflect it toward the calcaneus (Fig. 19-7). Just underneath the plantar aponeurosis, separate the flexor digitorum brevis muscle, which arises from the deep surface of the aponeurosis. Reflect the plantar aponeurosis posteriorly to its attachment to the calcaneus. Carefully dissect out the fibrous attachments between the plantar aponeurosis and the digits, and identify the digital branches of the medial plantar nerve (Fig. 19-8).

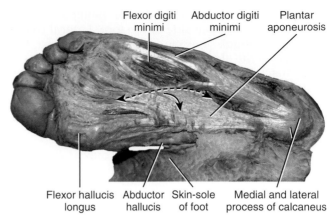

FIGURE 19-6. Fat removal exposes the plantar aponeurosis and fibrous slips to the digits.

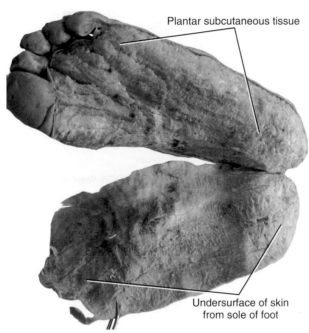

FIGURE 19-4. Skin completely reflected over plantar portion of foot, maintaining attachment to calcaneus.

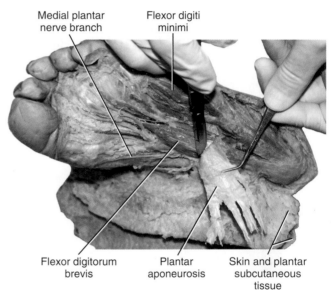

FIGURE 19-7. Abductor digiti minimi muscle and underlying flexor digiti minimi on lateral side of foot, with plantar aponeurosis reflected toward calcaneus, and flexor digitorum brevis muscle separated.

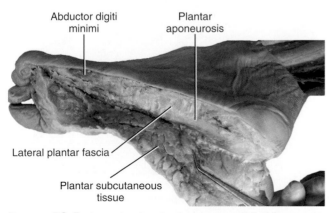

FIGURE 19-5. Lateral side of calcaneus incised, reflecting fat over plantar aponeurosis medially.

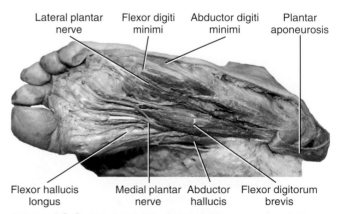

FIGURE 19-8. Dissected view between plantar aponeurosis and digits reveals digital branches of medial plantar nerve, abductor hallucis muscle, and tendons of flexor digitorum brevis and abductor digiti minimi muscles.

Identify and clean the abductor hallucis muscle located on the medial side of the foot. Lateral to the abductor hallucis muscle, clean and expose the tendons of the flexor digitorum brevis muscle. On this muscle's lateral side, identify and clean the abductor digiti minimi muscle (Fig. 19-8).

> ✋ *DISSECTION TIP:* These three muscles (abductor hallucis, flexor digitorum brevis, abductor digiti minimi) make up the 1st and most superficial layer of muscles of the plantar surface of the foot.

Between the abductor hallucis and flexor digitorum brevis muscles, identify and expose the *medial plantar nerve* (Fig. 19-9). Identify the distal part of the tendons of the flexor digitorum brevis muscle, and using scissors, cut and reflect them (with the belly of the flexor digitorum brevis) posteriorly (Fig. 19-10).

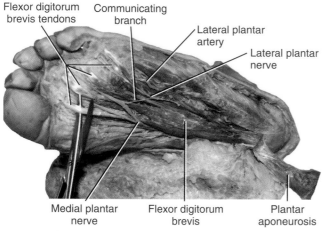

FIGURE 19-9. Medial plantar nerve exposed between abductor hallucis and flexor digitorum brevis muscles, with distal parts of flexor digitorum brevis tendons incised.

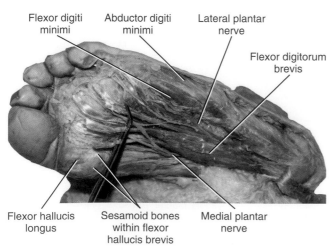

FIGURE 19-10. Tendons reflected posteriorly.

Just underneath the flexor digitorum brevis, clean and expose the *lateral plantar nerve* and lateral plantar artery as they travel to the lateral side of the foot (Fig. 19-11).

Identify and clean the tendon of the flexor hallucis longus muscle located on the medial side of the foot and inserting onto the base of the distal phalanx of the 1st digit (Fig. 19-12). Lateral to the flexor hallucis longus muscle, identify the tendons of the flexor digitorum longus muscle inserting onto the distal phalanges of the remaining four digits. Arising from the tendons of the flexor digitorum longus, note the four lumbrical muscles. Lateral to the main belly of the flexor digitorum longus, identify a small muscle arising from the calcaneus and inserting onto the flexor digitorum, the *quadratus plantae muscle.*

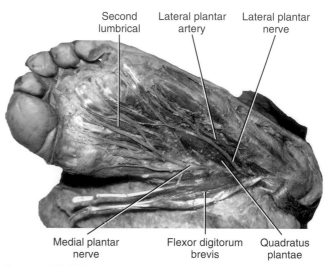

FIGURE 19-11. View of lateral plantar nerve and artery underneath flexor digitorum brevis muscle.

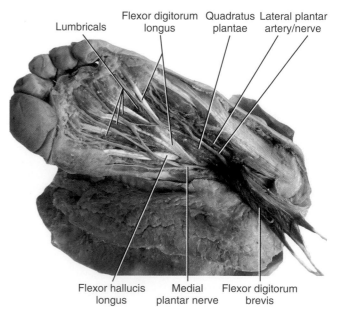

FIGURE 19-12. View highlighting tendon of flexor hallucis longus muscle on medial side of foot.

With scissors, cut the tendon of the flexor digitorum longus at the posterior aspect of the foot near the calcaneus (Fig. 19-13).

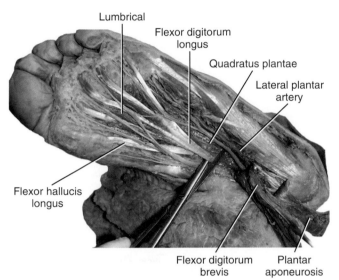

FIGURE 19-13. Tendon of flexor digitorum longus incised at posterior aspect of foot near calcaneus.

Continue the dissection by transecting the quadratus plantae muscle (Fig. 19-14). Reflect the transected muscle toward the toes (Fig. 19-15). Clean the small amounts of fascia and fat, then identify the two heads of the adductor hallucis muscle, the *oblique* and *transverse* heads (Fig. 19-16).

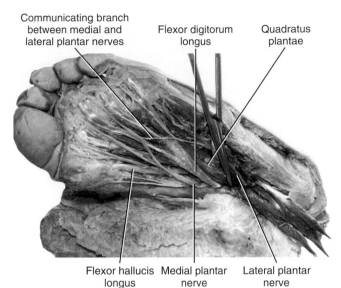

FIGURE 19-14. Quadratus plantae muscle transected.

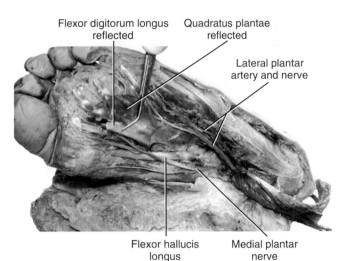

FIGURE 19-15. Quadratus plantae muscle reflected toward the toes.

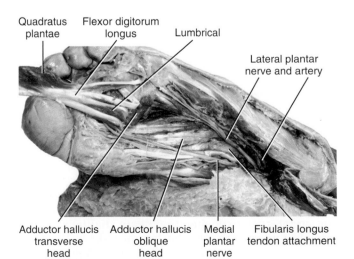

FIGURE 19-16. Further reflection demonstrates oblique and transverse heads of the adductor hallucis muscle.

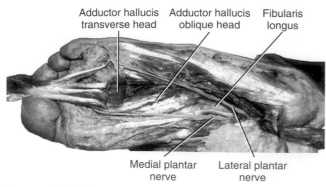

Adductor hallucis transverse head · Adductor hallucis oblique head · Fibularis longus

Medial plantar nerve · Lateral plantar nerve

FIGURE 19-17. Appreciate oblique and transverse heads of the adductor hallucis muscle (fibularis longus tendon lies posteriorly).

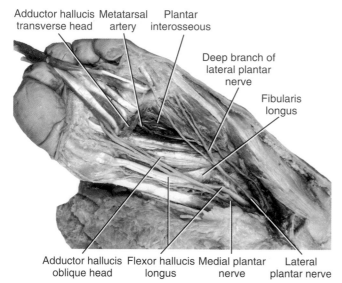

Adductor hallucis transverse head · Metatarsal artery · Plantar interosseous

Deep branch of lateral plantar nerve

Fibularis longus

Adductor hallucis oblique head · Flexor hallucis longus · Medial plantar nerve · Lateral plantar nerve

FIGURE 19-18. Tendon of flexor hallucis longus reflected toward the great toe, exposing the flexor hallucis brevis muscle; tendon of abductor digiti minimi reflected to locate the flexor digiti minimi brevis muscle.

> ✋ *DISSECTION TIP:* These muscles (adductor hallucis, flexor hallucis brevis, abductor digiti minimi, flexor digiti minimi brevis) occupy the 3rd layer of muscles of the plantar aspect of the foot.

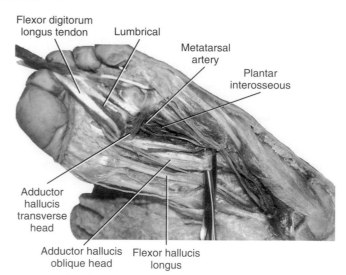

Flexor digitorum longus tendon · Lumbrical · Metatarsal artery · Plantar interosseous

Adductor hallucis transverse head

Adductor hallucis oblique head · Flexor hallucis longus

FIGURE 19-19. Plantar interosseous muscles exposed in space between the two heads of the adductor hallucis muscle, with the oblique head cut.

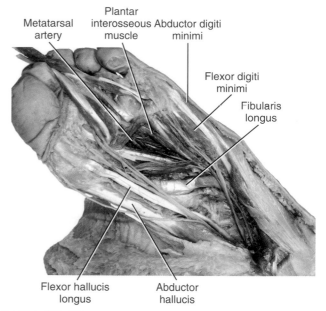

Metatarsal artery · Plantar interosseous muscle · Abductor digiti minimi

Flexor digiti minimi

Fibularis longus

Flexor hallucis longus · Abductor hallucis

FIGURE 19-20. Identify the fibularis longus tendon and insertion onto the 1st cuneiform and 1st metatarsal bones.

Posterior to the two heads of the adductor hallucis muscle, identify the peroneus longus tendon and its attachments (Figs. 19-17 and 19-18).

Retract or cut (toward calcaneus) the tendon of the flexor hallucis longus muscle, and reflect it toward the great toe, exposing the flexor hallucis brevis muscle underneath. On the lateral side of the foot, retract the tendon of the abductor digiti minimi muscle, and medially and deep to it, identify the flexor digiti minimi brevis muscle.

Trace the lateral plantar nerve from its origin to its final distribution, and identify its superficial and deep branches.

In the space between the two heads of the adductor hallucis muscle, expose the interosseous muscles (Fig. 19-19). With scissors, cut the oblique head of the adductor hallucis muscle; fully expose and trace the peroneus longus tendon to its insertion onto the 1st cuneiform and 1st metatarsal bones (Fig. 19-20).

OPTIONAL DISSECTION

Follow the lateral plantar artery along the lateral plantar nerve. Identify the deep branch of the lateral plantar nerve at the lateral side of the oblique head of the adductor hallucis muscle (see Fig. 19-18). At this point, the lateral plantar artery gives off a branch to form the deep plantar arterial arch, just underneath the oblique head of the adductor

hallucis muscle. Trace the branches from this arch, the *metatarsal branches,* which provide plantar digital vessels to the digits. Follow the deep plantar arch to the base of the 1st metatarsal. In the space between the 1st and 2nd metatarsals, the deep plantar arch joins the plantar branch of the dorsalis pedis artery.

LABORATORY IDENTIFICATION CHECKLIST

Nerves
- ❐ Medial plantar
  - ❐ Common plantar digital
    - ❐ Plantar digital nerves
- ❐ Lateral plantar
  - ❐ Common plantar digital
    - ❐ Plantar digital nerves
- ❐ Superficial fibular
  - ❐ Dorsal digital branches
- ❐ Deep fibular
  - ❐ Dorsal digital branches
- ❐ Medial calcaneal
- ❐ Lateral calcaneal

Arteries
- ❐ Dorsalis pedis
  - ❐ Lateral tarsal
  - ❐ Arcuate
  - ❐ Deep plantar
- ❐ Dorsal metatarsal arteries
  - ❐ Dorsal digital arteries
- ❐ Medial plantar
- ❐ Plantar metatarsal
  - ❐ Common plantar digital
    - ❐ Plantar digital
- ❐ Lateral plantar
- ❐ *Deep plantar arch*
  - ❐ Plantar metatarsal
    - ❐ Common plantar digital
      - ❐ Plantar digital

Veins
- ❐ Dorsal venous arch

Muscles
- ❐ *Dorsal muscles and tendons*
  - ❐ Extensor hallucis brevis
  - ❐ Extensor digitorum brevis
  - ❐ Extensor hallucis longus tendon
  - ❐ Extensor digitorum longus tendons
  - ❐ Tibialis anterior tendon
- ❐ *Plantar muscles and leg tendons*
  - ❐ Abductor hallucis
  - ❐ Flexor hallucis brevis
    - ❐ Medial head
    - ❐ Lateral head
  - ❐ Flexor hallucis longus tendon
  - ❐ Flexor digitorum brevis
  - ❐ Flexor digiti minimi brevis
  - ❐ Abductor digiti minimi
  - ❐ Flexor digitorum longus tendons
  - ❐ Quadratus plantae
  - ❐ Lumbricals
  - ❐ Fibularis longus tendon
  - ❐ Tibialis posterior tendon
  - ❐ Fibularis brevis tendon
  - ❐ Adductor hallucis
    - ❐ Transverse head
    - ❐ Oblique head
  - ❐ Plantar interossei
  - ❐ Dorsal interossei

Ligaments
- ❐ Plantar calcaneonavicular (spring) ligament
- ❐ Long plantar ligament
- ❐ Plantar calcaneocuboid (short plantar) ligament

Connective Tissue
- ❐ Plantar aponeurosis
- ❐ Inferior extensor retinaculum

Bones
- ❐ *Tarsal bones*
  - ❐ Calcaneus
  - ❐ Talus
  - ❐ Cuboid
  - ❐ Navicular
  - ❐ Medial cuneiform
  - ❐ Middle cuneiform
  - ❐ Lateral cuneiform
  - ❐ Metatarsals
  - ❐ Phalanges
    - ❐ Proximal
    - ❐ Middle
    - ❐ Distal

TROCHANTERIC BURSITIS INJECTION

Gray's Anatomy for Students: 549

Netter: 491

Clinical Application

Introduce local anesthetic using an intrabursal injection to relieve pain of inflamed trochanteric bursa.

Anatomic Landmarks (Figs. VII-1 and VII-2)

- Skin
- Subcutaneous tissue
- Iliotibial fascia
- Tensor fasciae latae
- Trochanteric bursa
- Greater trochanter

PREPATELLAR BURSITIS ASPIRATION/INJECTION

Gray's Anatomy for Students: 578

Netter: 499

Clinical Application

Introduce local anesthesia into prepatellar bursa to withdraw fluid and relieve pain from prepatellar bursa.

Anatomic Landmarks (Fig. VII-3)

- Skin
- Patella
- Subcutaneous tissue
- Prepatellar bursa

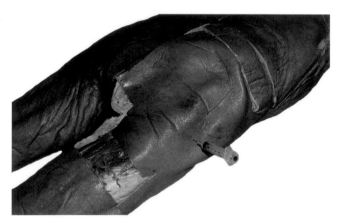

FIGURE VII-1.

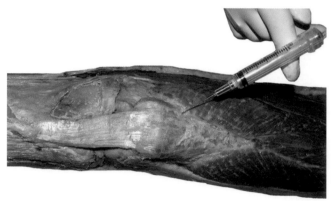

FIGURE VII-3.

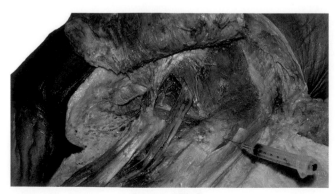

FIGURE VII-2.

SUPRAPATELLAR BURSITIS ASPIRATION/INJECTION

Gray's Anatomy for Students: 578

Netter: 499

Clinical Application

Introduce local anesthesia into suprapatellar bursa to relieve pain from prepatellar bursa.

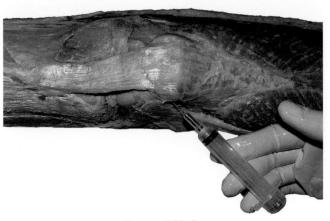

FIGURE VII-4.

Anatomic Landmarks (Fig. VII-4)

- Skin
- Subcutaneous tissue
- Suprapatellar bursa

PLANTAR FASCITIS INJECTION

Gray's Anatomy for Students: 578

Netter: 520

Clinical Application

Injection of local anesthetic at the point of maximal tenderness within the plantar fascia or plantar aponeurosis, often near its attachment to the medial process of the calcaneal tuberosity, to relieve pain caused by inflamed fascia.

Anatomic Landmarks (Figs. VII-5 and VII-6)

- Skin
- Subcutaneous tissue/fat pad
- Plantar fascia/aponeurosis
- Calcaneal tuberosity

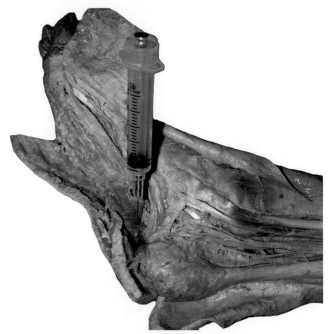

FIGURE VII-6.

ARTHROCENTESIS: KNEE

Gray's Anatomy for Students: 578

Netter: 495

Clinical Application

Introduce needle into the knee joint to withdraw fluid and to inject medication.

Anatomic Landmarks

- Skin
- Subcutaneous tissue
- Patella
- Intercondylar notch
- Joint cavity

GREAT SAPHENOUS VEIN CUTDOWN OR CANNULATION

Gray's Anatomy for Students: 542

Netter: 471

Clinical Application

Procedure to cannulate great saphenous vein for infusion of fluids.

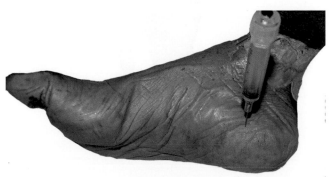

FIGURE VII-5.

Anatomic Landmarks (Figs. VII-7 and VII-8)

- Medial malleolus
- Skin
- Subcutaneous tissue
- Great saphenous vein
- Saphenous nerve

FEMUR AND KNEE REPLACEMENT

Figure VII-9 depicts a head of the femur replacement.
Figure VII-10 depicts a knee replacement.

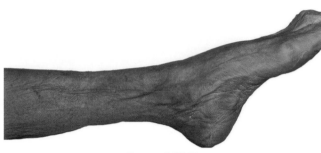

FIGURE VII-7.

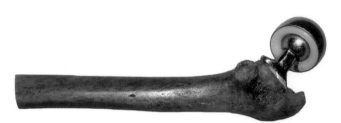

FIGURE VII-9.

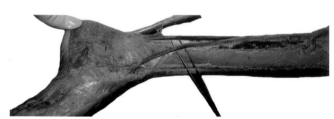

FIGURE VII-8.

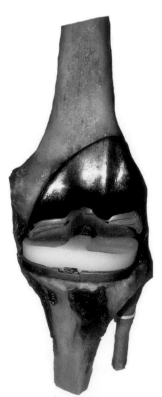

FIGURE VII-10.

NECK

Netter: 26–33, 74, 128–129

McMinn: 38–47

Gray's Atlas: 491–503, 508–509

BEFORE DISSECTION

Palpate the following landmarks on your neck or the cadaver:

- Mental protuberance
- Hyoid bone
- Laryngeal prominence ("Adam's apple")
- Cricoid cartilage
- Suprasternal notch
- Thyroid gland

ANATOMIC TRIANGLES

The neck may be divided into smaller topographic areas, the *triangles* of the neck. Specifically, the "carotid triangle" and the "root of the neck" are involved in many surgical procedures on the neck. There are two major triangles of the neck, the anterior and posterior cervical triangles (Fig. 20-1). The *anterior cervical triangle* is demarcated anteriorly by the midline of the neck; its base is the lower border of the mandible, and the posterior border is the anterior boundary of the sternocleidomastoid muscle. The *posterior cervical triangle* is bounded by the posterior border of the sternocleidomastoid muscle, the middle third of the clavicle, and the anterior border of the trapezius muscle. The cervical triangles may be subdivided as follows:

Anterior cervical triangle
1. Digastric triangle
2. Submental triangle
3. Carotid triangle
5. Muscular triangle
Posterior cervical triangle
5. Occipital triangle
6. Supraclavicular triangle

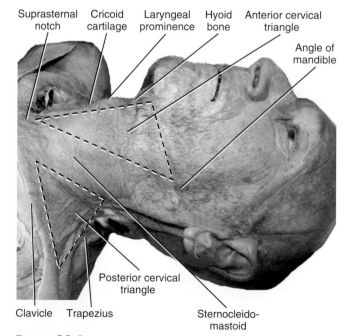

FIGURE 20-1. Anterolateral view of surface anatomy of the neck, highlighting hyoid bone, laryngeal prominence, sternal notch, angle of mandible, sternocleidomastoid muscle, and anterior and posterior triangles of the neck.

NECK DISSECTION

Make a midline incision through the skin from the suprasternal notch to the mental protuberance. A second incision should be made from the suprasternal notch laterally, along the clavicles bilaterally, to the acromion processes. Make a final incision from the mental protuberance along the inferior border of the mandible, toward the earlobe (Fig. 20-2). Carefully reflect the skin over the neck.

> 👆 *DISSECTION TIP:* The skin over the neck is thin. Pay special attention during its reflection for the subcutaneous tissue so that you do not reflect the platysma muscle with the skin.

Start the dissection by reflecting the subcutaneous tissue from the mental protuberance inferiorly and laterally toward the clavicles, to expose the platysma muscle (Fig. 20-3). The platysma is pierced by the transverse cervical and supraclavicular nerves of the cervical plexus. Reflect the subcutaneous tissue over the platysma muscle (Fig. 20-4). Separate the lateral border of the platysma from the subcutaneous tissue. Identify the sternocleidomastoid muscle posterior to the platysma muscle. At the level of the clavicle, cut and reflect the platysma upward, toward the mandible (Figs. 20-5 and 20-6). Similarly, at the angle of the mandible, cut and reflect the platysma anteriorly (Fig. 20-7).

> 👆 *DISSECTION TIP:* At this stage, it is possible to identify the cervical branch of the facial nerve, which innervates the platysma muscle, coursing from the inferior border of the parotid gland toward the platysma.

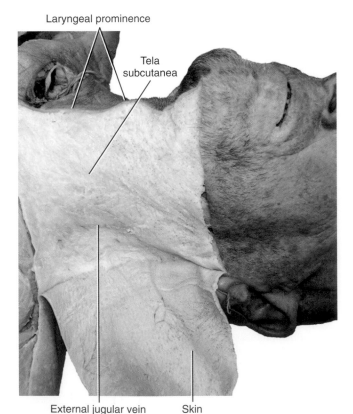

FIGURE 20-2. Skin of neck reflected laterally, revealing tela subcutanea (subcutaneous tissue), laryngeal prominence, superficial lobe of submandibular gland, external jugular vein, and midline of the neck.

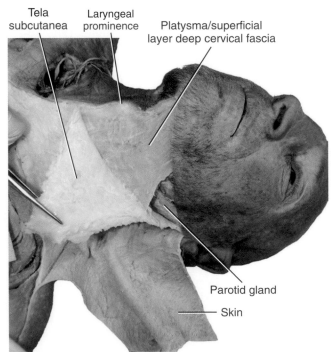

FIGURE 20-3. Skin and tela subcutanea reflected laterally, revealing platysma muscle, superficial layer of deep cervical fascia, superficial lobe of submandibular gland, and sternocleidomastoid muscle.

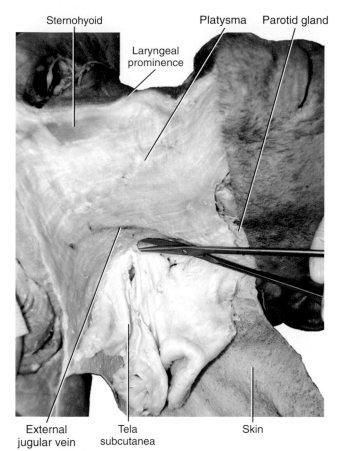

FIGURE 20-4. Separation of lateral border of platysma muscle from tela subcutanea.

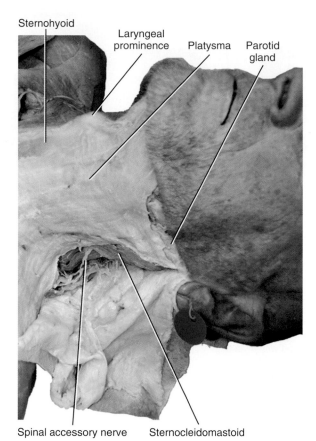

FIGURE 20-5. Identification of spinal accessory nerve at interval junction between platysma, sternocleidomastoid, and trapezius muscles.

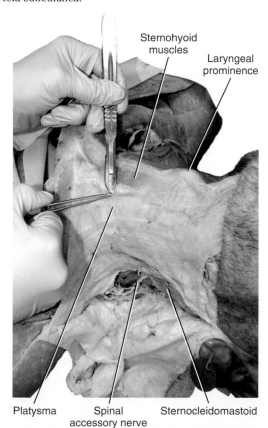

FIGURE 20-6. Dissection of medial border of platysma muscle from underlying tissues.

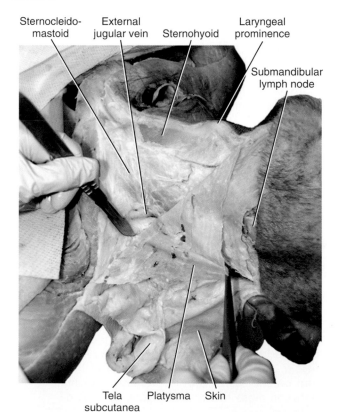

FIGURE 20-7. Anterolateral view of neck with skin, tela subcutanea, and platysma reflected laterally, revealing sternocleidomastoid muscle, external jugular vein, sternohyoid muscle, thyroid cartilage, and submandibular gland.

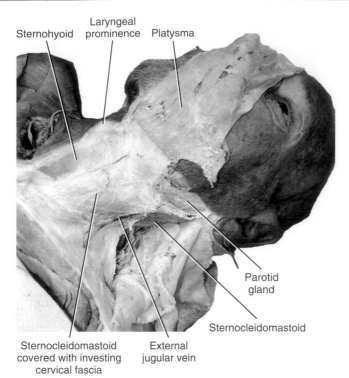

Sternohyoid — Laryngeal prominence — Platysma

Parotid gland

Sternocleidomastoid

Sternocleidomastoid covered with investing cervical fascia — External jugular vein

FIGURE 20-8. Complete reflection of platysma muscle and exposure of underlying structures.

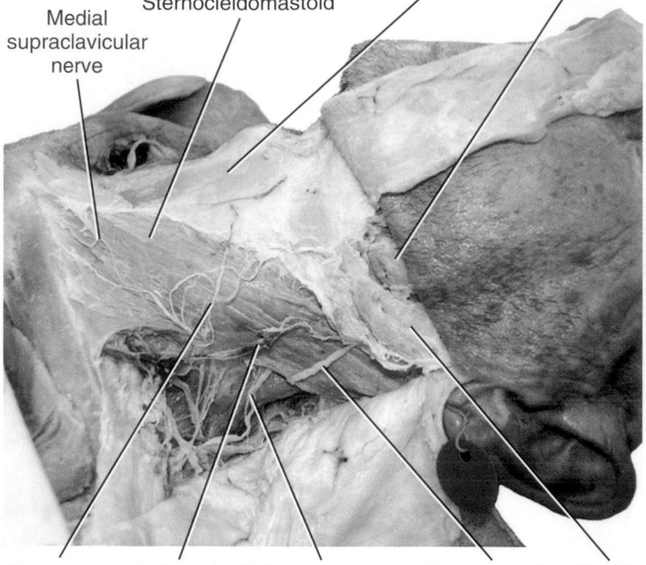

Medial supraclavicular nerve — Sternocleidomastoid — Sternohyoid — Submandibular lymph node

Transverse cervical nerve — External jugular vein — Spinal accessory nerve — Great auricular nerve — Parotid gland

FIGURE 20-9. Anterolateral view of neck with skin and tela subcutanea reflected laterally and platysma reflected superiorly, revealing sternocleidomastoid muscle, great auricular nerve, transverse cervical nerve, medial branch of supraclavicular nerve, sternohyoid muscle, thyroid cartilage, and submandibular and parotid glands.

Preserve the attachment of the platysma muscle along the mandible (Fig. 20-8).

About 1 cm (⅖ inch) inferior to the angle of the mandible, expose the marginal mandibular branch of the facial nerve. This nerve passes superficial to the facial vein and artery. The facial vein usually drains into the internal jugular vein through the retromandibular vein.

Notice the investing *cervical fascia* covering the sternocleidomastoid muscle (Fig. 20-8). Observe the external jugular vein running lateral to the sternocleidomastoid muscle.

Clean the superficial investing fascia over the sternocleidomastoid muscle (Fig. 20-9). Use care when you reflect the fascia so as not to sever any of the cutaneous nerves arising deep to the posterior edge of the sternocleidomastoid muscle. Identify the external jugular vein running superficial to the sternocleidomastoid muscle, as well as the following cutaneous nerve branches of the cervical plexus:

- Lesser occipital nerve (C2-C3)
- Great auricular nerve (C2-C3)
- Transverse cervical nerve (C2-C3)
- Supraclavicular nerves (C3-C4)

Once you expose these nerves, look for the spinal accessory nerve; it appears posterior to the sternocleidomastoid, about two-thirds the distance up its posterior edge, and then crosses the posterior triangle to reach the trapezius muscle. From top to bottom, along the sternocleidomastoid muscle, the lesser occipital, great auricular, and transverse cervical nerves emerge along its posterior border.

DISSECTION TIP: The investing cervical fascia encircles the trapezius and sternocleidomastoid muscles before reaching the midline of the neck. In the gap between these muscles, this fascia forms the "roof" of the posterior cervical triangle. The "floor" of the posterior cervical triangle is provided by another fascia, the *prevertebral fascia,* which covers the musculature of the lateral and anterior aspects of the vertebral column. Between these two fascial layers, there is a potential space.

DISSECTION TIP: In many specimens the transverse cervical nerve, which is a cutaneous nerve, communicates with the cervical branch of the facial nerve, which is a motor nerve.

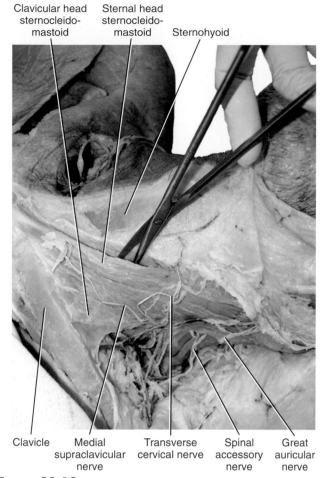

Clavicular head sternocleidomastoid   Sternal head sternocleidomastoid   Sternohyoid

Clavicle   Medial supraclavicular nerve   Transverse cervical nerve   Spinal accessory nerve   Great auricular nerve

FIGURE 20-10. Medial border of underlying tissues detached.

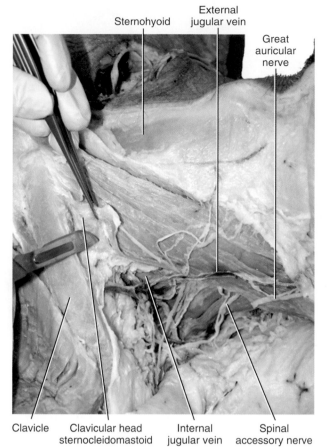

Sternohyoid   External jugular vein   Great auricular nerve

Clavicle   Clavicular head sternocleidomastoid   Internal jugular vein   Spinal accessory nerve

FIGURE 20-11. Sternocleidomastoid muscle detached from clavicle.

The external jugular vein arises at the junction of the posterior auricular vein and the posterior division of the retromandibular vein. This vein terminates in the subclavian vein.

> **☞ DISSECTION TIP:** The external jugular vein may be absent in the presence of a large anterior jugular vein.

With scissors, detach the medial border of the sternocleidomastoid muscle from its fascial investment (Fig. 20-10). Cut the origin of the sternocleidomastoid muscle from the clavicle and the manubrium of the sternum (Fig. 20-11).

Reflect the sternocleidomastoid muscle upward, away from it fascial investment (Figs. 20-12 and 20-13). Leave the posterior layer of the superficial cervical fascia intact. Trace the spinal accessory nerve from the posterior aspect of the sternocleidomastoid muscle, and preserve this nerve for later dissection.

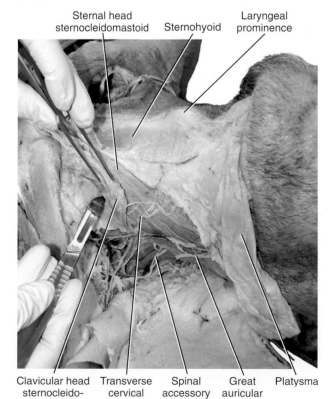

Sternal head sternocleidomastoid   Sternohyoid   Laryngeal prominence

Clavicular head sternocleidomastoid   Transverse cervical nerve   Spinal accessory nerve   Great auricular nerve   Platysma

FIGURE 20-12. Sternocleidomastoid further detached from clavicle and reflected laterally.

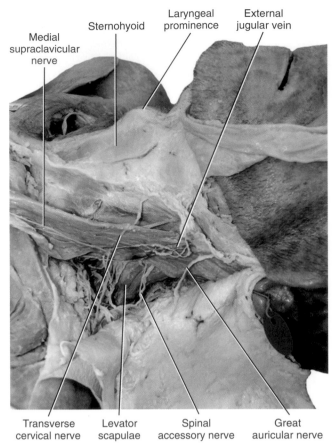

Medial supraclavicular nerve — Sternohyoid — Laryngeal prominence — External jugular vein

Transverse cervical nerve — Levator scapulae — Spinal accessory nerve — Great auricular nerve

FIGURE 20-13. Anterolateral view of neck with skin and tela subcutanea reflected laterally and platysma muscle reflected superiorly, revealing clavicle, sternocleidomastoid muscle and nerves, external jugular vein, submandibular gland, and levator scapulae muscle.

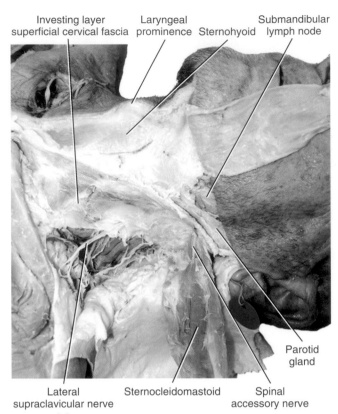

Investing layer superficial cervical fascia — Laryngeal prominence — Sternohyoid — Submandibular lymph node

Parotid gland

Lateral supraclavicular nerve — Sternocleidomastoid — Spinal accessory nerve

FIGURE 20-14. Anterolateral view of neck with skin, tela subcutanea and sternocleidomastoid muscle reflected laterally and platysma reflected superiorly, revealing investing layer of deep cervical fascia, sternohyoid muscle, thyroid cartilage, submandibular gland, spinal accessory nerve, and parotid gland.

Dissect out the fascia, and separate the parotid gland from the sternocleidomastoid muscle without damaging the great auricular and lesser occipital nerves.

Reflect the superficial layer of the investing fascia, and note its contribution to the formation of the carotid sheath (Fig. 20-15). Identify the carotid sheath, omohyoid muscle, and internal jugular vein. Clean the carotid sheath over the internal jugular vein, and identify the *ansa cervicalis*. The ansa cervicalis usually lies superficial to the internal jugular vein, outside the carotid sheath (Fig. 20-16).

☝ *DISSECTION TIP:* In some specimens the spinal accessory nerve will exhibit communications with C3 and C4 ventral rami. The spinal accessory nerve in the posterior triangle is found between the superficial investing fascia and the prevertebral fascia. In some cadavers the parotid gland may cover the most proximal portion of the sternocleidomastoid muscle (Fig. 20-14). It is important to separate the parotid gland from the sternocleidomastoid in order to reflect the muscle as laterally as possible. The more the sternocleidomastoid is reflected, the more space that will be available for later dissection.

☝ *DISSECTION TIP:* As you expose the internal jugular vein from the carotid sheath and superficial layer of the investing cervical fascia, look for the deep cervical lymph nodes. These lymph nodes are often prominent where the omohyoid crosses the internal jugular vein (jugulo-omohyoid node) and where the digastric muscle crosses the internal jugular vein (jugulodigastric node).

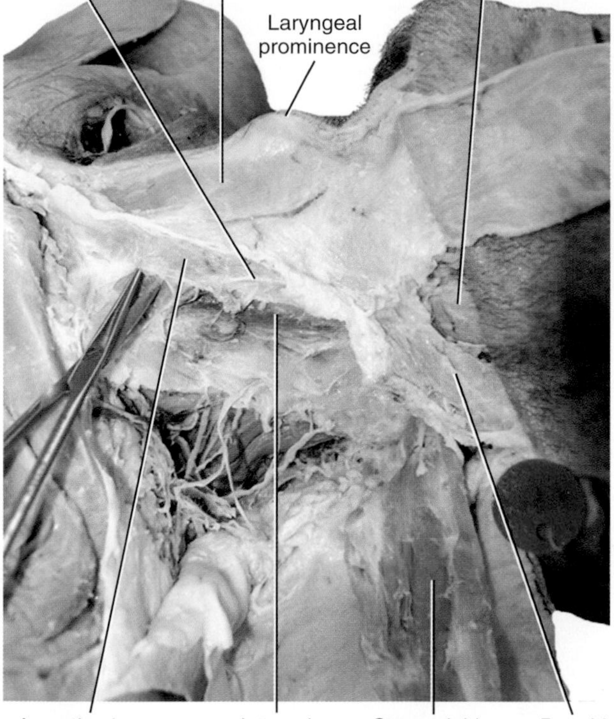

Carotid sheath   Sternohyoid   Submandibular lymph node

Laryngeal
prominence

Investing layer
superficial cervical
fascia

Internal
jugular vein

Sternocleido-
mastoid

Parotid
gland

FIGURE 20-15. Carotid sheath cleaned over internal jugular vein.

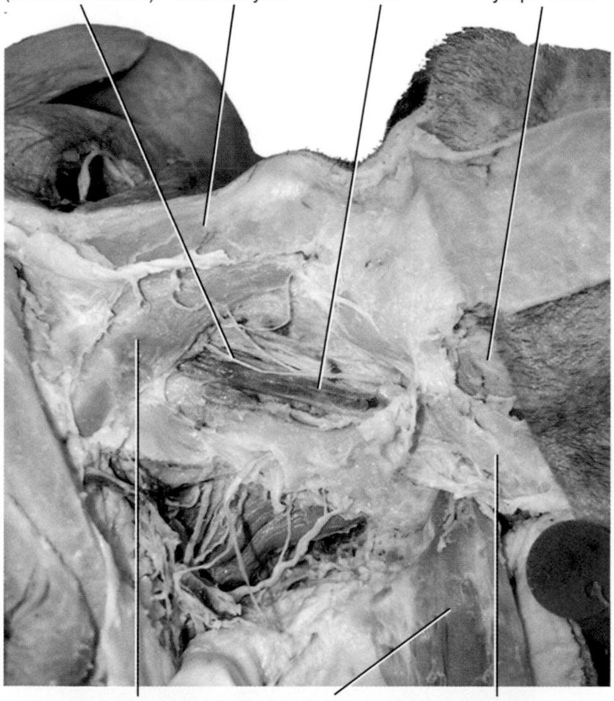

Descendens
hypoglossi
(ansa cervicalis)   Sternohyoid

Internal jugular
vein

Submandibular
lymph node

Superior belly
of omohyoid

Sternocleidomastoid

Parotid
gland

FIGURE 20-16. Superior belly of omohyoid muscle exposed, revealing ansa cervicalis superficial to internal jugular vein.

There are two techniques for the identification of the ansa cervicalis:

1. Look superficial and lateral to the internal jugular vein in the lower part of the part of the neck, and identify the ansa cervicalis.
2. Identify and clean the strap muscles. Follow their nerve supply backward, and trace it to the ansa cervicalis. Specifically, identify the sternohyoid muscle, and follow its small nerve branches proximally.

Pull the internal jugular vein laterally, and expose the other contents of the carotid sheath, the *vagus nerve* and *common carotid artery* (Fig. 20-17).

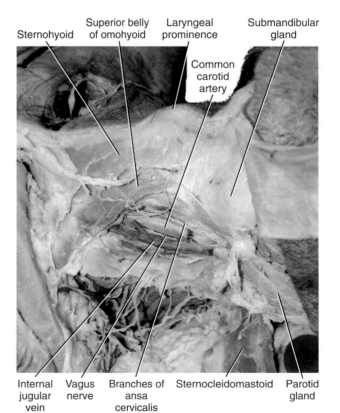

Sternohyoid

Superior belly
of omohyoid

Laryngeal
prominence

Submandibular
gland

Common
carotid
artery

Internal
jugular
vein

Vagus
nerve

Branches of
ansa
cervicalis

Sternocleidomastoid

Parotid
gland

FIGURE 20-17. Anterolateral view of neck with skin, tela subcutanea, and sternocleidomastoid muscle reflected laterally and platysma muscle reflected superiorly, revealing internal jugular vein, common carotid artery, vagus nerve, ansa cervicalis, superior belly of omohyoid muscle, sternohyoid muscle, thyroid cartilage, and parotid gland.

Ansa
cervicalis   Sternothyroid   Sternohyoid   Thyrohyoid   Submandibular gland

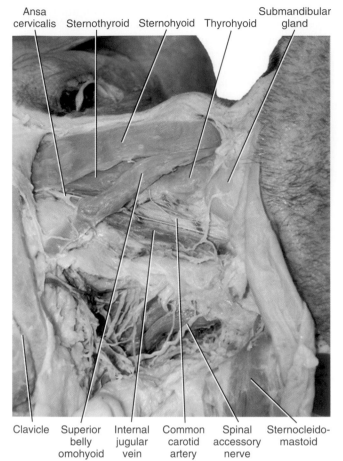

Clavicle   Superior   Internal   Common   Spinal   Sternocleido-
belly   jugular   carotid   accessory   mastoid
omohyoid   vein   artery   nerve

FIGURE 20-18. Connective tissue cleaned, highlighting strap muscles (omohyoid superior/inferior bellies, sternohyoid, sternothyroid, thyrohyoid).

Ansa   Superior belly   Submandibular
Sternohyoid   cervicalis   omohyoid   Thyrohyoid   gland

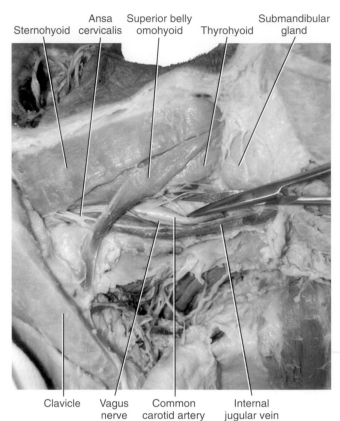

Clavicle   Vagus   Common   Internal
nerve   carotid artery   jugular vein

FIGURE 20-19. Remaining carotid sheath cleaned, fully exposing vagus nerve and carotid artery.

Clean the connective tissue, and identify the "strap muscles": the omohyoid (superior and inferior bellies), sternohyoid, sternothyroid, and thyrohyoid muscles (Fig. 20-18). Clear away the carotid sheath, and fully expose the internal jugular vein, common carotid artery, and vagus nerve (Fig. 20-19).

> ☞ *DISSECTION TIP:* With scissors, pull the common carotid artery from the carotid sheath (Fig. 20-19), to avoid severing important arteries and nerves.

Clean the connective tissue, fat, and carotid sheath, and expose the cervical plexus (Figs. 20-20 and 20-21). Continue the exposure of the contents of the carotid sheath toward the clavicle (Fig. 20-22). Identify the submandibular gland, and pull it toward the midline. Clean the carotid sheath toward the angle of the mandible, and identify (if prominent) the *jugulodigastric lymph nodes* (Fig. 20-23).

Common carotid   Submandibular
Sternohyoid   artery   Thyrohyoid   gland

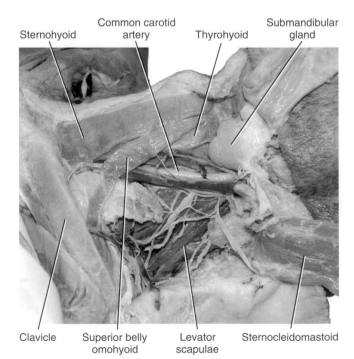

Clavicle   Superior belly   Levator   Sternocleidomastoid
omohyoid   scapulae

FIGURE 20-20. Adipose tissue removed from posterior cervical triangle, leaving intact nerves and arteries.

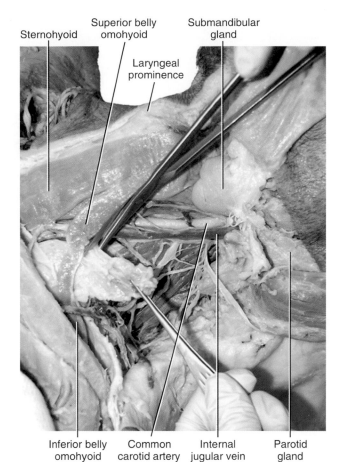

Sternohyoid

Superior belly omohyoid

Submandibular gland

Laryngeal prominence

Inferior belly omohyoid

Common carotid artery

Internal jugular vein

Parotid gland

FIGURE 20-21. Fat cleaned underneath omohyoid muscle, revealing key musculature and vasculature.

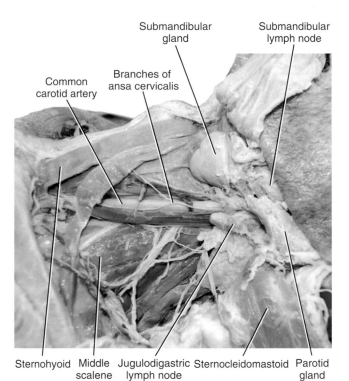

Submandibular gland

Submandibular lymph node

Common carotid artery

Branches of ansa cervicalis

Sternohyoid Middle scalene Jugulodigastric lymph node Sternocleidomastoid Parotid gland

FIGURE 20-23. Appreciate jugulodigastric lymph nodes and parotid and submandibular glands.

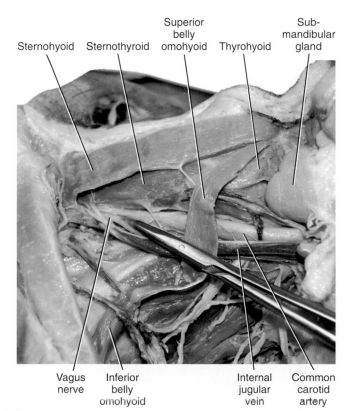

Sternohyoid Sternothyroid Superior belly omohyoid Thyrohyoid Sub-mandibular gland

Vagus nerve Inferior belly omohyoid Internal jugular vein Common carotid artery

FIGURE 20-22. Carotid sheath cleaned inferiorly, revealing vagus verve and carotid artery toward root of neck.

Sternohyoid | Superior belly omohyoid | Superior thyroid artery | Submandibular gland

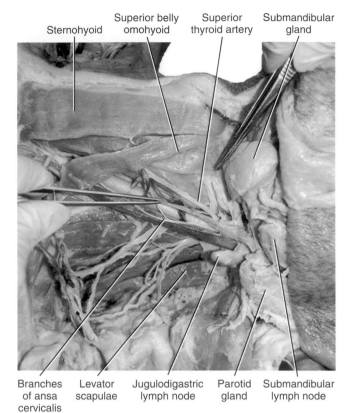

Branches of ansa cervicalis | Levator scapulae | Jugulodigastric lymph node | Parotid gland | Submandibular lymph node

FIGURE 20-24. Fat and connective tissue removed around common carotid artery and medial to carotid sheath to highlight superior thyroid artery.

Anterior belly digastric | Posterior belly of digastric | Stylohyoid | Submandibular gland | Parotid gland | Spinal accessory nerve

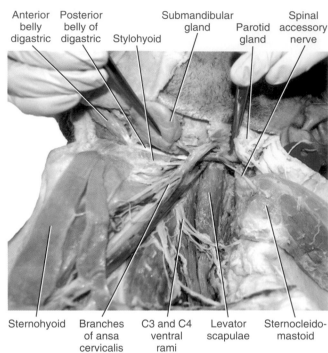

Sternohyoid | Branches of ansa cervicalis | C3 and C4 ventral rami | Levator scapulae | Sternocleido-mastoid

FIGURE 20-26. Submandibular and parotid glands lifted to expose external and internal carotid arteries.

Sternohyoid | Superior belly omohyoid | Branches of ansa cervicalis | Superior thyroid artery | Superficial lobe submandibular gland | Parotid gland

Inferior belly omohyoid | Middle scalene | C3 and C4 ventral rami | Jugulodigastric lymph node | Sternocleidomastoid | Submandibular lymph node

FIGURE 20-25. Fat and lymphatics cleaned at angle of mandible to expose external and internal carotid arteries.

Clean away fat and connective tissue around the common carotid artery and medial to the carotid sheath and identify the superior thyroid artery (Figs. 20-24 and 20-25). This artery runs between the thyrohyoid muscle and the carotid sheath. Do not try to identify the origin of this artery yet.

Remove the jugulodigastric lymph nodes, and by pulling the parotid gland laterally, expose the posterior belly of the digastric muscle (Fig. 20-26) Expose the digastric muscle, with its posterior and anterior bellies, and the stylohyoid muscle. Observe the tendon insertion of the stylohyoid muscle onto the hyoid and its relationship with the posterior belly of the digastric muscle. Identify the hyoid bone, and expose the mylohyoid muscle, which is partially hidden by the anterior belly of the digastric muscle (Fig. 20-26).

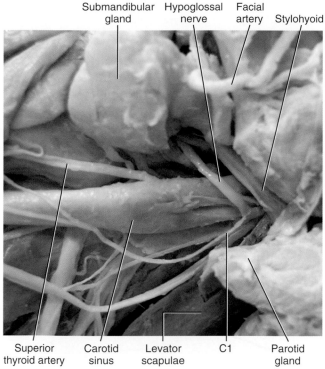

Submandibular gland Hypoglossal nerve Facial artery Stylohyoid

Superior thyroid artery Carotid sinus Levator scapulae C1 Parotid gland

FIGURE 20-32. Anterolateral close-up view of neck in region of carotid bifurcation, revealing common carotid artery, external carotid artery, internal carotid artery, carotid sinus, stylohyoid, hypoglossal nerve, parotid gland, levator scapulae, and vagus nerve.

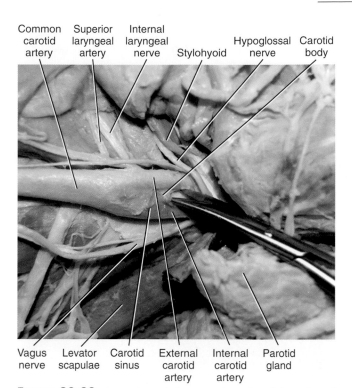

Common carotid artery Superior laryngeal artery Internal laryngeal nerve Stylohyoid Hypoglossal nerve Carotid body

Vagus nerve Levator scapulae Carotid sinus External carotid artery Internal carotid artery Parotid gland

FIGURE 20-33. Anterolateral close-up view of neck in region of carotid bifurcation, revealing superficial lobe of submandibular gland, facial artery, hypoglossal nerve, stylohyoid, ansa cervicalis, parotid gland, levator scapulae, ascending pharyngeal artery, carotid sinus, and superior thyroid artery.

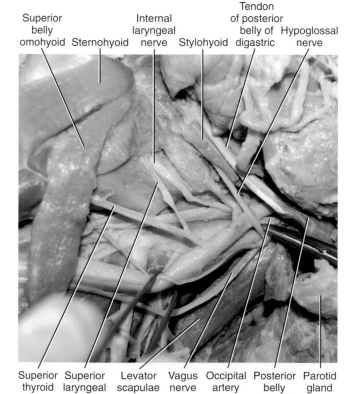

Superior belly omohyoid Sternohyoid Internal laryngeal nerve Stylohyoid Tendon of posterior belly of digastric Hypoglossal nerve

Superior thyroid artery Superior laryngeal artery Levator scapulae Vagus nerve Occipital artery Posterior belly digastric Parotid gland

FIGURE 20-34. Anterolateral view of neck with skin, tela subcutanea, sternocleidomastoid reflected laterally and platysma reflected superiorly, revealing the sternohyoid, superior belly of omohyoid, superficial lobe of submandibular gland, intermediate tendon of digastric, stylohyoid, hypoglossal nerve, posterior belly of digastric, parotid gland, ansa cervicalis, and vagus nerve.

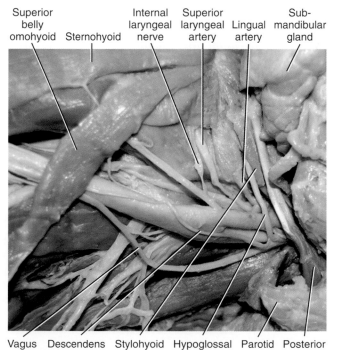

Superior belly omohyoid Sternohyoid Internal laryngeal nerve Superior laryngeal artery Lingual artery Submandibular gland

Vagus nerve Descendens hypoglossi Stylohyoid Hypoglossal nerve Parotid gland Posterior belly digastric

FIGURE 20-35. Anterolateral view of neck with skin, tela subcutanea, sternocleidomastoid, and platysma removed, revealing sternohyoid, superior belly of omohyoid, superficial lobe of submandibular gland, superior laryngeal artery and nerve, hypoglossal nerve, ansa cervicalis, parotid gland, vagus nerve, and superior thyroid artery.

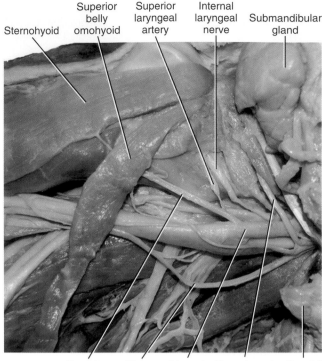

FIGURE 20-36. Anterolateral view of neck with skin, tela subcutanea, sternocleidomastoid, platysma, sternohyoid, sternothyroid, omohyoid, and carotid sheath removed, revealing superior pole of thyroid gland, ansa cervicalis, superficial lobe of submandibular gland, mandible, facial artery, superior laryngeal nerve and artery, hypoglossal nerve, parotid gland, superior thyroid artery, and vagus nerve.

FIGURE 20-37. Anteroinferior view of midline of neck with skin, tela subcutanea, and platysma reflected, revealing anterior belly of digastric, mylohyoid, mandible, submental artery, facial artery, parotid gland, superficial lobe of submandibular gland, digastric tendon, thyroid cartilage, and cricothyroid ligament.

At the lateral border of the external carotid artery, expose the *occipital artery*, which passes posteriorly, crossing over the hypoglossal nerve (Fig. 20-34). In the majority of cases, the occipital artery will give rise to the artery of the sternocleidomastoid muscle.

Opposite the occipital artery, at the medial border of the external carotid artery and superior to the lingual artery, identify the *facial artery*, and trace it to the submandibular gland at the angle of the mandible (Fig. 20-37).

Clean any muscle attachments and connective tissue from the clavicle to expose the *brachial plexus* in the supraclavicular area (Figs. 20-38 and 20-39). Cover the neck and thorax with paper towels (Fig. 20-40).

With an electric saw, cut the clavicle at the suprasternal notch and at its distal one third (Fig. 20-41).

> **DISSECTION TIP:** In some cadavers the facial and lingual arteries may have a common origin, the *faciolingual trunk.* Similarly, the lingual and the superior thyroid arteries may originate as a common trunk. Posterior to the origin of the external carotid artery, identify the ascending pharyngeal artery, which travels between the internal carotid and the lateral aspect of the pharynx.

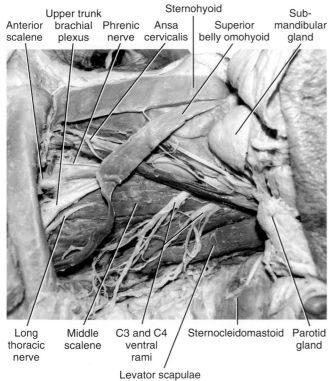

Anterior scalene · Upper trunk brachial plexus · Phrenic nerve · Ansa cervicalis · Sternohyoid · Superior belly omohyoid · Sub-mandibular gland

Long thoracic nerve · Middle scalene · C3 and C4 ventral rami · Levator scapulae · Sternocleidomastoid · Parotid gland

FIGURE 20-38. Anterolateral view of neck with skin, tela subcutanea, and sternocleidomastoid reflected laterally from midline and platysma reflected superiorly, revealing sternohyoid, sternothyroid, superficial lobe of submandibular gland, superior thyroid artery, parotid gland, levator scapulae, superior belly of omohyoid, middle scalene, subclavian artery, anterior scalene, phrenic nerve, ansa cervicalis, and clavicle.

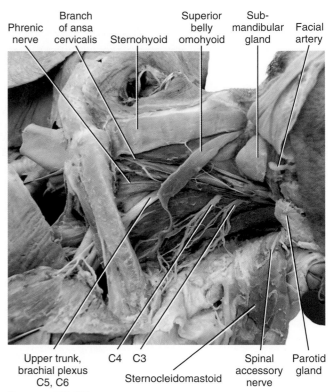

Phrenic nerve · Branch of ansa cervicalis · Sternohyoid · Superior belly omohyoid · Sub-mandibular gland · Facial artery

Upper trunk, brachial plexus C5, C6 · C4 · C3 · Sternocleidomastoid · Spinal accessory nerve · Parotid gland

FIGURE 20-39. Cleaned clavicle and adipose tissue, further revealing key neurovascular structures.

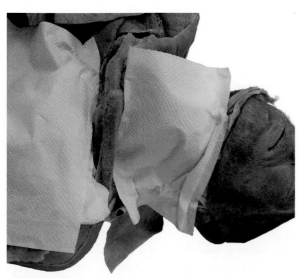

FIGURE 20-40. Cover the neck and thorax with paper towels to protect the dissected structures from bone dust.

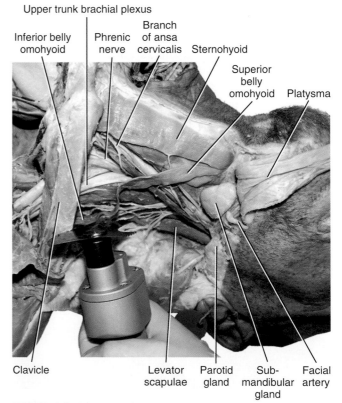

Upper trunk brachial plexus

Inferior belly omohyoid · Phrenic nerve · Branch of ansa cervicalis · Sternohyoid · Superior belly omohyoid · Platysma

Clavicle · Levator scapulae · Parotid gland · Sub-mandibular gland · Facial artery

FIGURE 20-41. Clavicle cut at suprasternal notch and its distal one third.

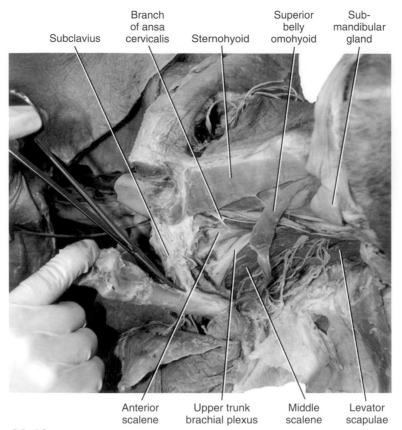

Subclavius Branch of ansa cervicalis Sternohyoid Superior belly omohyoid Sub-mandibular gland

Anterior scalene Upper trunk brachial plexus Middle scalene Levator scapulae

FIGURE 20-42. Clavicle detached from underlying connective tissue and subclavius muscle.

With scissors, detach the clavicle from the underlying connective tissue and subclavius muscle (Figs. 20-42 and 20-43). Reflect the subclavius muscle laterally, and expose the root of the neck and the brachial plexus (Fig. 20-44). Identify the anterior scalene muscle (Fig. 20-45), and on its surface identify the phrenic nerve (Fig. 20-46).

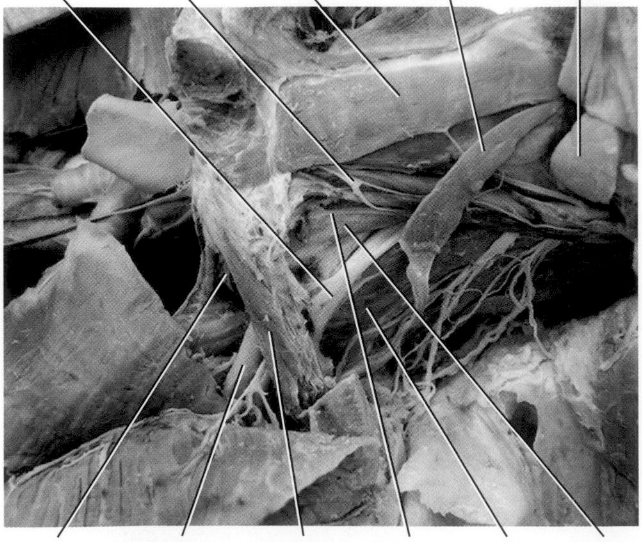

With scissors, cut the internal jugular vein at the level of the bifurcation of the common carotid artery, and remove it from the neck (Fig. 20-46). Trace the supraclavicular nerves, noting their origin from

Upper trunk brachial plexus Branch of ansa cervicalis Sternohyoid Superior belly omohyoid Sub-mandibular gland

Subclavian vein Subclavian artery Subclavius Phrenic nerve Middle scalene Anterior scalene

FIGURE 20-43. Appreciate subclavius muscle and brachial plexus at root of neck.

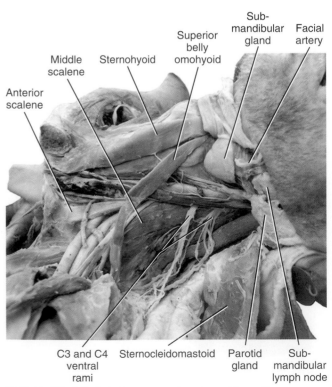

Anterior scalene Middle scalene Sternohyoid Superior belly omohyoid Sub-mandibular gland Facial artery

C3 and C4 ventral rami Sternocleidomastoid Parotid gland Sub-mandibular lymph node

FIGURE 20-44. Subclavius muscle reflected laterally to expose root of neck, brachial plexus, first rib, anterior scalene muscle, and phrenic nerve.

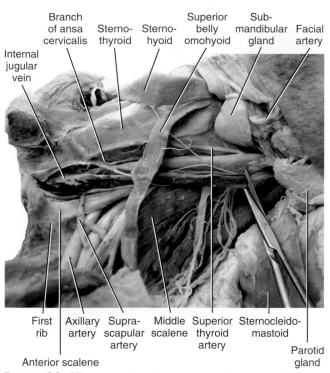

FIGURE 20-45. Internal jugular vein incised at level of bifurcation of common carotid artery and removed from the neck.

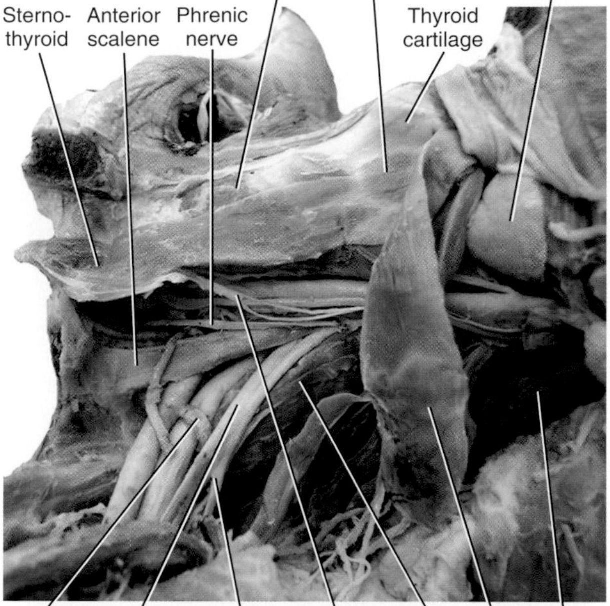

FIGURE 20-47. Inferior attachments of sternohyoid and sternothyroid muscles reflected upward to expose thyroid gland.

cervical nerves 3 and 4 (C3, C4). On the anterior surface of the anterior scalene muscle, note the phrenic nerve is crossed by branches of the thyrocervical trunk, the transverse cervical and suprascapular arteries (see Fig. 20-49).

Cut the inferior attachments of the sternohyoid and sternothyroid muscles, and reflect them upward to expose the *thyroid gland* (Figs. 20-47 and 20-48). Notice the branches from the ansa cervicalis innervating the strap muscles.

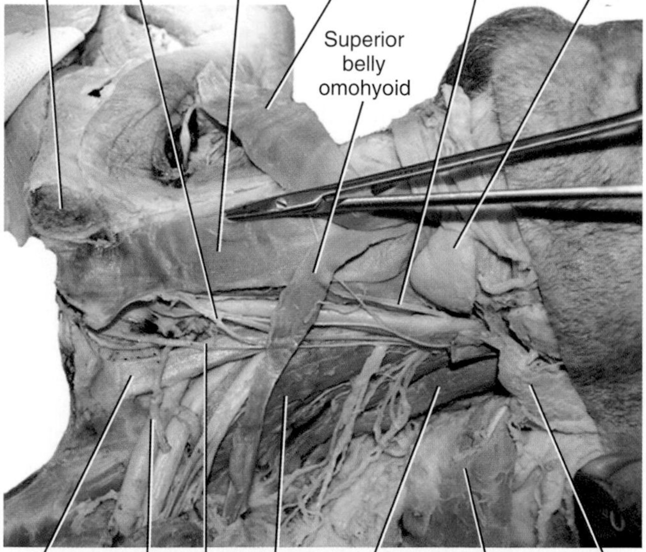

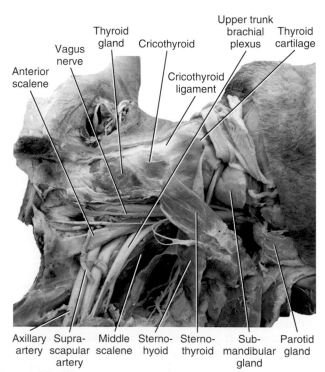

FIGURE 20-46. Appreciate supraclavicular nerves and phrenic nerve crossed by branches of thyrocervical trunk.

FIGURE 20-48. Thyroid gland and cricothyroid muscle exposed.

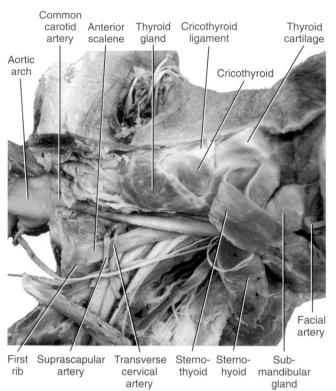

Aortic arch — Common carotid artery — Anterior scalene — Thyroid gland — Cricothyroid ligament — Cricothyroid — Thyroid cartilage

First rib — Suprascapular artery — Transverse cervical artery — Sterno-thyroid — Sterno-hyoid — Sub-mandibular gland — Facial artery

FIGURE 20-49. Appreciate the trachea with fat cleaned, highlighting key landmarks.

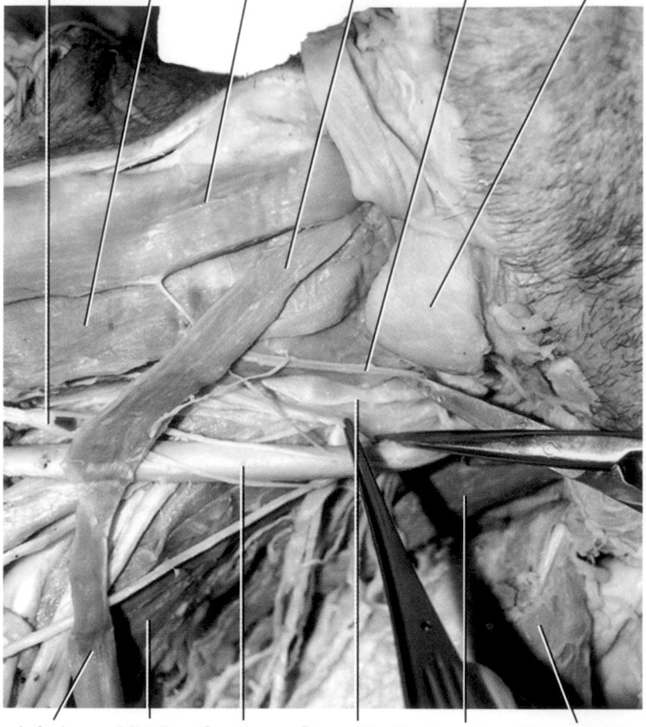

Branch of ansa cervicalis — Sterno-thyroid — Sterno-hyoid — Superior belly omohyoid — Superior thyroid artery — Sub-mandibular gland

Inferior belly omohyoid — Middle scalene — Common carotid artery — Sympathetic chain — Levator scapulae — Sternocleido-mastoid

FIGURE 20-50. Common carotid artery pulled laterally to trace superior thyroid artery, internal laryngeal nerve, superior laryngeal artery, and external laryngeal nerve.

Follow the superior thyroid artery medial to its termination into the thyroid gland. Identify the cricothyroid muscle superior to the thyroid gland (Fig. 20-49). Note the two lobes of the thyroid gland connected by the isthmus.

> ✋ *DISSECTION TIP:* A pyramidal lobe may be present, traveling from the thyroid gland toward the hyoid bone. If time permits, cut the isthmus of the thyroid gland, and reflect the gland laterally from the trachea. Look on the posterior surface of the thyroid gland for the *parathyroid glands,* typically found close to the posterior branches of the superior and inferior thyroid arteries. If time permits, identify the superior and middle thyroid veins, and trace them back to the internal jugular vein.

Pull the common carotid artery laterally, and trace the superior thyroid artery (Fig. 20-50). Locate the internal laryngeal nerve, and trace its origin back to the superior laryngeal nerve. Pull the internal

laryngeal nerve away from its origin, and identify the external laryngeal branch. Follow this nerve as it descends into the neck medial to the common carotid artery, running alongside the superior thyroid artery. Clean the superior thyroid artery, and find the external laryngeal nerve piercing the cricothyroid muscle.

Pull the common carotid artery laterally to expose the space between the anterior scalene muscle and trachea (Fig. 20-51). Clean the connective tissue between this gap, and identify and the inferior thyroid artery, thyrocervical trunk, and recurrent laryngeal nerve (Fig. 20-52). The *inferior thyroid artery* is a branch of the thyrocervical trunk that supplies the inferior pole of the thyroid gland.

Dissect the fat and connective tissue medial to the trachea (tracheoesophageal groove), and identify the *recurrent laryngeal nerve* (Fig. 20-53). The left recurrent laryngeal nerve arises from the left vagus nerve in the thorax as the vagus nerve crosses the arch of the aorta. The right recurrent laryngeal nerve arises from the right vagus nerve as it crosses the right subclavian artery.

The *inferior thyroid artery* crosses the recurrent laryngeal nerve at the inferior pole of the thyroid artery (Fig. 20-54). This is an important surgical landmark.

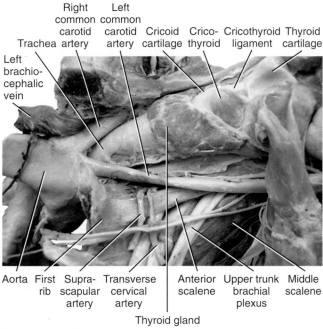

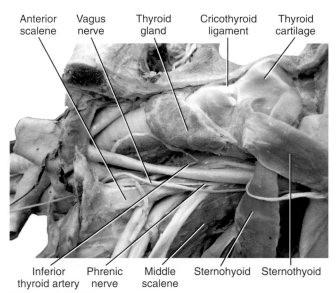

FIGURE 20-51. Appreciate the common carotid artery in the tracheoesophageal region, with recurrent laryngeal nerve along the tracheoesophageal groove.

FIGURE 20-52. Appreciate the inferior thyroid artery, a key surgical landmark.

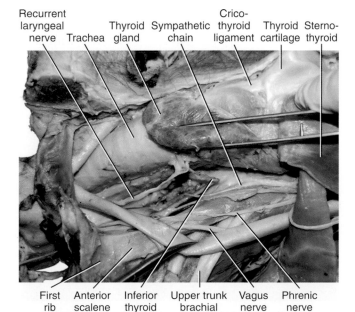

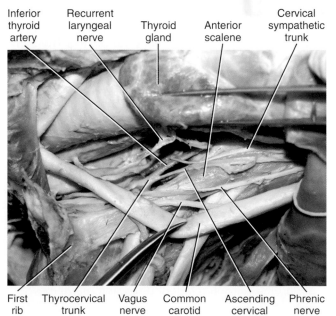

FIGURE 20-53. Common carotid artery pulled laterally, revealing branches of thyrocervical trunk. Note the relationship between the recurrent laryngeal nerve and inferior thyroid artery.

FIGURE 20-54. Medial to the thyrocervical trunk, identify the vertebral artery arising as the first branch of the subclavian artery.

When the inferior thyroid artery arises from the aortic arch, brachiocephalic trunk, or common carotid or vertebral artery, it is called the *thyroidea ima* (lowest thyroid) artery. This variation is present in approximately 5% of the population.

> ☝ *DISSECTION TIP:* In some specimens a nonrecurrent laryngeal nerve is present. This variation is caused by a delay in the development of the aortic arches, resulting in the right vagus nerve giving off a transversely oriented, nonrecurrent laryngeal nerve, which passes directly toward the larynx without reaching the thorax. This anatomic situation is usually associated with a retroesophageal right subclavian artery.

Trace the previously identified transverse cervical and suprascapular arteries deep to their origin from the thyrocervical trunk (Fig. 20-54).

> ☝ *DISSECTION TIP:* The transverse cervical or suprascapular arteries may be absent. In such cases the dorsal scapular artery may be large and may arise from the subclavian artery, crossing over the first rib.

Lift the contents of the carotid sheath (internal jugular vein, common carotid artery, vagus nerve), and look posterior for the cervical part of the sympathetic trunk, or sympathetic chain (see Fig. 20-50). Note that the sympathetic chain and the roots of the cervical plexus lie behind the carotid sheath. The sympathetic chain lies within a dense fascial layer, the prevertebral fascia. Clean the prevertebral fascia (and remnants of carotid sheath) posterior to the common carotid artery. Trace the sympathetic chain inferiorly, and identify the superior, middle, and inferior cervical ganglia (Figs. 20-53 and 20-54).

> ☝ *DISSECTION TIP:* The middle cervical ganglion is variable in origin and is often not present. The superior cervical ganglion can be identified at the level of the angle of the mandible. However, during the retropharyngeal dissection, it will be fully exposed.

Once the thyrocervical trunk is identified and its branches exposed, pull it laterally and look for the *vertebral artery,* which ascends medial and deep to it

(Fig. 20-55). Near the origin of the vertebral artery, identify the inferior cervical ganglion and/or the stellate ganglion (Figs. 20-56 and 20-57). The inferior cervical ganglion is large and often fused with the first thoracic chain ganglion, forming the stellate (cervicothoracic) ganglion (Fig. 20-58).

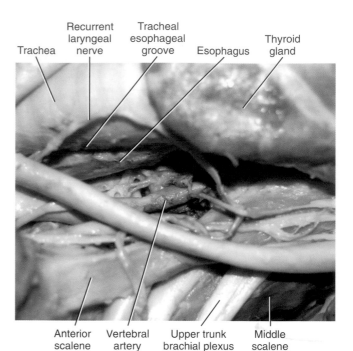

FIGURE 20-55. Common carotid artery and thyrocervical trunk pulled laterally to identify the vertebral artery and sympathetic chain.

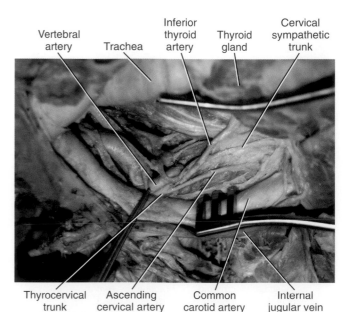

FIGURE 20-56. Retractors used (as necessary) to keep common carotid artery and thyrocervical trunk reflected laterally, highlighting the sympathetic chain with its stellate ganglion and vertebral artery.

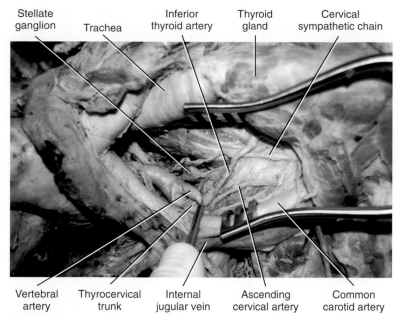

Stellate ganglion | Trachea | Inferior thyroid artery | Thyroid gland | Cervical sympathetic chain

Vertebral artery | Thyrocervical trunk | Internal jugular vein | Ascending cervical artery | Common carotid artery

FIGURE 20-57. Appreciate the stellate ganglion, vertebral artery, and sympathetic chain fully exposed.

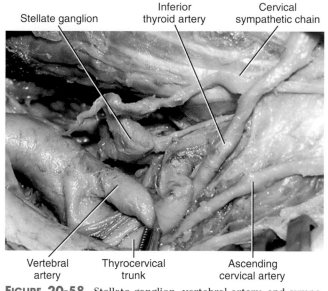

Stellate ganglion | Inferior thyroid artery | Cervical sympathetic chain

Vertebral artery | Thyrocervical trunk | Ascending cervical artery

FIGURE 20-58. Stellate ganglion, vertebral artery, and sympathetic chain fully dissected and exposed.

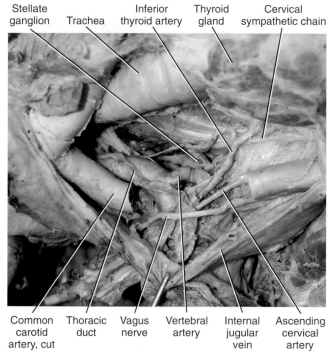

Stellate ganglion | Trachea | Inferior thyroid artery | Thyroid gland | Cervical sympathetic chain

Common carotid artery, cut | Thoracic duct | Vagus nerve | Vertebral artery | Internal jugular vein | Ascending cervical artery

FIGURE 20-59. Common carotid artery cut, exposing thoracic duct.

After identifying the stellate ganglion or inferior cervical ganglion, cut 2 to 3 cm of the inferior portion of the common carotid artery (Fig. 20-59). Immediately beneath this artery, identify the *thoracic duct.* On the left side, the thoracic duct will empty into the junction between the internal jugular and subclavian veins. On the right side, the smaller right lymphatic duct will terminate at the junction of the right internal jugular and right subclavian veins.

DISSECTION TIP: The thoracic duct is located close to the stellate or inferior cervical ganglion and is often severed during this dissection.

Optional Dissection

The subclavian artery gives rise to the following branches:

1. Thyrocervical trunk
2. Vertebral artery
3. Internal thoracic artery
4. Costocervical trunk

The *costocervical trunk* is located on the deep surface of the subclavian artery posterior to the anterior scalene muscle. It usually gives off the highest intercostal artery, which supplies the uppermost intercostal spaces. Cut the anterior scalene muscle midway from its attachment to the first rib (Fig. 20-60). Look at the posterior surface of subclavian artery, and trace the costocervical trunk (Fig. 20-61). This dissection can also take place from the internal surface of the already-dissected thorax. The other branch of the costocervical trunk is the deep cervical artery, which ascends in the neck posterior to the transverse processes of the cervical vertebrae.

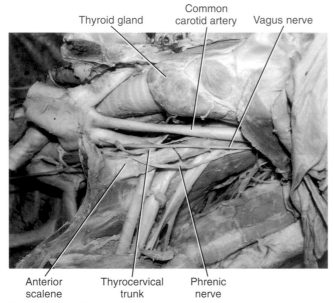

FIGURE 20-60. Anterior scalene muscle cut midway from its attachment onto first rib.

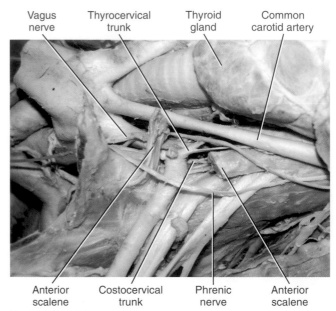

FIGURE 20-61. Anterior scalene muscle and posterior surface of subclavian artery lifted, revealing origin of costocervical trunk.

LABORATORY IDENTIFICATION CHECKLIST

Nerves
Cervical plexus
- ❏ Great auricular
- ❏ Transverse cervical
- ❏ Supraclavicular nerves
- ❏ Lesser occipital
- ❏ C1 fibers to thyrohyoid muscle
- ❏ Ansa cervicalis (C1-C3)
  - ❏ Superior root (C1)
  - ❏ Inferior root (C2 and C3)
  - ❏ Trunk (C1-C3)
- ❏ Phrenic (C3-C5)

Cranial nerves (CN)
- ❏ Spinal accessory (CN XI)
- ❏ Hypoglossal nerve (CN XII)
- ❏ Vagus nerve (CN X)
- ❏ Nerve to mylohyoid/anterior digastric muscle (CN V; from inferior alveolar nerve)
- ❏ Cervical branch from facial (CN VII)

Autonomic nerves
- ❏ Vagus
- ❏ Superior laryngeal
  - ❏ External laryngeal
  - ❏ Internal laryngeal
  - ❏ Recurrent laryngeal
  - ❏ Inferior laryngeal
- ❏ Cervical sympathetic chain/ trunk

Ganglia
- ❏ Superior cervical
- ❏ Middle cervical
- ❏ Stellate

Arteries
- ❏ Common carotid
  - ❏ Internal carotid
  - ❏ External carotid
- ❏ Superior thyroid
  - ❏ Superior laryngeal

Arteries—cont'd
- ❏ Lingual
- ❏ Facial
- ❏ Occipital
- ❏ Ascending pharyngeal
- ❏ Subclavian
- ❏ Vertebral
- ❏ Thyrocervical trunk
  - ❏ Inferior thyroid
  - ❏ Transverse scapular
  - ❏ Suprascapular
- ❏ Dorsal scapular

Veins
- ❏ External jugular
- ❏ Anterior jugular
- ❏ Internal jugular
  - ❏ Superior thyroid
  - ❏ Middle thyroid
- ❏ Subclavian
- ❏ Inferior thyroid veins

Muscles
- ❏ Platysma
- ❏ Sternocleidomastoid
  - ❏ Sternal head
  - ❏ Clavicular head
- ❏ Sternohyoid
- ❏ Omohyoid
- ❏ Sternothyroid
- ❏ Thyrohyoid
- ❏ Anterior belly of digastric
- ❏ Mylohyoid
- ❏ Posterior belly of digastric
- ❏ Stylohyoid
- ❏ Splenius capitis
- ❏ Levator scapulae
- ❏ Posterior scalene
- ❏ Middle scalene
- ❏ Anterior scalene
- ❏ Trapezius

Fascia
- ❏ Superficial fascia
- ❏ Tela subcutanea
- ❏ Deep fascia
  - ❏ Investing layer
  - ❏ Pretracheal layer
  - ❏ Prevertebral layer

Bones
- ❏ Mandible
- ❏ Hyoid
- ❏ Manubrium
- ❏ Clavicle
- ❏ Cervical vertebrae (C1-C7)
  - ❏ Atlas (C1)
  - ❏ Axis (C2)
- ❏ Occipital
- ❏ Temporal
  - ❏ Mastoid process
  - ❏ Styloid process

Connective Tissue
- ❏ Thyroid cartilage
- ❏ Cricoid cartilage
- ❏ Cricothyroid ligament
- ❏ Stylohyoid ligament
- ❏ Stylomandibular ligament
- ❏ Thyrohyoid membrane

Glands
- ❏ Submandibular gland
- ❏ Thyroid gland
  - ❏ Right lobe
  - ❏ Left lobe
  - ❏ ±Pyramidal lobe
- ❏ Parathyroid glands

CHAPTER 21

FACE

Netter: 2–3, 24–25, 35

McMinn: 49–50

Gray's Atlas: 455–459

BEFORE DISSECTION

Palpate the following facial landmarks on the cadaver:

- Suprasternal notch
- Mental protuberance
- Nasion, glabella, vertex, and external occipital protuberance (inion)
- Mastoid process
- Ramus, angle, and body of mandible

- Zygomatic arch
- Infraorbital margin
- Supraorbital margin
- Superciliary ridge

With a marker, outline the dissection for the cadaver as follows (Fig. 21-1):
1. Make a line from the mental protuberance to the vertex. The line should encircle the lips, nostrils, and eyelids.
2. Make a second line from the mental protuberance to the lobule of the ear.
3. Make a third line from the vertex to the upper part of the helix of the ear.

Based on the lines drawn, make an incision between the angle of the mandible and the mental protuberance (Fig. 21-2). Carefully reflect the flaps of skin (from medial to lateral) created by the incisions (Figs. 21-3 and 21-4). Beneath the skin, notice the surface of the face covered almost entirely by fat. This fibrofatty tissue is also known as the *superficial musculoaponeurotic space* or *system* (SMAS).

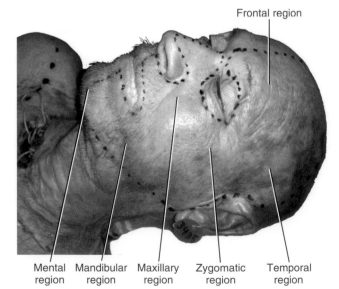

Frontal region

Mental region   Mandibular region   Maxillary region   Zygomatic region   Temporal region

FIGURE 21-1. Anterolateral facial view with stippled lines for incisions, showing six major surface regions (temporal, frontal, zygomatic, maxillary, mandibular, mental).

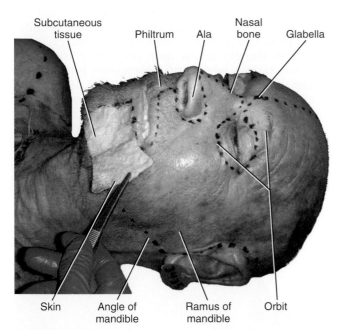

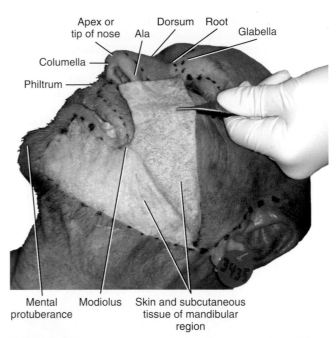

FIGURE 21-2. Anterolateral facial view with skin reflected from the mental region and facial landmarks highlighted (orbit, glabella, nasal bone, ala, ramus of mandible, philtrum, angle of mandible).

FIGURE 21-3. Anterolateral facial view with skin reflected from the mandibular region, revealing subcutaneous tissue, glabella, root of nose, dorsum of nose, tip of nose, ala, columella nasi, philtrum, mental protuberance, and modiolus (columella cochleae).

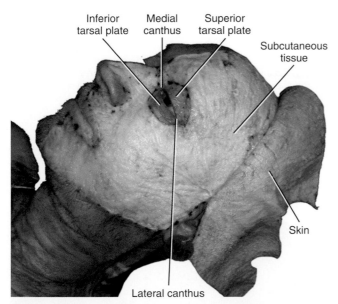

FIGURE 21-4. Lateral facial view with skin reflected from mandibular, maxillary, zygomatic, frontal, and temporal regions, revealing subcutaneous tissue, superior/inferior tarsal plate, and medial/lateral canthus.

DISSECTION TIP: The muscles of facial expression vary in thickness. To identify these mimetic muscles, remove the skin over the SMAS. Pay special attention with this technique to avoid cutting any muscles, because many attach directly into the skin. While cleaning the mimetic muscles and removing the superficial fascia, preserve the branches of the facial nerve, which innervate them.

Situated in front of the ear (auricle), the *parotid gland* is covered with variable amounts of fat. Using the separating technique with your scissors, reflect as much fat as possible until you identify the substance of the parotid gland (Fig. 21-5). The parotid gland typically extends into the space between the zygomatic arch and the angle of the mandible (Fig. 21-6). The parotid gland is covered by a dense fibrous capsule, which sends septae into the gland, dividing it into lobules.

As the SMAS is reflected more medially, identify the *parotid duct,* usually found emerging from the anterior edge of the parotid gland, about 1 inch (2.5 cm) inferior to the zygomatic arch (Figs. 21-7 and 21-8). From this point, the parotid duct passes horizontally across the masseter muscle, then turns around the anterior edge of the masseter and pierces the buccinator muscle (Fig. 21-9). Identify the superficial temporal artery just superior to the zygomatic arch in front of the ear. The auriculotemporal nerve can be found just posterior to this artery.

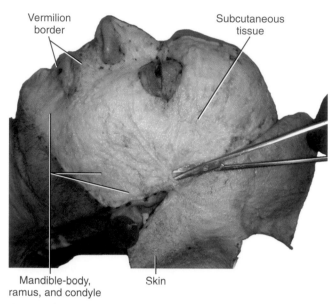

FIGURE 21-5. Lateral facial view with skin reflected from mandibular, maxillary, zygomatic, frontal, and temporal regions, revealing subcutaneous tissue, vermilion border, and body, ramus, and condyle of mandible.

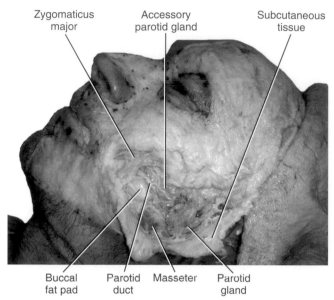

FIGURE 21-7. Lateral facial view with skin reflected and subcutaneous tissue removed from the mandibular region, revealing parotid gland, parotid duct, accessory parotid gland, zygomaticus major muscle, buccal fat pad, and masseter muscle.

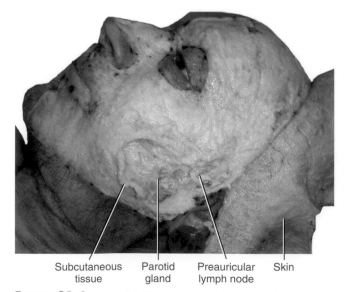

FIGURE 21-6. Lateral facial view with skin reflected and subcutaneous tissue removed from the mandibular region, revealing parotid gland and preauricular nodes.

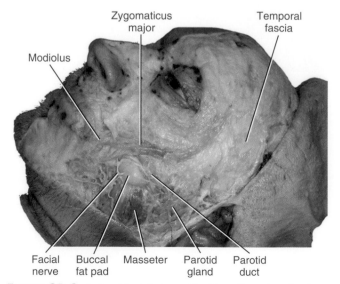

FIGURE 21-8. Lateral facial view with skin reflected and subcutaneous tissue removed from mandibular, maxillary, and temporal regions, revealing temporal fascia, parotid duct, parotid gland, masseter, buccal fat pad, facial nerve, modiolus, and zygomaticus major muscle.

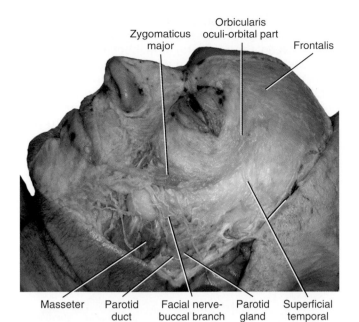

FIGURE 21-9. Lateral facial view with skin reflected and subcutaneous tissue removed from the mandibular, maxillary, and orbital regions, revealing frontalis muscle, orbicularis oculi muscle (orbital section), superficial temporal artery, parotid duct, parotid gland, buccal branch of facial nerve, masseter muscle, and zygomaticus major muscle.

FIGURE 21-10. Anterolateral view of face with skin and subcutaneous tissue removed, revealing parotid gland and accessory parotid gland, parotid duct, facial nerve branches (buccal, zygomatic, temporal), and superior labial artery.

✋ *DISSECTION TIP:* Accessory glandular tissue (the socia parotidis) can often be identified along the parotid duct in its course across the masseter muscle (Fig. 21-9). Pay special attention to the buccal branch of the facial nerve, which usually runs alongside the parotid duct. In some specimens, some of the parotid lymph nodes may be encountered as the gland is dissected. The transverse facial artery runs superior to the parotid duct, but because of its small size, identifying this artery is often difficult.

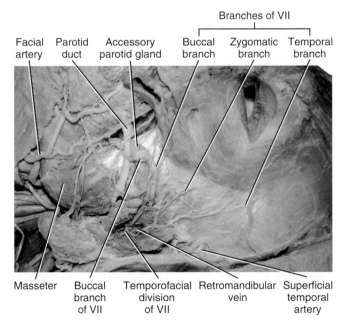

FIGURE 21-11. Anterolateral view of face with skin and subcutaneous tissue removed, revealing parotid structures and temporofacial division of facial nerve and its branches (buccal, zygomatic, temporal) with facial and superficial temporal arteries.

Tracing the branches of the facial nerve can be challenging. Identify the *buccal branch,* which runs alongside the parotid duct (Fig. 21-10). After you have exposed the buccal branch of the facial nerve, carefully trace it into the substance of the parotid gland until you find its junction(s) with other branches, then dissect them out to their target muscles (Fig. 21-11).

The parotid gland may be completely removed when the trunk of the facial nerve and its branches are exposed. The facial nerve typically bifurcates into *temporofacial* and *cervicofacial* divisions (Fig. 21-10). Identify the terminal branches of the facial nerve: temporal, zygomatic, buccal, mandibular, and cervical. The terminal branches of the facial nerve often connect to one another or with infraorbital branches of the trigeminal nerve.

✍ DISSECTION TIP: Several branches of the facial nerve are not identified with the cadaver in the supine position, including the *posterior auricular nerve,* which innervates musculature of the external ear and the occipitalis muscle, and the *digastric* branch, which supplies the posterior belly of the digastric muscle and the stylohyoid muscle. Landmarks for other branches of the facial nerve follow:
- *Temporal* branch: dissect near the posterior part of the zygomatic arch.
- *Zygomatic* branch: dissect around the zygomaticus major muscle at the base of the zygomatic bone.
- *Buccal* branch: runs parallel to the parotid duct and crosses the masseter muscle.
- *Mandibular* branch: dissect at the posteroinferior margin of the mandible.
- *Cervical* branch: dissect deep to the platysma muscle, approximately one fingerbreadth posterior to the angle of the mandible.

The *facial artery* is hidden along part of its course by the submandibular gland and by several mimetic muscles. The facial artery becomes superficial at the inferior border of the mandible near its angle. It then crosses the cheek, passes near the angle of the mouth, and ends near the medial angle of the eye as the *angular artery.* Identify the superior labial artery within the substance of the orbicularis oris muscle.

Expose the *superior labial artery,* and trace it backward toward the angle of the mandible (Fig. 21-10). Medially reflect any of the mimetic muscles covering the facial artery. Once the facial artery is exposed, continue exposing the terminal part, the angular artery.

✍ DISSECTION TIP: The facial artery will terminate in approximately 50% of the specimens as an angular artery. The course of the facial artery is tortuous and in contact with the facial vein, which lies just posterior to it.

After you expose all terminal branches of the facial nerve, identify and remove the *buccal fat pad* (see Fig. 21-8), an encapsulated mass of adipose tissue, which lies between the masseter and buccinator muscles (Fig. 21-12). The parotid duct can be clearly traced to its point of penetration into the buccinator muscle.

Lift the buccal fat bad with forceps, and use scissors to cut its attachments to nearby structures (Figs. 21-13 and 21-14). Pay special attention to preserve the neurovascular structures in the area as you remove the fat pad.

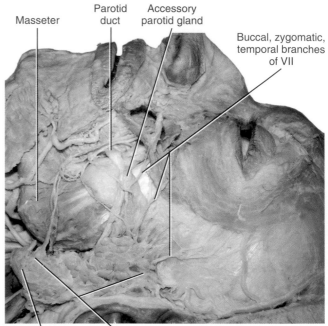

FIGURE 21-12. Anterolateral view of face with skin and subcutaneous tissue removed, revealing parotid capsule (superficial fascia), parotid gland, accessory parotid gland, parotid duct, temporofacial division of the facial nerve and its branches (buccal, zygomatic, temporal).

✍ DISSECTION TIP: As you remove the buccal fat pad, you will probably notice branches of the buccal artery and nerve. The buccal nerve is usually located between the masseter and buccinator muscles and follows the anterior border of the temporalis muscle to its insertion onto the coronoid process of the mandible. Do not spend time completely exposing the temporalis now; this occurs during the infratemporal area dissection (Chapter 22).

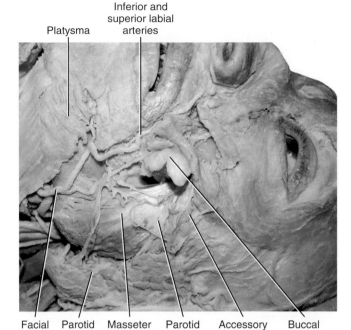

FIGURE 21-13. Anterolateral view of face with skin and subcutaneous tissue removed, revealing parotid structures, masseter and platysma muscles, and arteries (facial, inferior labial, superior labial).

Remove the SMAS and identify several mimetic muscles. The muscle surrounding the lips is the *orbicularis oris*. The muscle identified around the eyelids is the *orbicularis oculi,* comprising orbital, palpebral, and lacrimal parts. The platysma muscle has been identified in the dissection of the neck (see Chapter 20). Some platysma fibers pass up over the lower border of the mandible and mingle with the depressor muscles of the lips and with the risorius muscle more laterally. Identify the zygomaticus major and minor, depressor anguli oris, and depressor labii inferioris muscles as well as the buccinator muscle (Figs. 21-15 to 21-17).

> ☝ *DISSECTION TIP:* Often you will need to remove additional skin from the margins of the lips to expose the orbicularis oris fully. Fibers from several other facial muscles merge with the orbicularis oris, including the buccinator and the elevators and depressors of the angles of the mouth.

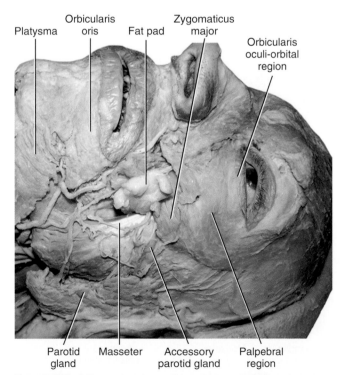

FIGURE 21-14. Anterolateral view of face with skin and subcutaneous tissue removed, revealing parotid gland, accessory parotid gland, buccal fat pad, and muscles (masseter, platysma, orbicularis oris, orbicularis oculi with orbital/palpebral parts).

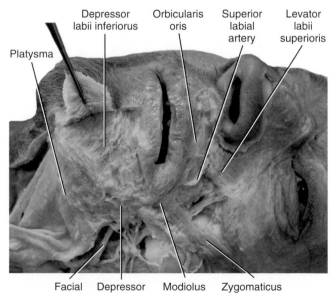

FIGURE 21-15. Anterior view of mandible and neck with skin removed, revealing key arteries (facial, superior labial) and muscles (depressor anguli oris, zygomaticus major, levator labii superioris, orbicularis oris, depressor labii inferiorus, platysma).

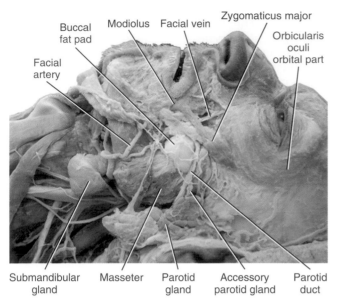

FIGURE 21-16. Anterior view of face with skin reflected over mental and neck regions, highlighting submandibular gland, masseter, parotid gland, accessory parotid gland, parotid duct, orbicularis oculi (orbital part), zygomaticus major, facial vein, modiolus, buccal fat pad, and facial artery.

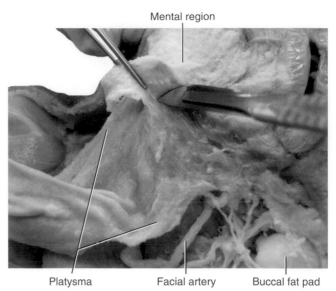

FIGURE 21-18. Anterolateral view of the face and neck with skin and subcutaneous tissue removed, revealing platysma muscle, facial artery, and buccal fat pad.

Expose the fibers of the platysma muscle (Fig. 21-18). With scissors, remove the platysma, depressor labii inferioris, and depressor anguli oris muscles medially over the periosteum of the mandible (Fig. 21-19). Identify the mental foramen and the mental nerve (Fig. 21-20).

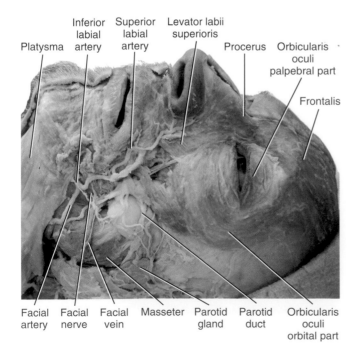

FIGURE 21-17. Anterolateral view of face and neck with skin and subcutaneous tissue removed, revealing facial artery, nerve, and vein; masseter muscle; parotid gland and duct; orbicularis oculi (orbital/palpebral), frontalis, procerus, levator labii superioris, and platysma muscles; and superior/inferior labial arteries.

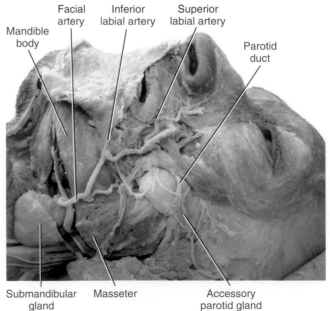

FIGURE 21-19. Anterolateral view of face and neck with skin and subcutaneous tissue removed, revealing masseter, parotid duct, accessory parotid gland, superior labial artery, inferior labial artery, mandibular body, facial artery, and submandibular gland.

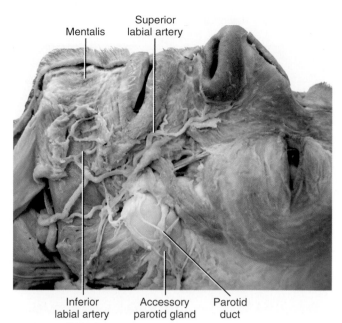

Mentalis   Superior labial artery

Inferior labial artery   Accessory parotid gland   Parotid duct

FIGURE 21-20. Anterolateral view of face and neck with skin and subcutaneous tissue removed, revealing parotid duct, accessory parotid gland, superior labial artery, mentalis muscle, and inferior labial artery.

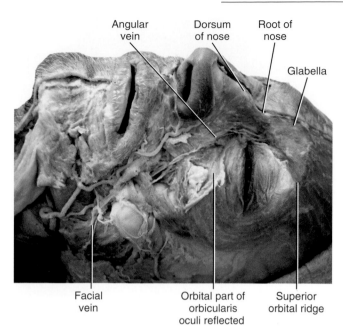

Angular vein   Dorsum of nose   Root of nose

Glabella

Facial vein   Orbital part of orbicularis oculi reflected   Superior orbital ridge

FIGURE 21-22. Anterolateral view of face and neck with skin and subcutaneous tissue removed, revealing orbital part of orbicularis oculi reflected, supraorbital ridge, glabella, root and dorsum of nose, and angular vein.

One way to identify the infraorbital and mental nerves is to draw an imaginary line from the supraorbital notch vertically to the mandible, which will pass over, or near, the infraorbital and mental foramina. Detach the inferior part of the orbicularis oris superiorly from the inferior orbital rim (medial to zygomaticus major muscle) (Fig. 21-21). Detach the levator labii superioris alaeque nasi medially, and identify the infraorbital nerve (Figs. 21-22 to 21-24)

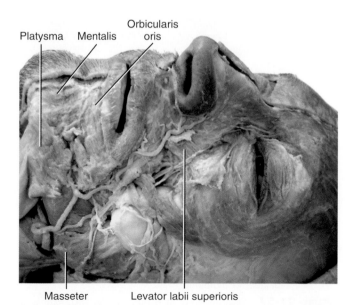

Platysma   Mentalis   Orbicularis oris

Masseter   Levator labii superioris

FIGURE 21-21. Anterolateral view of face and neck with skin and subcutaneous tissue removed, revealing mentalis, orbicularis oris, platysma, masseter, and levator labii superioris muscles.

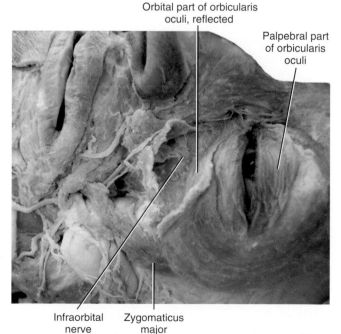

Orbital part of orbicularis oculi, reflected

Palpebral part of orbicularis oculi

Infraorbital nerve   Zygomaticus major

FIGURE 21-23. Anteromedial view of nasal, orbital, and maxillary region with skin and subcutaneous tissue removed, revealing palpebral part of orbicularis oculi, zygomaticus major muscle, and infraorbital nerve.

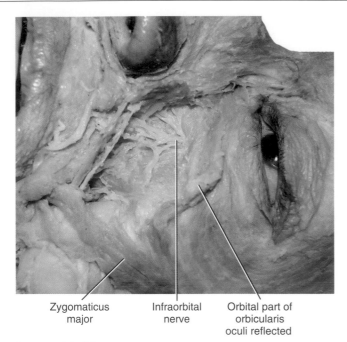

FIGURE 21-24. Anteroinferior view of orbital region with skin and subcutaneous tissue removed, revealing orbital part of orbicularis oculi reflected, infraorbital nerve, and zygomaticus major muscle.

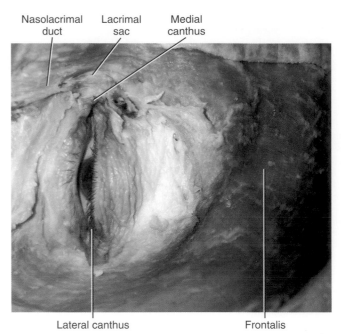

FIGURE 21-26. Anterior view of orbital region with skin and subcutaneous tissue removed, revealing frontalis, tarsal plate, lateral canthus, nasolacrimal duct, lacrimal sac, and medial canthus.

Reflect the superior part of the orbicularis oculi muscle, and identify the superior tarsal plate (Figs. 21-25 and 21-26). Reflect the superior tarsal plate, and notice the fascia of the levator palpebrae superioris muscle (Fig. 21-27). Palpate the supraorbital notch, and with scissors, separate the muscle fibers and the connective tissue superficial (inferior and superior) to the notch to expose the *supraorbital nerve* (Fig. 21-28).

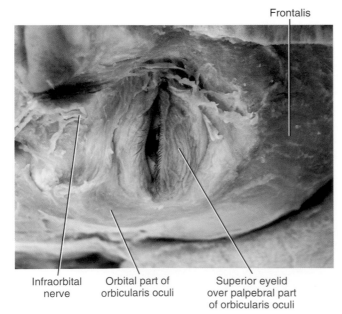

FIGURE 21-25. Anteroinferior view of orbital region with skin and subcutaneous tissue removed, revealing frontalis muscle, palpebral and orbital parts of orbicularis oculi muscle, and infraorbital nerve.

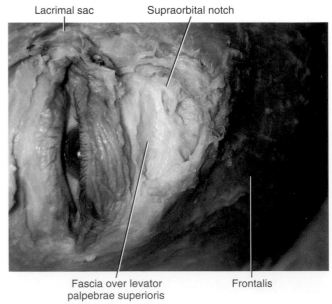

FIGURE 21-27. Anterior view of orbital region with skin and subcutaneous tissue removed, revealing frontalis, fascia over levator palpebrae superioris, superior tarsal plate, supraorbital notch, and lacrimal sac.

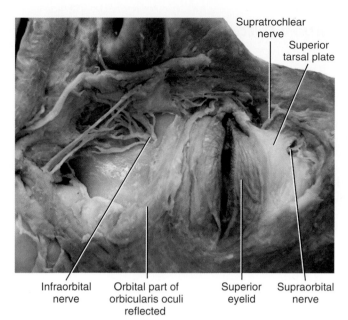

Supratrochlear
nerve

Superior
tarsal plate

Infraorbital   Orbital part of   Superior   Supraorbital
nerve   orbicularis oculi   eyelid   nerve
            reflected

FIGURE 21-28. Anterior superior view of orbital region with skin removed, revealing subcutaneous tissue and supratrochlear nerve, supraorbital nerve, superior tarsal plate, orbicularis oculi (orbital) reflected, and infraorbital nerve.

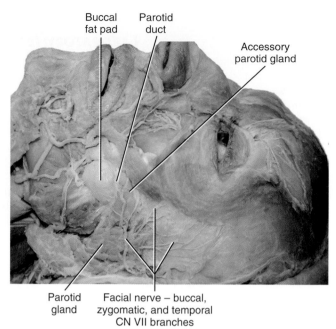

Buccal   Parotid
fat pad   duct

Accessory
parotid gland

Parotid   Facial nerve – buccal,
gland   zygomatic, and temporal
        CN VII branches

FIGURE 21-30. Anterolateral view of face with skin and subcutaneous tissue removed, revealing parotid gland, accessory parotid gland, parotid duct, buccal fat pad, and facial nerve (buccal, zygomatic, and temporal branches).

DISSECTION TIP: In most specimens the supraorbital nerve, artery, and vein emerge through the orbital septum and superior tarsal plate (Fig. 21-28), whereas the supratrochlear nerve emerges medially (Fig. 21-29).

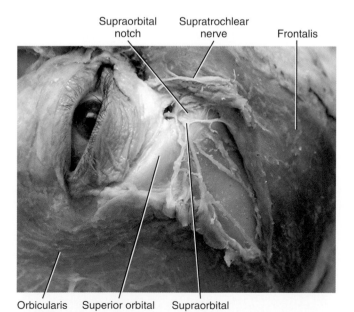

Supraorbital   Supratrochlear
notch   nerve   Frontalis

Orbicularis   Superior orbital   Supraorbital
oculi   ridge   nerve

FIGURE 21-29. Anterosuperior view of orbital region with skin and subcutaneous tissue removed, revealing supraorbital notch and ridge, supratrochlear and supraorbital nerves, and orbicularis oculi and frontalis muscles.

Identify the superficial temporal vein. This vein joins the maxillary vein to form the retromandibular vein.

You may remove the parotid gland now (Fig. 21-30), or during the dissection of the infratemporal fossa (Chapter 22).

Identify the *retromandibular vein* deep to the facial nerve. The retromandibular vein splits into anterior and posterior divisions; the posterior division joins the posterior auricular vein to form the external jugular vein, and the anterior division joins the facial vein to form the common facial vein.

Identify and trace the *facial vein,* and look for its drainage into the common facial vein (see Fig. 21-17). The facial vein begins at the medial orbit as the angular vein, then courses with the facial artery toward the angle of the mandible (see Fig. 21-22). Identify the junction of the posterior division of the retromandibular vein with the posterior auricular vein, forming the external jugular vein. Lastly, trace the facial veins drain into the anterior division of the retromandibular vein, creating the common facial vein, which drains into the internal jugular vein.

LABORATORY IDENTIFICATION CHECKLIST

Nerves

Trigeminal nerve branches (cutaneous)

❐ Supratrochlear nerve
❐ Supraorbital nerve
❐ Zygomaticotemporal nerve
❐ Zygomaticofacial nerve
❐ Auriculotemporal nerve
❐ Infratrochlear nerve
❐ Infraorbital nerve
❐ Mental nerve

Facial nerve branches (motor)

❐ Facial nerve trunk (deep within parotid gland)
❐ Temporal branches
❐ Zygomatic branches
❐ Buccal branches
❐ Marginal mandibular branches
❐ Cervical branches

Arteries

❐ External carotid (within parotid gland)
❐ Superficial temporal
❐ Maxillary
❐ Transverse facial
❐ Facial
  ❐ Superior labial
  ❐ Inferior labial
❐ Angular

Veins

❐ Facial
❐ Angular
❐ Retromandibular (within parotid gland)

Muscles

❐ Occipitofrontalis
  ❐ Frontalis belly
  ❐ Galea aponeurotica
  ❐ Occipitalis belly
❐ Procerus
❐ Orbicularis oculi
  ❐ Orbital part
  ❐ Palpebral part
  ❐ Lacrimal part
❐ Levator labii superioris alaeque nasi
❐ Levator labii superioris
❐ Levator anguli oris
❐ Risorius
❐ Zygomaticus major/minor
❐ Buccinator
❐ Orbicularis oris
❐ Depressor anguli oris
❐ Depressor labii inferioris
❐ Mentalis
❐ Platysma

Bones

❐ Frontal
❐ Zygomatic
❐ Temporal
❐ Maxillary
❐ Mandible

Gland

❐ Parotid
  ❐ Parotid duct (Stensen's duct)

CHAPTER 22

INFRATEMPORAL FOSSA

Netter: 39, 45, 54, 55

McMinn: 52, 86

Gray's Atlas: 478–485

The infratemporal fossa dissection requires the use of an electric saw or a hammer and chisel. Make sure that you wear eye protection when you use these tools.

Cut the terminal branches of the facial nerve, and reflect the nerves posteriorly toward the parotid gland. Similarly, cut the parotid duct as it penetrates the buccinator muscle (Fig. 22-1), and reflect it posteriorly toward the parotid gland (Fig. 22-2).

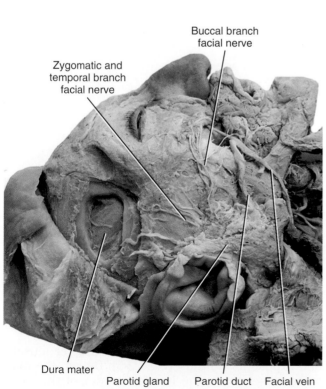

FIGURE 22-1. Lateral view of face with skin reflected, revealing superficial structures.

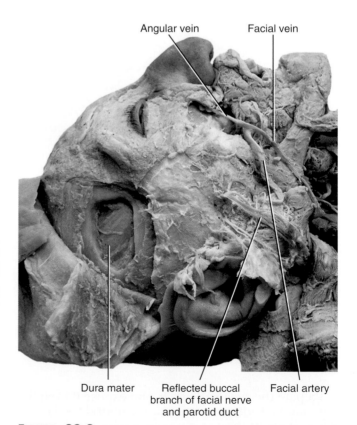

FIGURE 22-2. Lateral view of face, with parotid duct and branches of facial nerve reflected.

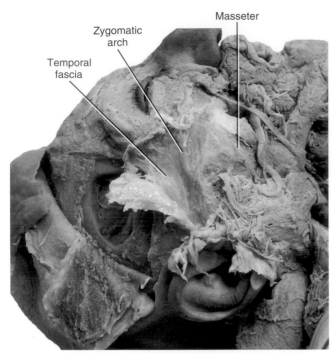

FIGURE 22-3. Lateral view of face, with skin and subcutaneous tissue removed and temporal fascia reflected.

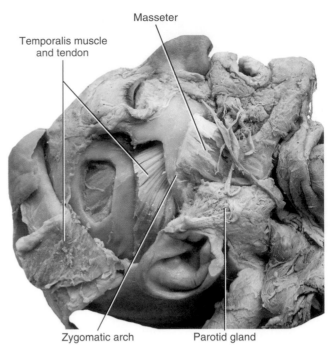

FIGURE 22-5. Lateral view with skin and subcutaneous tissue removed, revealing temporalis and masseter musculature, as well as zygomatic arch.

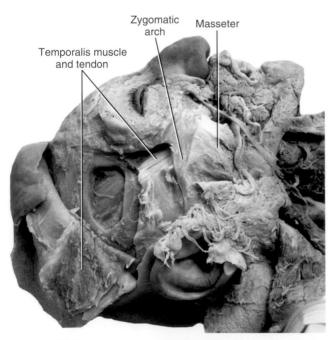

FIGURE 22-4. Lateral view of face, with skin, subcutaneous tissue, and temporal fascia removed, exposing temporalis muscle and zygomatic arch.

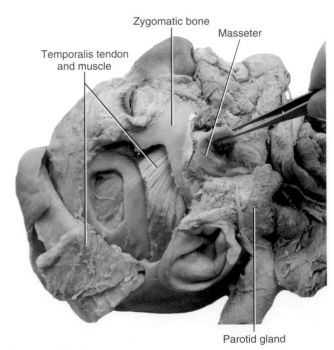

FIGURE 22-6. Reflection of masseter muscle from inferior border of zygomatic arch.

Palpate the zygomatic arch, and expose it from the surrounding adipose tissue and temporal fascia (Fig. 22-3). Identify the temporalis muscle, and trace its course underneath the zygomatic arch (Fig. 22-4).

Clean the lateral surface of the masseter muscle, and expose its borders (Fig. 22-5). Detach the masseter muscle from the inferior border of the zygomatic arch (Fig. 22-6), and reflect it inferiorly toward the angle of the mandible (Figs. 22-7 and 22-8).

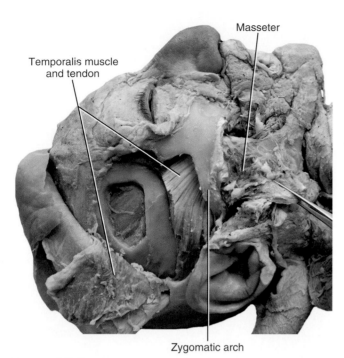

Masseter

Temporalis muscle and tendon

Zygomatic arch

FIGURE 22-7. Further reflection of masseter muscle from inferior zygomatic arch.

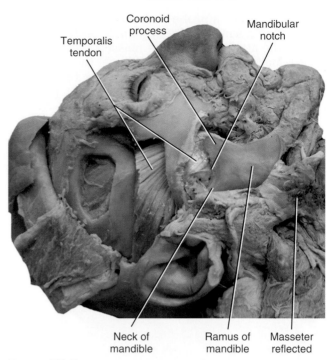

Coronoid process

Temporalis tendon

Mandibular notch

Neck of mandible

Ramus of mandible

Masseter reflected

FIGURE 22-9. Lateral view of face with superficial skin and subcutaneous skin removed and masseter muscle reflected, revealing temporal, zygomatic, and mandibular bony regions.

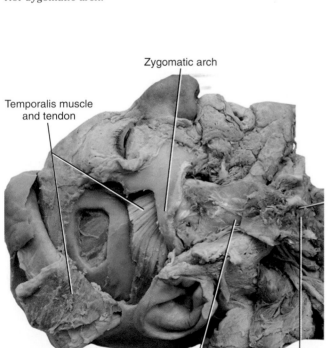

Zygomatic arch

Temporalis muscle and tendon

Mandible

Masseter reflected

FIGURE 22-8. Complete reflection of masseter muscle from inferior zygomatic border, exposing mandible.

Clean the remaining soft tissues over the mandible, and expose its surface (Fig. 22-9).

> ✎ *DISSECTION TIP:* Just deep to the anterior border of the ramus of the mandible, in the fat and connective tissue of the anterior edge of the temporalis muscle, identify and clean the *buccal nerve,* a branch of the mandibular division (V3) of the trigeminal nerve (Fig. 22-9).

Place scissors or a probe underneath the zygomatic arch. Using a saw, cut the zygomatic arch just anterior to the attachment of the masseter muscle (Fig. 22-10) Make a second cut through the arch just posterior to the masseter and anterior to the temporomandibular joint, and detach the cut piece of zygomatic bone (Figs. 22-11 and 22-12).

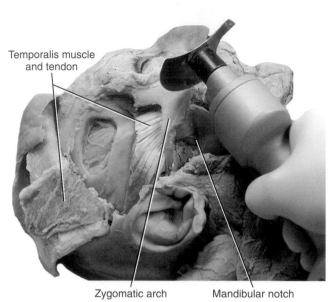

FIGURE 22-10. Saw cut of zygomatic arch just anterior to attachment of masseter muscle.

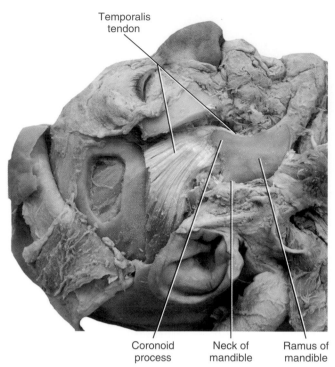

FIGURE 22-12. Removal of zygomatic arch, exposing attachments of temporalis muscle and bony landmarks of mandible.

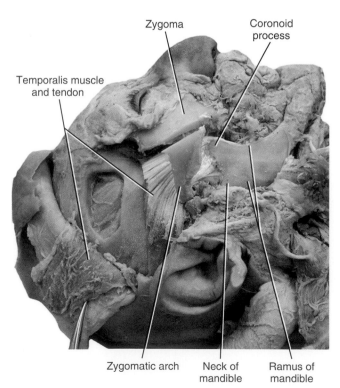

FIGURE 22-11. Lateral view of face, revealing zygomatic arch osteotomy anterior to masseter attachment, with a second cut anterior to temporomandibular joint.

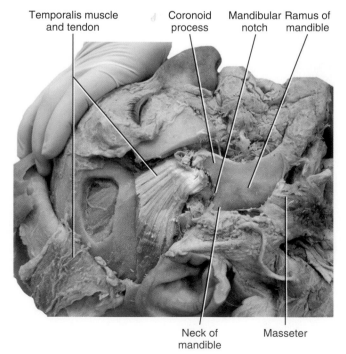

FIGURE 22-13. Detachment of temporalis muscle from coronoid process and mandibular notch.

With scissors, cut the *temporalis muscle* from the coronoid process and ramus of the mandible (Fig. 22-13). Reflect the temporalis upward, and clean the soft tissues and fat over the mandibular notch (Fig. 22-14).

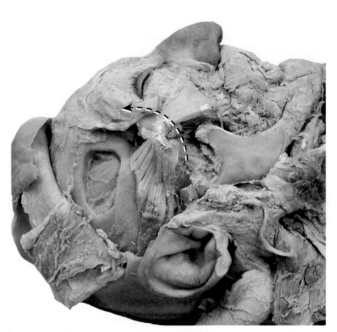

FIGURE 22-14. Reflection of temporalis muscle upward *(broken arrow)*.

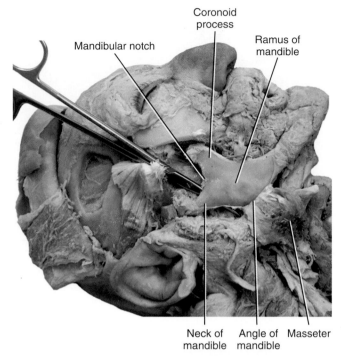

FIGURE 22-15. Placing scissors underneath ramus of mandible, pushing soft tissues, muscles, and vessels inferiorly, preserves underlying structure when mandible is cut with electric saw.

Place your scissors or a probe or scalpel handle immediately beneath the ramus of the mandible, and push the soft tissues and musculature and the vessels inferiorly (Fig. 22-15).

> ✋ *DISSECTION TIP:* This maneuver (Fig. 22-15) is important for preserving underlying structures when the mandible is cut. You may leave the probe or scissors in place to protect the inferior alveolar neurovascular bundle and lingual nerve when you perform the cut (see next).

With an electric saw, cut horizontally through the ramus of the mandible 2 to 3 inches (5-7.5 cm) below the coronoid process, leaving the articular process in place (Fig. 22-16).

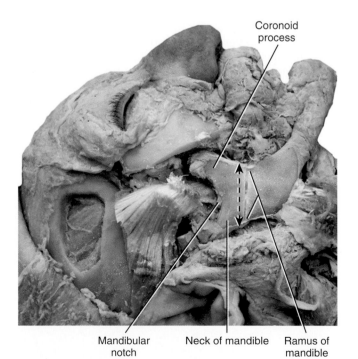

FIGURE 22-16. Saw cut horizontally through ramus of mandible below coronoid process.

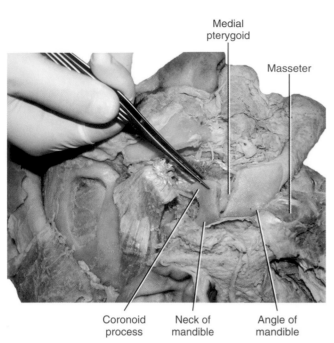

FIGURE 22-17. Severed coronoid process and the temporalis muscle reflected superiorly, to open up dissection area.

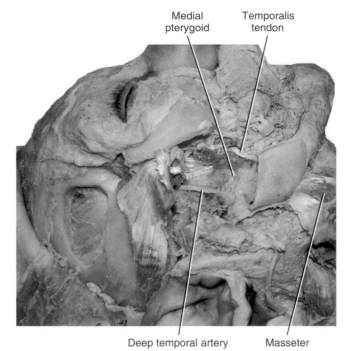

FIGURE 22-18. Appreciate medial pterygoid muscle with all soft tissues removed.

> ✋ *DISSECTION TIP:* Take special care when you reflect the coronoid process and the temporalis muscle so as not to injure the buccal nerve.

Reflect the severed coronoid process and the temporalis muscle superiorly (Fig. 22-17).

As the temporalis is reflected superiorly, observe the deep temporal arteries supplying this muscle. You can choose either to sever the arteries or to keep them. In this dissection, we choose to keep the deep temporal vessels (Figs. 22-18 and 22-19).

Once the temporalis muscle is reflected and the soft tissues are cleaned, identify and expose the *lateral pterygoid muscle,* which lies just beneath the temporalis. The lateral pterygoid muscle arises from the lateral pterygoid plate and passes horizontally to insert onto the articular disc of the temporomandibular joint (Figs. 22-20 and 22-21).

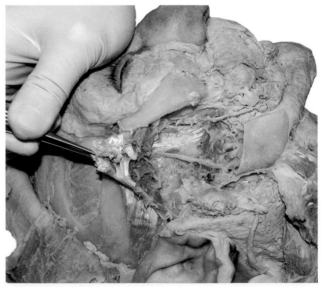

FIGURE 22-19. Further reflection of temporalis muscle to expose contents of the infratemporal fossa.

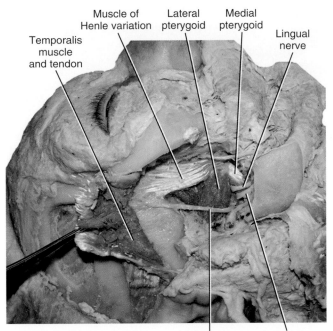

Muscle of Henle variation   Lateral pterygoid   Medial pterygoid   Lingual nerve

Temporalis muscle and tendon

Posterior deep temporal artery   Inferior alveolar nerve

FIGURE 22-20. Appreciate medial and lateral pterygoid muscles. Maxillary artery is located deep to lateral pterygoid in this specimen; note also the rare pterygoideus proprius (muscle of Henle).

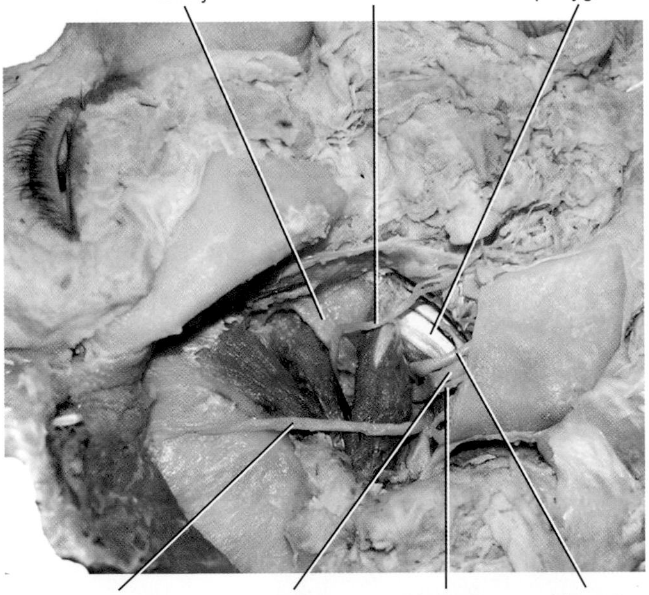

> *DISSECTION TIP:* In some cadavers, a variant muscle may be seen in the infratemporal fossa. In this specimen, a *pterygoideus proprius* was identified (muscle of Henle). This muscle originates from the anterior infratemporal crest, runs vertically downward to insert onto the lateral pterygoid plate, and crosses superficially to the lateral pterygoid muscle (Fig. 22-20). Typically, the muscle of Henle has no functional significance, but it may compress the mandibular nerve, resulting in possible trigeminal neuralgia.

Clean the soft tissues and fat at the inferior border of the lateral pterygoid muscle, and identify the *inferior alveolar nerve* and inferior alveolar artery superficial to the medial pterygoid muscle (Fig. 22-21). Clean the inferior alveolar nerve and trace it to the mandibular foramen.

Look at the lateral surface of the inferior alveolar nerve, and note the small branch that runs parallel with it, the nerve to the mylohyoid muscle. This nerve arises just before the inferior alveolar nerve enters the mandibular foramen. The nerve to the mylohyoid travels inferiorly, beneath the ramus and body of the mandible, to innervate the mylohyoid muscle and the anterior belly of the digastric muscle.

Lateral to the inferior alveolar nerve, identify the *lingual nerve* (Figs. 22-22 and 22-23). Medial to the inferior alveolar nerve, identify the *buccal nerve.*

Maxillary artery   Buccal nerve   Medial pterygoid

Posterior deep temporal artery   Inferior alveolar nerve   Nerve to mylohyoid   Lingual nerve

FIGURE 22-21. Soft tissue in space between medial and lateral pterygoid muscles cleaned, exposing inferior alveolar artery and nerve, lingual nerve, and nerve to mylohyoid; *V3,* mandibular division of trigeminal nerve.

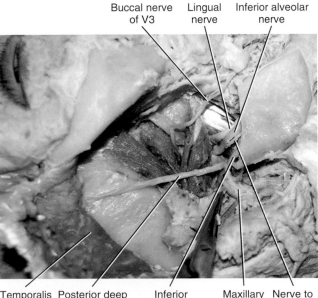

Buccal nerve of V3   Lingual nerve   Inferior alveolar nerve

Temporalis   Posterior deep temporal artery   Inferior alveolar artery   Maxillary artery   Nerve to mylohyoid

FIGURE 22-22. Maxillary artery exposed to trace its branches.

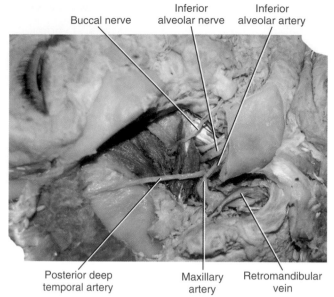

FIGURE 22-23. Further exposure of maxillary artery and accompanying maxillary and retromandibular veins.

FIGURE 22-24. Lateral pterygoid muscle removed with scissors and forceps.

Immediately underneath these nerves, observe the medial pterygoid muscle passing from the pterygoid plate to its insertion onto the inferior and posterior parts of the medial surface of the mandibular ramus. Proceed by carefully detaching the lateral pterygoid muscle from its origin on the pterygoid plate (Fig. 22-24).

✍ DISSECTION TIP: Removing the lateral pterygoid muscle can be a challenge. Be patient, and detach its muscle fibers carefully, paying special attention to the branches of the maxillary artery underneath it (Fig. 22-25). In the majority of cadavers, the lateral pterygoid muscle is crossed superficially by branches of the maxillary artery; in the remaining specimens, the artery travels deep to the muscle.

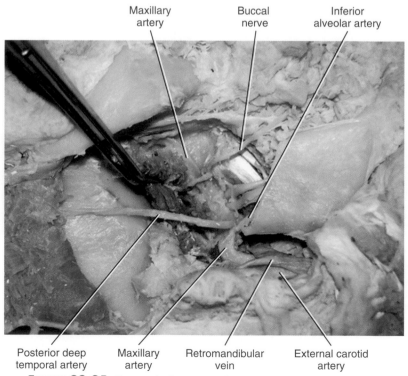

FIGURE 22-25. Removal of remaining lateral pterygoid muscle fibers.

Posterior to the inferior alveolar artery and nerve and anterior to the medial pterygoid muscle, identify the sphenomandibular ligament. This ligament is thin and may resemble a nerve, often confused with the inferior alveolar nerve.

Once the lateral pterygoid muscle is removed, expose the maxillary artery and its branches (Fig. 22-26). Note the retromandibular vein formed by the junction of the superficial temporal and maxillary veins. Identify the middle meningeal artery, which typically runs vertically toward the sphenoid bone, to enter the foramen spinosum. In the majority of cases, you will find the middle meningeal artery encircled by two roots of the *auriculotemporal nerve* (Figs. 22-27 and 22-28).

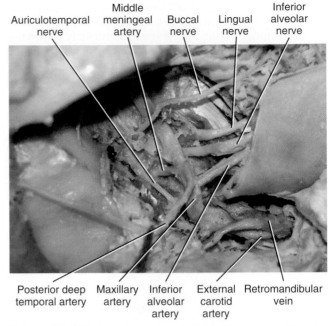

FIGURE 22-27. Complete removal of soft tissues, revealing neurovascular structures.

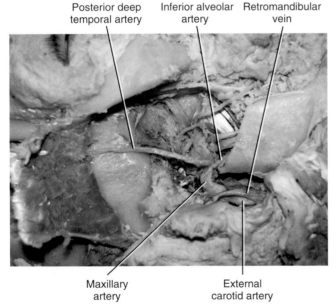

FIGURE 22-26. Complete removal of lateral pterygoid muscle. Note soft tissues around maxillary artery; carefully remove all soft tissues.

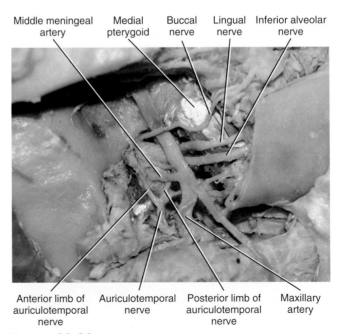

FIGURE 22-28. Lateral view of infratemporal fossa, revealing medial pterygoid muscle and neurovascular structures.

Clean all the soft tissues deep to the infratemporal fossa, and expose the nerves and arteries (Fig. 22-29). Lift the lingual nerve, and trace it superiorly until you see it joined on its posterior surface by a small nerve, the *chorda tympani,* which is a branch of the facial nerve (Fig. 22-30). Clean the lingual and inferior alveolar nerves, and trace their passage deep to the medial pterygoid muscle (Fig. 22-31).

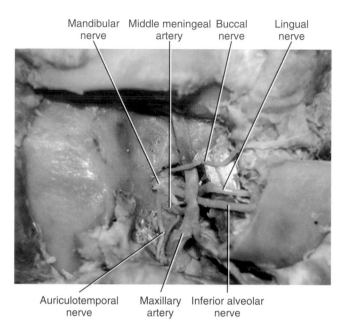

FIGURE 22-29. Lateral view of infratemporal fossa, revealing the medial pterygoid muscle and neurovascular structures.

Mandibular nerve · Middle meningeal artery · Buccal nerve · Lingual nerve

Auriculotemporal nerve · Maxillary artery · Inferior alveolar nerve

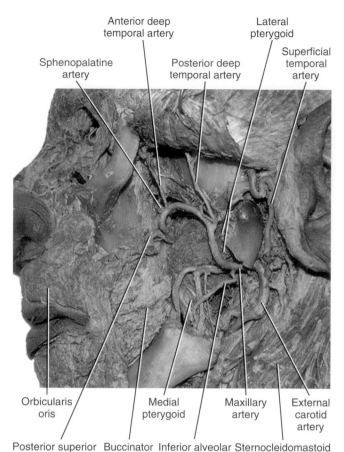

FIGURE 22-31. A different specimen, with branches of maxillary artery exposed superficial to lateral pterygoid muscle.

Anterior deep temporal artery · Lateral pterygoid · Sphenopalatine artery · Posterior deep temporal artery · Superficial temporal artery

Orbicularis oris · Medial pterygoid · Maxillary artery · External carotid artery

Posterior superior alveolar artery · Buccinator · Inferior alveolar artery · Sternocleidomastoid

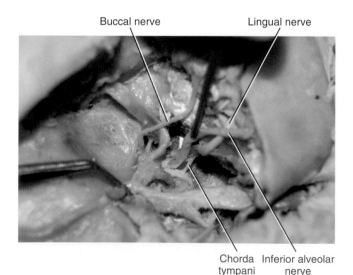

FIGURE 22-30. Lingual nerve lifted and followed posteriorly to its connection with chorda tympani nerve. If this nerve is not evident, clean the soft tissue around the lingual nerve more posteriorly.

Buccal nerve · Lingual nerve

Chorda tympani · Inferior alveolar nerve

Deep to the infratemporal fossa, trace and follow the termination of the maxillary artery, the *sphenopalatine artery,* toward the sphenopalatine foramen. Typically, two additional branches are easily identifiable. The *infraorbital artery* ascends to enter the infraorbital canal, and the *posterior superior alveolar artery* descends to enter the infratemporal surface of the maxilla (Fig. 22-32).

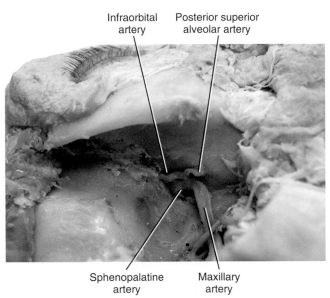

FIGURE 22-32. Deep view of infratemporal fossa, revealing termination of maxillary artery. Note three important branches: sphenopalatine, posterior superior alveolar, and infraorbital arteries.

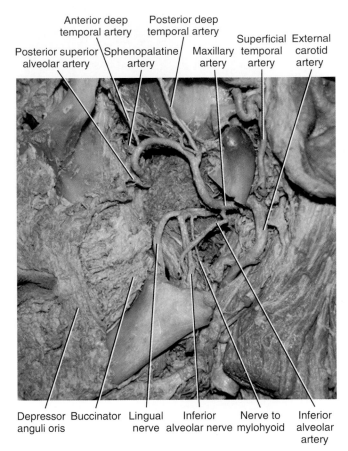

FIGURE 22-33. Lateral view of infratemporal fossa, revealing medial and lateral pterygoid muscles, temporomandibular joint, and neurovascular structures.

With an electric drill, cut the mandible in a direction demarcating a line between the mandibular canal and mental foramen. Expose the mandibular canal and the inferior alveolar nerve (Figs. 22-33 to 22-35). With fine forceps, lift the small branches of the inferior alveolar nerve terminating on the teeth (Fig. 22-36).

Using a bone saw, make a shallow parasagittal cut through the temporomandibular joint to expose the articular disc, the two synovial cavities, and the articular capsule of that joint.

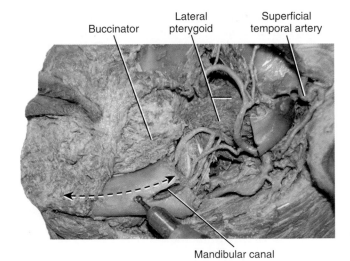

FIGURE 22-34. Mandible drilled in direction demarcated *(broken line)* between mandibular canal and mental foramen.

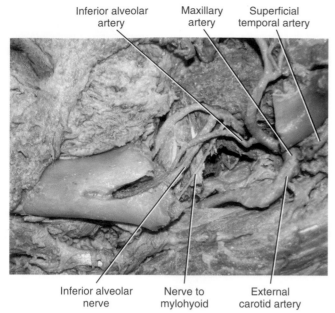

Inferior alveolar artery   Maxillary artery   Superficial temporal artery

Inferior alveolar nerve   Nerve to mylohyoid   External carotid artery

FIGURE 22-35. Exposure of contents of mandibular canal, including inferior alveolar nerve and artery.

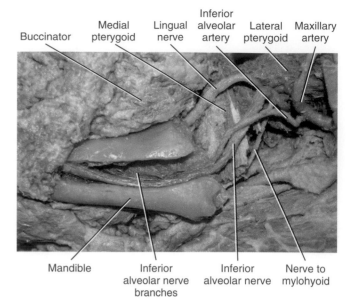

Buccinator   Medial pterygoid   Lingual nerve   Inferior alveolar artery   Lateral pterygoid   Maxillary artery

Mandible   Inferior alveolar nerve branches   Inferior alveolar nerve   Nerve to mylohyoid

FIGURE 22-36. Further exposure of inferior alveolar nerve within mandibular canal. Note small branches to the teeth.

LABORATORY IDENTIFICATION CHECKLIST

Nerves
❏ Trigeminal, mandibular division (V3)
❏ Auriculotemporal
❏ Inferior alveolar
❏ Nerve to mylohyoid
❏ Lingual
❏ Chorda tympani
❏ Buccal (long buccal of trigeminal)

Arteries
❏ Maxillary
   ❏ Middle meningeal
   ❏ Inferior alveolar
   ❏ Deep temporal arteries
      ❏ Muscular branches
         ❏ Masseteric artery
         ❏ Artery to medial pterygoid
         ❏ Artery to lateral pterygoid

Arteries—cont'd
   ❏ Sphenopalatine (terminal branch of maxillary artery)
   ❏ Posterior superior alveolar
   ❏ Infraorbital
   ❏ Buccal

Veins
❏ Pterygoid plexus (often difficult to isolate in cadaveric tissue)

Muscles
❏ Masseter
❏ Temporalis
❏ Lateral pterygoid
❏ Medial pterygoid

Bones
❏ Temporal
❏ Sphenoid
❏ Mandible
   ❏ Head
   ❏ Coronoid process
   ❏ Notch
   ❏ Ramus
   ❏ Angle

Connective Tissue
❏ Temporomandibular joint capsule
❏ Temporomandibular joint (articular) disc
❏ Stylomandibular ligament

CHAPTER 23

CALVARIA, DURAL VENOUS SINUSES, BRAIN, AND CRANIAL NERVES

Netter: 4–13, 99–107, 135–143

McMinn: 61–63, 72–82

Gray's Atlas: 428–437, 442–454, 528–529

The skin of the face has been previously removed (see Chapter 21). Continue the removal of the facial skin toward the occipital region, and separate the skin from the subcutaneous tissue (Fig. 23-1).

Identify and expose the superficial temporal artery and its branches (Fig. 23-2). Once the superficial temporal artery has been fully exposed, separate the subcutaneous tissue and fat from the underlying galea aponeurotica, or *epicranial aponeurosis* (Fig. 23-2). This aponeurosis is a flattened tendon that connects the occipitalis and frontalis muscles, forming the occipitofrontalis muscle.

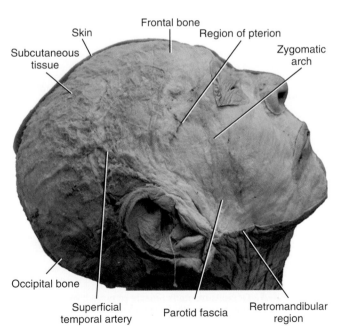

FIGURE 23-1. Lateral view of external cranium and face, revealing skin, subcutaneous tissue, parotid fascia, and regions (frontal, temporal, zygomatic, occipital, retromandibular).

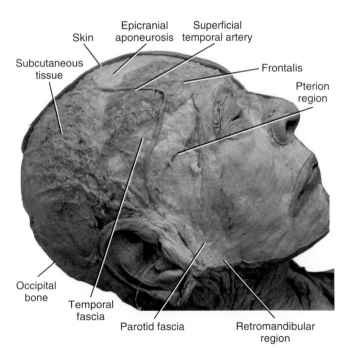

FIGURE 23-2. Lateral view of exposed superficial temporal artery and branches.

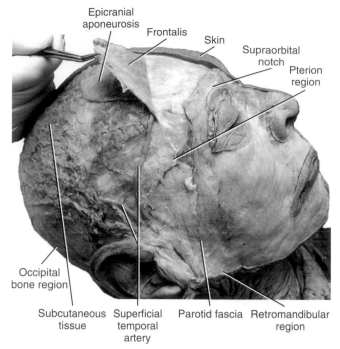

FIGURE 23-3. Frontalis muscle detached from frontal bone and reflected posteriorly.

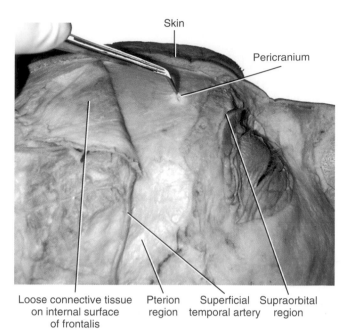

FIGURE 23-4. Appreciate the loose areolar tissue at the internal surface of frontalis muscle and the pericranium on cranial surface.

Cut and detach the frontalis muscle from the frontal bone. With forceps, grasp the frontalis muscle and reflect it posteriorly (Fig. 23-3). On the internal surface of the frontalis muscle, note the loose areolar tissue, and on the surface of the cranium, note the *pericranium* (Fig. 23-4).

⬥ DISSECTION TIP: At this part of the dissection, identify all the previously dissected layers of the *scalp:*

*S*kin
*C*onnective tissue (subcutaneous tissue)
*A*poneurotic layer
*L*oose areolar tissue
*P*ericranium

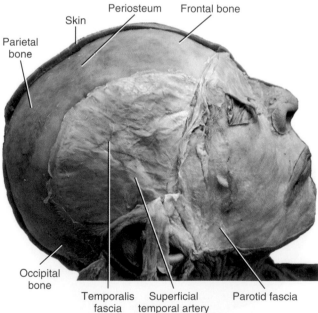

FIGURE 23-5. Occipitofrontalis muscle removed, exposing pericranium and leaving temporalis fascia intact.

To expose the brain, the *calvaria,* or skullcap, needs to be removed. The calvaria consists primarily of the parietal, frontal, and occipital bones. Dissect away the occipitofrontalis muscle and expose the pericranium, leaving the temporalis fascia intact (Fig. 23-5). With a scalpel, reflect the temporal fascia and expose the temporalis muscle (Fig. 23-6).

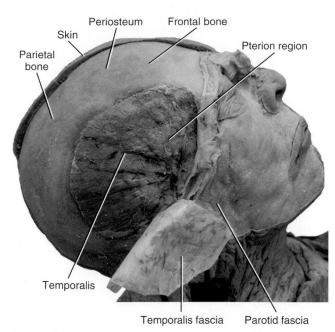

FIGURE 23-6. Temporalis fascia reflected, exposing temporalis muscle.

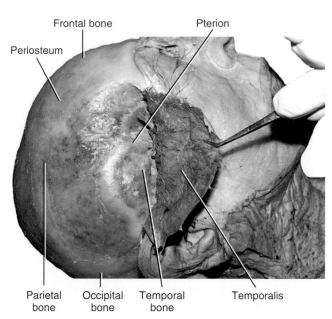

FIGURE 23-8. Temporalis muscle reflected toward zygomatic bone, exposing pterion.

Clean the temporalis muscle and note its tendinous fibers (Fig. 23-7). Reflect the temporalis toward the zygomatic bone, and expose the *pterion* (Fig. 23-8). Once the temporalis muscle is completely reflected and the calvaria fully exposed, identify the frontal, parietal, temporal, and occipital bones, as well as the sagittal, coronal, and lambdoid sutures.

> ✐ *DISSECTION TIP:* Place paper towels around the face and temporalis muscles to protect them from bone dust (Fig. 23-9).

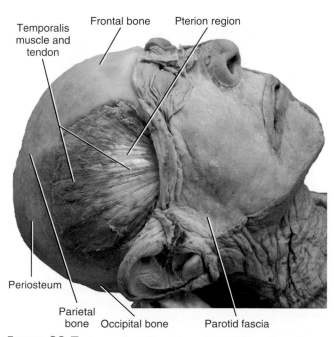

FIGURE 23-7. Appreciate the temporalis muscle and tendinous fibers.

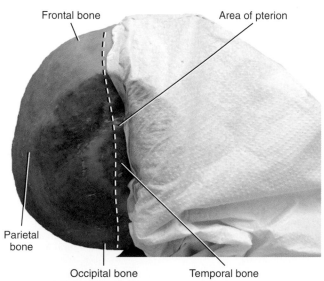

FIGURE 23-9. Lateral view of external cranium and face (covered), revealing frontal, parietal, temporal, and occipital bones and pterion; dashed line indicates craniotomy cut.

DISSECTION OF THE SKULL

We use two different techniques to expose the contents of the skull.

Technique 1

Keep the cadaver in the supine position. Place a plastic or wooden block under the head or shoulders to elevate the body from the dissection table. With a marker, draw a stippled midsagittal line from the nasion to the external occipital protuberance. Draw a second, circumferential line passing 1 to 2 cm above the superciliary ridges and ears to reach 1 to 2 cm above the external occipital protuberance posteriorly (Fig. 23-9).

With an electric saw, cut along this line (Fig. 23-10). Leave 2 to 3 cm (~1 inch) of bone intact at the midline. In this way, the superior sagittal sinus and the falx cerebri will remain intact.

Use the electric saw carefully. Make a shallow, circumferential cut of approximately 1 cm. Do not place the saw too deeply, because you will cut the dura and the brain. To complete the cut toward the external occipital protuberance, it is necessary to rotate the cadaver.

Once the first cut is complete, use the chisel and mallet to break through the bone and detach the two bone flaps.

> ☝ *DISSECTION TIP:* Detaching the bone flap from the underlying dura mater can be challenging. Place the forceps or a chisel into the gap (created by the saw cut) between the two adjacent bones, and use it to lift it up from the dura. If the dura is attached to the calvaria, use a probe to reflect the endosteal layer away from the calvaria, leaving the dura mater intact.

After removal of the calvaria, examine the dura mater and identify the middle meningeal artery and its branches (Figs. 23-11 to 23-13). Cut and reflect the dura, and expose the subdural space. Observe the arachnoid layer covering the brain and the cerebral veins penetrating the arachnoid mater (Fig. 23-12).

Place your hands on one of the cerebral hemispheres and retract it laterally (Fig. 23-14). Notice the midline connection between the two hemispheres, the corpus callosum (Fig. 23-15). With a scalpel, make a midsagittal cut, and reflect one of the brain hemispheres, leaving intact the dural venous sinuses (Fig. 23-16).

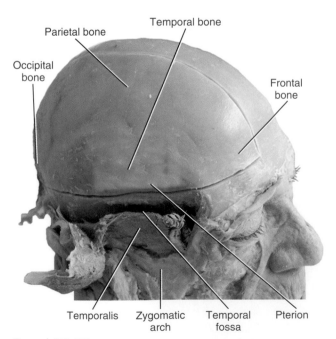

FIGURE 23-10. Anterolateral view of external cranium and face, revealing bones, pterion, temporalis muscle, temporal fossa, and zygomatic arch.

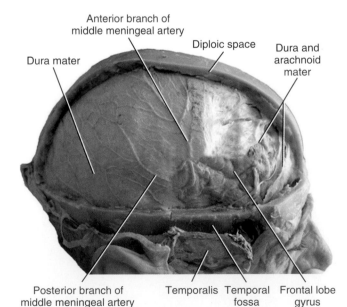

FIGURE 23-11. Lateral view of right hemisphere after craniotomy revealing the calvaria (with diploic space of the skull), anterior and posterior branches of middle meningeal artery, scalp, dura mater, arachnoid mater, temporalis muscle, and temporal fossa.

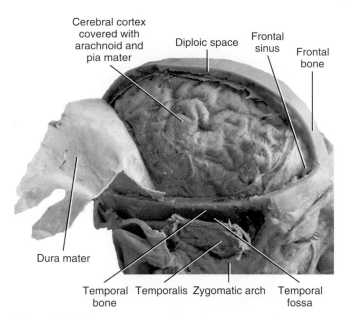

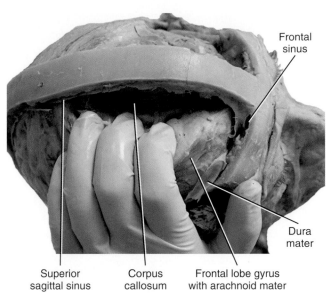

FIGURE 23-12. Dura mater reflected, exposing subdural space. Observe arachnoid layer covering the brain and cerebral veins penetrating it.

FIGURE 23-14. Cerebral hemisphere retracted laterally; note the frontal and superior sagittal sinuses and corpus callosum.

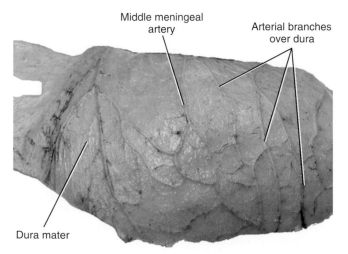

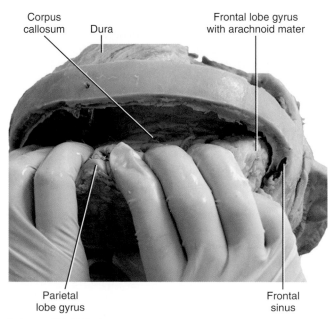

FIGURE 23-13. External surface of removed dura mater, revealing the middle meningeal artery and arterial branches to dura mater.

FIGURE 23-15. Appreciate connection between the two hemispheres, the corpus callosum.

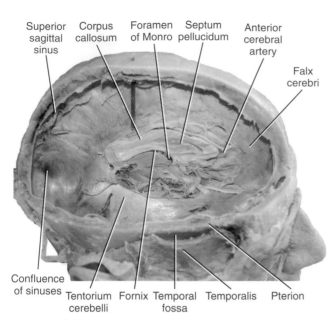

Superior sagittal sinus Corpus callosum Foramen of Monro Septum pellucidum Anterior cerebral artery Falx cerebri

Confluence of sinuses Tentorium cerebelli Fornix Temporal fossa Temporalis Pterion

FIGURE 23-16. With a midsagittal cut, the brain hemisphere is reflected, leaving the dural venous sinuses intact.

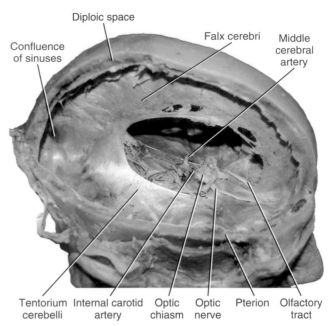

Diploic space Confluence of sinuses Falx cerebri Middle cerebral artery

Tentorium cerebelli Internal carotid artery Optic chiasm Optic nerve Pterion Olfactory tract

FIGURE 23-17. Lateral view of right hemisphere after craniotomy, revealing falx cerebri, diploic space, confluence of sinuses, tentorium cerebelli, pterion, olfactory tract, optic nerve, optic chiasm, internal carotid artery, and middle cerebral artery.

Perform the same technique to the contralateral side, and expose the sinuses bilaterally (Figs. 23-17 to 23-19).

Identify the *falx cerebri,* a dural partition separating the right from the left cerebral hemispheres. Superior to the falx cerebri, identify the *superior sagittal sinus,* which joins the two transverse sinuses at the confluence of sinuses ("torcular herophili," or wine-press of Herophilus). Inferolateral to the falx cerebri, look for the *tentorium cerebelli,* a large, dural infolding separating the occipital lobes from the cerebellar hemispheres.

> ✋ *DISSECTION TIP:* If time permits, remove the midportion of the calvaria, and expose the superior sagittal sinus. Incise the dura forming the sinus, and notice its internal structure. In the majority of specimens the superior sagittal sinus will drain into the right transverse sinus.

At this point, the dissection can continue as outlined later.

Technique 2

Keep the body in the supine position. Place a plastic or wooden block under the head to elevate it from the dissection table. With a pen, draw a circumferential

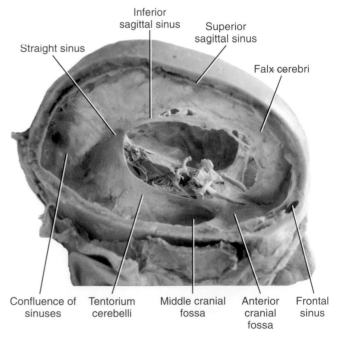

Inferior sagittal sinus Superior sagittal sinus Straight sinus Falx cerebri

Confluence of sinuses Tentorium cerebelli Middle cranial fossa Anterior cranial fossa Frontal sinus

FIGURE 23-18. Postcraniotomy lateral view of right hemisphere revealing falx cerebri, superior/inferior sagittal sinuses, straight sinus, confluence of sinuses, tentorium cerebelli, anterior/middle cranial fossae, and frontal sinus.

line passing 1 to 2 cm above the superciliary ridges and ears to reach 1 to 2 cm above the external occipital protuberance posteriorly (Figs. 23-20 and 23-21). With an electric saw, cut along this line (Figs. 23-22 and 23-23).

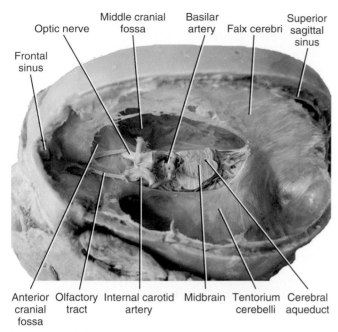

FIGURE 23-19. Lateral view of left hemisphere after craniotomy, showing frontal sinus, anterior cranial fossa, olfactory tract, internal carotid artery, basilar artery, middle cranial fossa, midbrain, cerebral aqueduct, falx cerebri, tentorium cerebelli, and superior sagittal sinus.

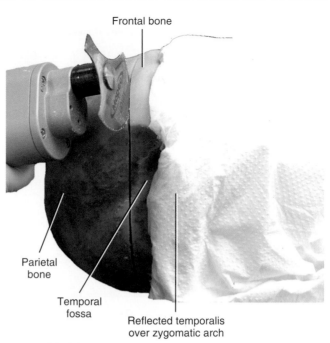

FIGURE 23-20. Postcraniotomy lateral view of external cranium, revealing frontal bone, parietal bone, temporal bone/fossa, and temporalis muscle reflected inferiorly over zygomatic arch.

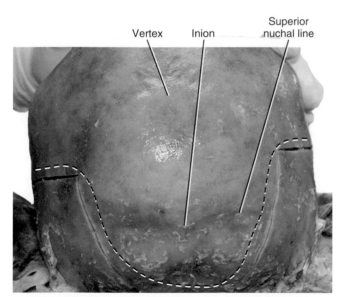

FIGURE 23-21. Superoposterior view of external cranium revealing the superior nuchal line, inion, posterior craniotomy *(dashed line),* and vertex.

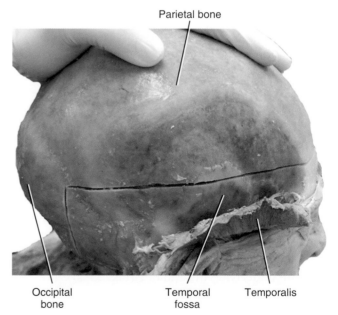

FIGURE 23-22. Posterolateral view of external cranium, revealing wedge resection cut; parietal, temporal, and occipital bones; and temporalis muscle.

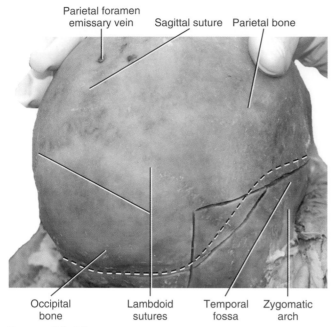

FIGURE 23-23. Posterolateral view of external cranium revealing parietal foramen, emissary vein, sutures (sagittal, lambdoid), and bony landmarks (parietal, temporal, zygomatic, occipital).

FIGURE 23-24. Posterior view of external cranium shows wedge resection of the cranium *(dashed line),* lambdoid suture, and occipital bone.

✋ *DISSECTION TIP:* The bone cut can extend below the external occipital protuberance, to the posterolateral aspects of the foramen magnum, including the posterior portions of the atlas and axis (Fig. 23-24). With this extension, removal of the brain and spinal cord is easier. However, this extension will sever the muscles of the suboccipital triangle.

Use the electric saw carefully. First, make a shallow, circumferential cut of about 1 cm. Do not insert the saw too deeply, or you may sever the dura mater and the brain (Fig. 23-25). To complete the cut at the external occipital protuberance, the cadaver needs to be rotated.

Second, complete the bone removal with a chisel and mallet to break through the bone, and detach it from the underlying dura mater (Fig. 23-26).

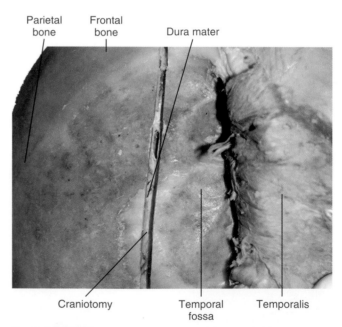

FIGURE 23-25. Once first cut is complete, use chisel and mallet to break through the bone and detach it from the dura.

✋ *DISSECTION TIP:* Detaching the bone from the underlying dura can be challenging. Place the chisel in the gap (created by saw cut) between the adjacent bones, slightly rotating it to lift the bone from the dura. If the dura is still connected to the calvaria, use a probe to reflect the endosteal layer from the calvaria, leaving the dura intact.

Inspect the internal surface of the calvaria and identify the small openings for emissary veins. Note the small pits (granular *fovea*) produced by the *arachnoid granulations* (large arachnoid *villi* that protrude into dural venous sinuses) (Fig. 23-27). Look for the frontal sinus extending into the calvaria. Note the spongy bone occupying the space between the outer

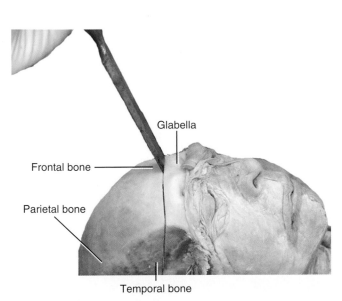

FIGURE 23-26. Anterolateral view of external cranium and face revealing sagittal suture line for craniotomy, with chisel inserted into scoring line and glabella.

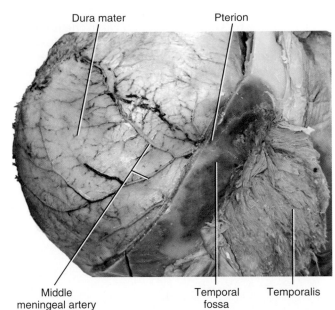

FIGURE 23-28. Lateral view showing dura mater, middle meningeal artery branches, pterion, temporal fossa, and temporalis muscle.

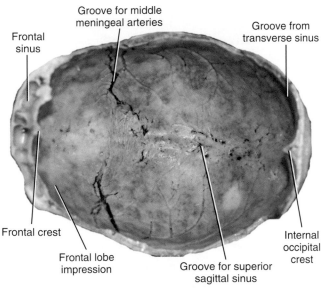

FIGURE 23-27. Craniotomy with calvaria removed, revealing internal surface and frontal lobe impressions, frontal sinus, grooves, frontal crest, and internal occipital crest.

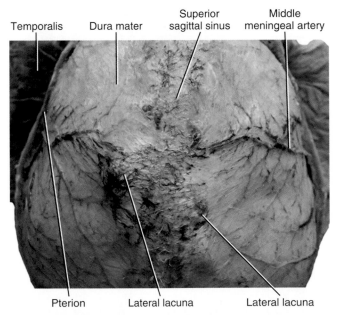

FIGURE 23-29. Superior view of craniotomy, revealing superior sagittal sinus, middle meningeal artery, lateral lacuna, dura mater, temporalis muscle, and pterion.

and inner compact bony layers (tables), the *diploic space.* Identify the impressions made by the superior sagittal sinus and the middle meningeal arteries.

Inspect the dura mater and identify the middle meningeal artery and its branches (Fig. 23-28). Identify the superior sagittal sinus and look for the *lateral lacunae* (Fig. 23-29). The lateral lacunae are lateral venous extensions of the superior sagittal sinus.

> ✋ *DISSECTION TIP:* If time permits, with a scalpel make an incision into the lateral lacunae, and note their opening to the superior sagittal sinus.

Dissection Continued

Cut the dura 2 to 3 cm (~1 inch) lateral to the midline, and reflect it inferiorly (Figs. 23-30 and 23-31). Inspect the subdural space and the arachnoid layer pierced with cerebral veins. Identify the arachnoid mater, and make a small incision to expose the pia mater. Notice how the cerebral arteries and veins are covered with pia mater.

On the brain, identify the central sulcus, precentral gyrus, postcentral gyrus, and the frontal and occipital lobes (Fig. 23-32). On the other side of the brain, remove the pia mater (Fig. 23-33). With forceps, pull the superior sagittal sinus and the falx cerebri laterally, and observe the corpus callosum (Fig. 23-34).

Observe the superior sagittal sinus, and identify the lacunae joining it. Look for the tuftlike projections, the arachnoid granulations (Fig. 23-35).

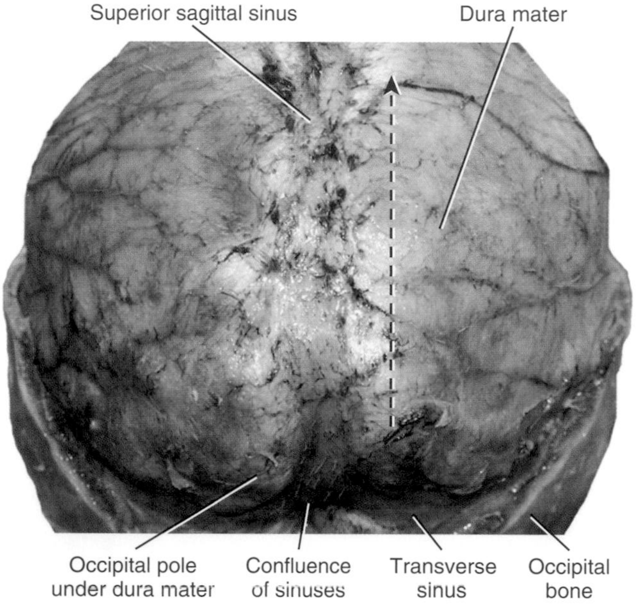

FIGURE 23-30. Dura mater cut laterally from midline *(dashed arrow)* and reflected inferiorly.

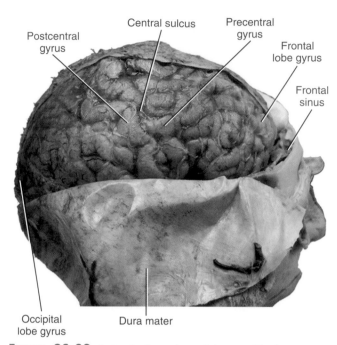

FIGURE 23-32. Lateral view of craniotomy with dura mater reflected laterally, revealing key gyri, central sulcus, and frontal sinus.

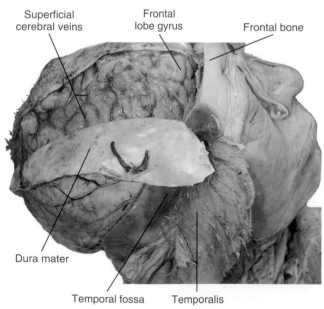

FIGURE 23-31. Anterolateral view of craniotomy revealing reflected dura mater, temporal bone region, temporalis muscle, frontal bone region, frontal lobe gyri covered with arachnoid and pia mater, and superior cerebral veins of parietal lobe.

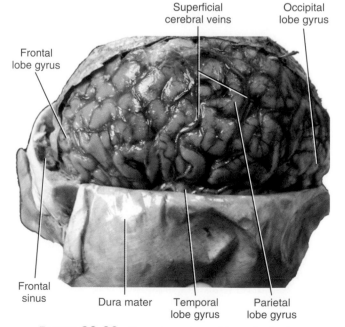

FIGURE 23-33. Pia mater removed from the brain.

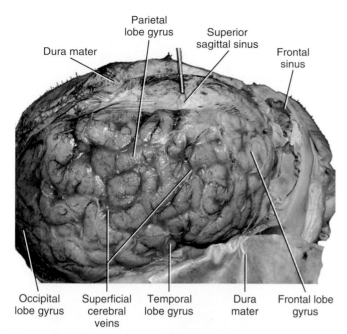

FIGURE 23-34. Superior sagittal sinus and falx cerebri pulled laterally, revealing corpus callosum.

✋ *DISSECTION TIP:* Appreciate the relationships of the following:
The *falx cerebri* separates the two cerebral hemispheres.
The *falx cerebelli* separates the two cerebellar hemispheres.
The *tentorium cerebelli* separates the cerebellum from the occipital lobes.

Gently lift the cerebral hemispheres and inferior to the frontal lobes identify the attachment of the falx cerebri at the *crista galli.* Cut this attachment from the crista galli and from the cerebral veins draining into the superior sagittal sinus. Pull the detached falx cerebri and superior sagittal sinus posteriorly (Fig. 23-36). Gently lift the cerebral hemispheres by placing your fingertips underneath the frontal lobes of the brain (Fig. 23-37).

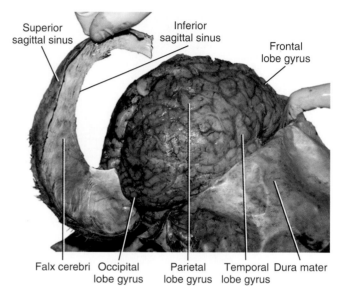

FIGURE 23-36. Anterolateral view with dura mater reflected laterally.

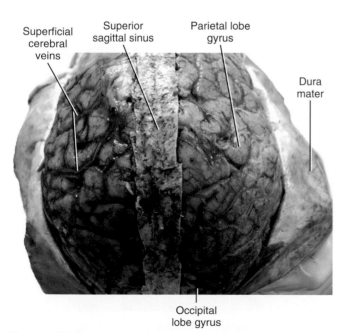

FIGURE 23-35. Appreciate the superior sagittal sinus, lacunae, and tuftlike arachnoid granulations.

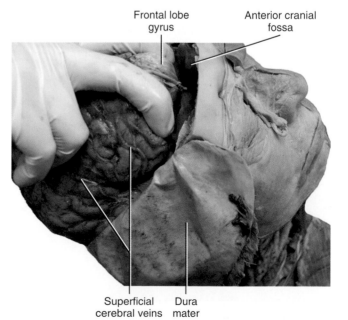

FIGURE 23-37. Gently lift cerebral hemispheres by placing fingertips underneath frontal lobes.

Look at the space between the cribriform plate of the ethmoid bone and the frontal lobes for the internal carotid artery, olfactory tracts, olfactory bulbs, optic nerve, optic chiasm, and anterior cerebral artery (Fig. 23-38). With scissors, cut the aforementioned structures (Fig. 23-39). Gently keep lifting the frontal lobes upward, and expose the brainstem and the basilar artery (Figs. 23-40 and 23-41).

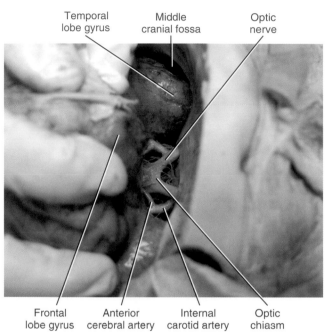

FIGURE 23-38. In space between cribriform plate of ethmoid bone and frontal lobes, appreciate the internal carotid artery, olfactory tracts/bulbs, optic nerve/chiasm, and anterior cerebral artery.

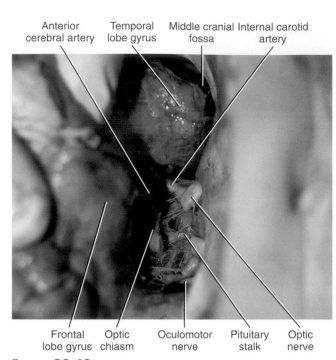

FIGURE 23-40. View with frontal lobes reflected superoposteriorly revealing temporal lobe, middle cranial fossa, cut optic nerves, internal carotid artery, anterior cerebral artery, optic chiasm cut, oculomotor nerve, and pituitary stalk.

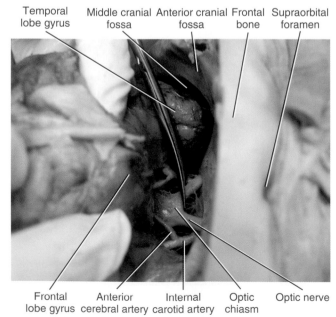

FIGURE 23-39. Insert a pair of scissors and cut the optic nerve and internal carotid artery.

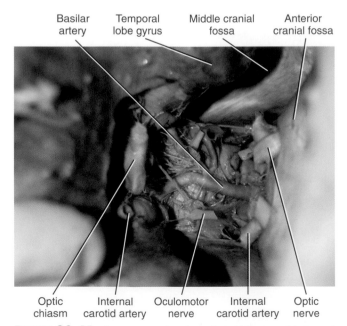

FIGURE 23-41. Anterosuperior view of craniotomy with frontal lobes reflected superiorly and posteriorly, revealing anterior/middle cranial fossae, temporal lobe, optic nerve cut, internal carotid artery cut, basilar artery, optic chiasm cut, and oculomotor nerve.

At this point, lift the occipital lobes of the cerebral hemisphere, and appreciate the tentorium cerebelli and the straight sinus (Fig. 23-42). With a scalpel, carefully make a circumferential cut along the lateral attachment of the tentorium cerebelli.

Return to the frontal lobes and pull them upward (Fig. 23-43). Cut the facial, vestibulocochlear, trigeminal, abducens, and trochlear nerves. Because the tentorium cerebelli has been cut, pull the brain farther back and note the vertebral arteries forming the basilar artery (Fig. 23-44).

DISSECTION TIP: The point at which you need to stop pulling the brain backward is when you visualize the junction where the vertebral arteries form the basilar artery.

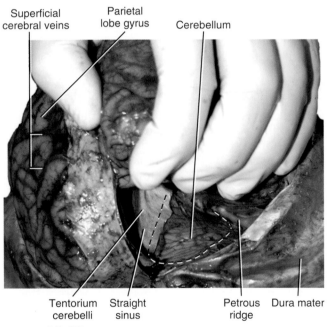

FIGURE 23-42. Occipital lobes lifted to visualize tentorium cerebelli and straight sinus; circumferential cut from lateral attachment of tentorium cerebelli alongside transverse sinus toward petrous ridge to tentorial notch.

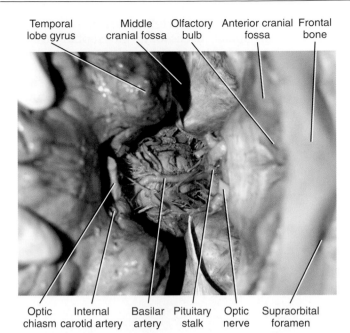

FIGURE 23-43. Anterosuperior view of craniotomy with frontal lobes reflected superiorly and posteriorly revealing frontal bone, supraorbital foramen, anterior cranial fossa, olfactory tract cut, optic nerve cut, middle cranial fossa, temporal lobe, internal carotid artery cut, optic nerves cut, pituitary stalk cut, and basilar artery.

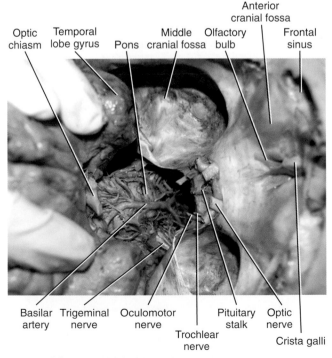

FIGURE 23-44. Appreciate facial, vestibulocochlear, trigeminal, abducens, and trochlear nerves; brain pulled farther back to visualize vertebral arteries forming basilar artery.

Once you observe the vertebral arteries, cut the hypoglossal, spinal accessory, glossopharyngeal, and vagus nerves. At this point, place a scalpel as deeply as possible within the foramen magnum, and cut the spinal cord (Fig. 23-45). Retract the brain from the base of the skull, leaving intact the dural venous sinuses (Fig. 23-46).

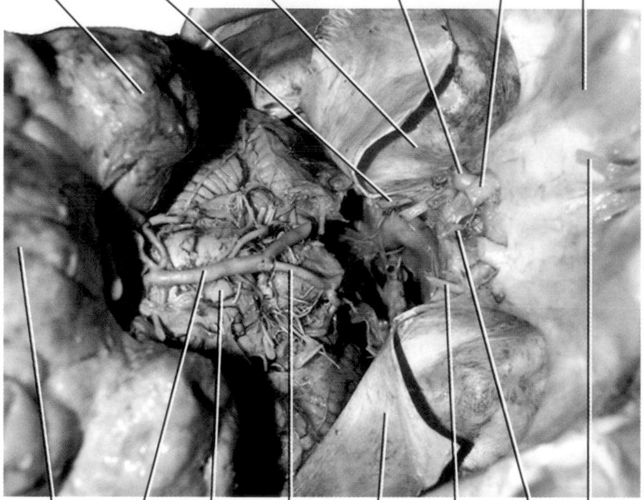
Temporal lobe gyrus
Trigeminal nerve
Anterior cranial fossa
Internal carotid artery
Optic nerve
Anterior cranial fossa
Frontal lobe gyrus
Basilar artery
Pons
Vertebral artery
Tentorium cerebelli reflected
Oculomotor nerve
Pituitary stalk
Olfactory bulb

FIGURE 23-45. With tentorium cerebelli reflected, appreciate hypoglossal, spinal accessory, glossopharyngeal, and vagus nerves.

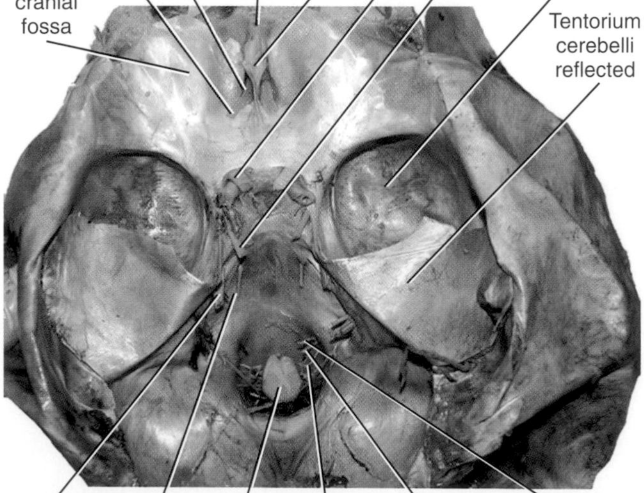
Olfactory tract
Foramen cecum
Oculomotor nerve
Olfactory bulb
Crista galli
Optic nerve
Middle cranial fossa
Anterior cranial fossa
Tentorium cerebelli reflected
Trigeminal nerve
Abducens nerve
Brainstem
Accessory nerve
Vagus nerve
Glossopharyngeal nerve

FIGURE 23-46. Brain retracted from base of skull leaving dural venous sinuses intact.

Once the brain is removed, identify the different dural venous sinuses, the superior sagittal sinus, inferior sagittal sinus, confluence of the sinuses, straight sinus, transverse sinus, sigmoid sinus, and the great vein of Galen (see Fig. 23-18).

EXAMINATION OF THE BRAIN

Once the brain is removed, dissect away the arachnoid and pia mater from its ventral surface. First, identify the cranial nerves on the brain (Figs. 23-47 and 23-48), as follows:

Cranial nerve I: The *olfactory bulbs and tracts* are usually found in contact with the frontal lobes of the brain.

Cranial nerve II: The *optic nerves* and the *optic chiasm* are usually well preserved in most cadavers. Posterior to the optic chiasm, identify the pituitary stalk.

Cranial nerve III: The *oculomotor nerve* passes between the posterior cerebral and superior cerebellar arteries, near the termination of the basilar artery.

Cranial nerve IV: The *trochlear nerve* is the smallest cranial nerve (less the olfactory nerves) and is often cut during brain removal. It passes anteriorly around the sides of the midbrain.

Cranial nerve V: The *trigeminal nerve* arises from the middle of the lateral aspect of the pons.

Cranial nerve VI: The *abducens nerve* arises from the inferior border of the pons, immediately superior to the medullary pyramids.

Cranial nerve VII: The *facial nerve* arises on the lateral aspect of the junction of the pons and the medulla oblongata, medial to the origin of cranial nerve VIII.

Cranial nerve VIII: The *vestibulocochlear nerve* arises lateral to the facial nerve.

Cranial nerve IX: The *glossopharyngeal nerve* arises at the groove posterior to the olive on the medulla oblongata.

Cranial nerve X: The *vagus nerve* arises from the medulla oblongata by 8 to 10 rootlets between the olive and the inferior cerebellar peduncle.

Cranial nerve XI: The *accessory nerve* arises from cranial rootlets from the medulla oblongata and from rootlets of the upper five cervical levels of the spinal cord.

> *POINT OF DEBATE:* Some anatomists do not consider the spinal accessory nerve a "cranial nerve" because (1) it does not arise from the brain and (2) it enters the skull through the foramen magnum. The definition of a cranial nerve states that it should arise from the brain and exit through one of the skull foramina.

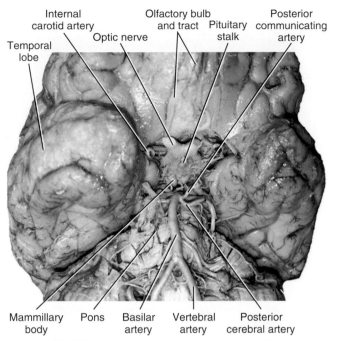

FIGURE 23-47. Inferior aspect of brain, revealing olfactory bulb and tract, optic nerve, pituitary stalk, temporal lobe, mammillary bodies (corpus mammillare), and arteries (internal carotid, posterior communicating, basilar, vertebral, posterior cerebral).

Cranial nerve XII: The *hypoglossal nerve* arises by a series of rootlets from the medulla oblongata on the ventrolateral sulcus between the pyramid and the olive.

Identify the following arteries contributing to the formation of the arterial circle of Willis (Figs. 23-47 and 23-48):

- The *anterior cerebral* arteries, connected by the anterior communicating artery.
- The *internal carotid* arteries, connected by posterior communicating arteries to the posterior cerebral arteries.

> ❦ *DISSECTION TIP:* Common variations encountered in the formation of the circle of Willis include the following:
> - Absent anterior communicating artery
> - Absent posterior communicating artery
> - Large posterior communicating artery
> - Posterior cerebral artery arises from the internal carotid (fetal posterior cerebral artery).

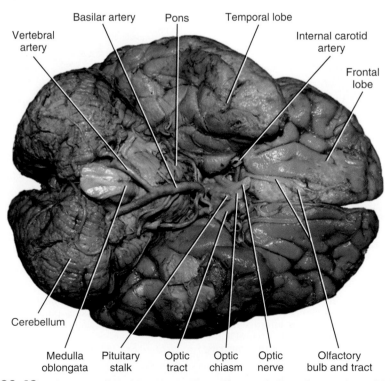

FIGURE 23-48. Inferior aspect of brain, revealing olfactory bulb and tract, frontal lobe, optic chiasm, optic nerve, optic tract, internal carotid artery, pituitary stalk, temporal lobe, pons, medulla oblongata, basilar artery, vertebral artery, and cerebellum.

Useful Landmarks

1. The *anterior choroidal artery* arises near the origin of the posterior communicating artery and passes posterolaterally along the optic tract.
2. The *trochlear nerve* and *oculomotor nerve* pass between the superior cerebellar and posterior cerebral arteries.

Make a midsagittal incision through the brain, separating the right from the left hemisphere. Identify the thalamus, hypothalamus, and the three parts of the brainstem—midbrain, pons, and medulla oblongata (Fig. 23-49). Identify the corpus callosum and fornix. Note the lateral ventricles, which open into the 3rd ventricle through the foramen of Monro. The 3rd ventricle is continuous inferiorly with the cerebral aqueduct, connecting the 3rd with the 4th ventricles. Identify the foramen of Monro (Fig. 23-49).

Identify the tentorium cerebelli and the anterior clinoid process. Visualize the dura covering the trigeminal nerve as it passes into the middle cranial fossa. With scissors, make a small cut in the dura covering the trigeminal nerve, and pull it upward (Fig. 23-50). Pull the dura covering the trigeminal nerve away from the middle cranial fossa, and expose *Meckel's cave,* the area where the trigeminal (semilunar) ganglion resides (Fig. 23-51).

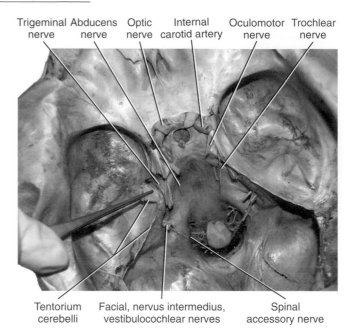

FIGURE 23-50. Appreciate the tentorium cerebelli, anterior clinoid process, and dura covering the trigeminal nerve pulled upward.

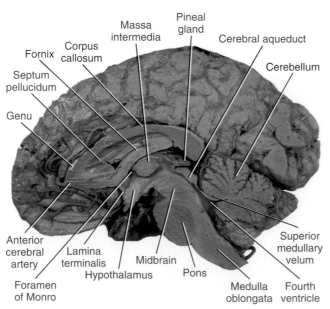

FIGURE 23-49. Sagittal section of cerebellum and brainstem revealing corpus callosum, genu, anterior cerebral artery, septum pellucidum, fornix, massa intermedia (adhesio interthalamica), foramen of Monro, lamina terminalis, pineal gland, cerebral aqueduct, cerebellum, superior medullary velum, fourth ventricle, hypothalamus, midbrain, pons, and medulla oblongata.

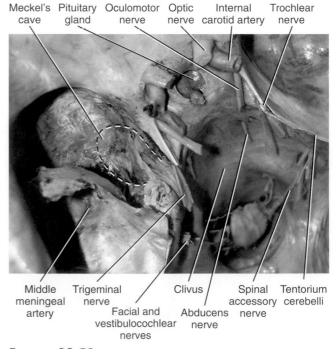

FIGURE 23-51. Trigeminal nerve dura pulled from middle cranial fossa, exposing pituitary gland, Meckel's cave *(dashed arch),* and clivus (bony surface of posterior cranial fossa).

Gently dissect out the soft tissues around Meckel's (trigeminal) cave and expose the trigeminal ganglion (Fig. 23-52) Continue the dissection distally to the trigeminal ganglion and identify the ophthalmic (V1), maxillary (V2), and mandibular (V3) divisions of the trigeminal nerve entering into the superior orbital fissure, foramen rotundum, and foramen ovale, respectively (Figs. 23-52 and 23-53).

Continue laterally by identifying the internal carotid arteries passing underneath the optic nerves. Posterior to the optic chiasm and optic nerves, identify the infundibulum of the pituitary gland *(hypophysis)* and the diaphragma sella (Fig. 23-54).

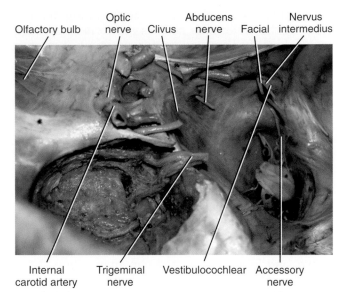

FIGURE 23-53. Anterolateral view of anterior, middle, and posterior cranial fossae revealing olfactory bulb, optic nerve, internal carotid artery, oculomotor nerve, abducens nerve, clivus, trigeminal nerve, facial nerve, nervus intermedius (intermediate nerve), vestibulocochlear nerve, and spinal accessory nerve.

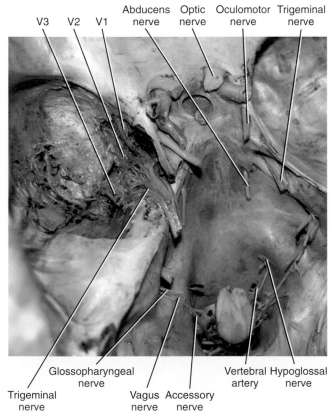

FIGURE 23-52. Dissection continued distally to trigeminal ganglion revealing ophthalmic *(V1)*, maxillary *(V2)*, and mandibular *(V3)* divisions of trigeminal nerve and key neurovascular structures.

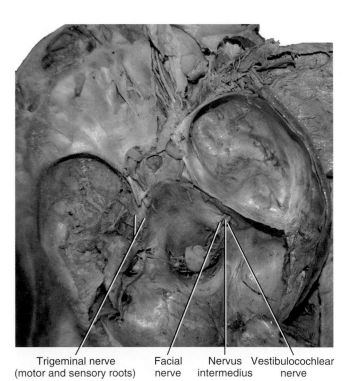

FIGURE 23-54. Appreciate foramina for trigeminal nerve branches and facial, intermediate, and vestibulocochlear nerves.

Identify the cavernous sinus, appreciating that the walls of the cavernous sinuses are formed by dura mater. Identify the oculomotor nerve as it passes underneath the free edge of the tentorium toward the posterior clinoid process. At the posterior clinoid process, identify the trochlear nerve. Inferior to the sella turcica, note the *abducens nerve* penetrating the dura wall of the cavernous sinus (Fig. 23-55).

Remove the dura from the middle cranial fossa as well as from the medial side of the cavernous sinus (Fig. 23-56). Separate the soft tissue around the oculomotor nerve and internal carotid artery. Notice the S-shaped course of the internal carotid artery (carotid siphon) within the cavernous sinus.

Identify the abducens nerve running lateral to the internal carotid artery within the cavernous sinus. Incise the dura at the entrance of the abducens nerve, and follow it into the cavernous sinus. Note that the internal carotid artery and the abducens nerve are covered by a layer that separates them from adjacent venous blood (Fig. 23-57).

Identify the sigmoid sinus, and cut open the dura that covers it. Pull the dura covering off the superior and inferior petrosal sinuses. Identify the internal acoustic meatus, and trace the facial and vestibulocochlear nerves as they enter the foramen. Look inferior to the internal acoustic meatus for the jugular foramen, and trace the glossopharyngeal, vagus, and spinal accessory nerves (see Fig. 23-50).

Note the upper cervical spinal fibers of the spinal accessory nerve entering through the foramen magnum. Inferior to the jugular foramen and superior to the foramen magnum, identify the hypoglossal canal with the hypoglossal nerve (see Fig. 23-50).

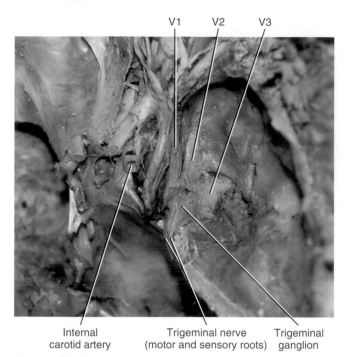

V1 V2 V3

Internal carotid artery | Trigeminal nerve (motor and sensory roots) | Trigeminal ganglion

FIGURE 23-56. Dura removed from middle cranial fossa and medial side of the cavernous sinus and soft tissue separated around the internal carotid artery.

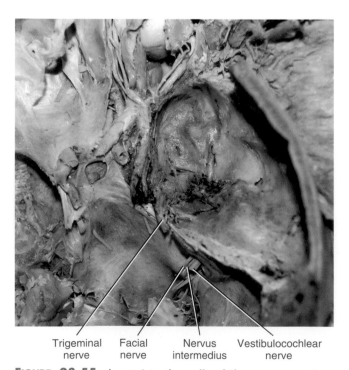

Trigeminal nerve | Facial nerve | Nervus intermedius | Vestibulocochlear nerve

FIGURE 23-55. Appreciate the walls of the cavernous sinus formed by dura; note neurovascular foramina.

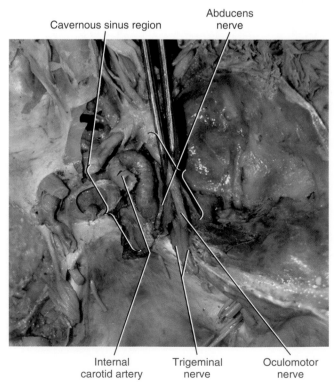

Cavernous sinus region | Abducens nerve

Internal carotid artery | Trigeminal nerve | Oculomotor nerve

FIGURE 23-57. Brackets show cavernous sinus region with abducens nerve running lateral to internal carotid artery.

LABORATORY IDENTIFICATION CHECKLIST

Brain/Brainstem
- ❏ Frontal lobe
  - ❏ Precentral gyrus
- ❏ Central sulcus
- ❏ Parietal lobe
  - ❏ Postcentral gyrus
- ❏ Occipital lobe
  - ❏ Occipital lobe gyri
- ❏ Temporal lobe
  - ❏ Temporal lobe gyri
- ❏ Corpus callosum
  - ❏ Genu
- ❏ Septum pellucidum
- ❏ Fornix
- ❏ Midbrain
- ❏ Hypothalamus
- ❏ Lamina terminalis
- ❏ Pineal gland
- ❏ Medulla oblongata
- ❏ Fourth ventricle
- ❏ Pons
- ❏ Mammillary body
- ❏ Foramen of Monro
- ❏ Cerebral aqueduct
- ❏ Pituitary stalk/gland
- ❏ Cerebellum

Nerves
- ❏ Olfactory bulb
- ❏ Olfactory tract
- ❏ Optic nerve
- ❏ Optic chiasm
- ❏ Oculomotor nerve
- ❏ Trochlear nerve
- ❏ Trigeminal nerve
  - ❏ V1 (ophthalmic) division
  - ❏ V2 (maxillary) division
  - ❏ V3 (mandibular) division

Nerves—cont'd
- ❏ Abducens nerve
- ❏ Facial nerve
- ❏ Nervus intermedius
- ❏ Vestibulocochlear nerve
- ❏ Glossopharyngeal nerve
- ❏ Vagus nerve
- ❏ Spinal accessory nerve
- ❏ Hypoglossal nerve

Arteries
- ❏ Internal carotid
- ❏ Basilar
- ❏ Middle meningeal
  - ❏ Anterior branch
  - ❏ Posterior branch
- ❏ Superficial temporal
- ❏ Anterior cerebral
- ❏ Middle cerebral
- ❏ Posterior cerebral
- ❏ Posterior communicating
- ❏ Vertebral

Veins/Sinuses
- ❏ Confluence of sinuses
- ❏ Superior sagittal sinus
- ❏ Inferior sagittal sinus
- ❏ Transverse sinus
- ❏ Straight sinus
- ❏ Emissary veins
- ❏ Superficial cerebral veins
- ❏ Cavernous sinus

Muscle
- ❏ Temporalis

Connective Tissue
- ❏ Skin
- ❏ Subcutaneous tissue

Connective Tissue—cont'd
- ❏ Epicranial aponeurosis
- ❏ Dura mater
- ❏ Lateral lacunae
- ❏ Falx cerebri
- ❏ Tentorium cerebelli
- ❏ Arachnoid mater
- ❏ Pia mater
- ❏ Temporalis fascia
- ❏ Parotid fascia

Bones/Fossae/Sinuses
- ❏ Frontal bone
  - ❏ Frontal sinus
  - ❏ Crista galli
  - ❏ Supraorbital notch/foramen
  - ❏ Glabella
- ❏ Temporal bone
- ❏ Parietal bone
- ❏ Occipital bone
  - ❏ Internal occipital crest
  - ❏ Frontal crest
- ❏ Periosteum
  - ❏ Vertex
  - ❏ Inion
  - ❏ Superior nuchal line
- ❏ Zygomatic arch
  - ❏ Diploic space
  - ❏ Pterion
  - ❏ Sagittal suture
  - ❏ Lambdoid suture
  - ❏ Parietal foramen
- ❏ Temporal fossa
- ❏ Anterior cranial fossa
- ❏ Middle cranial fossa
- ❏ Posterior cranial fossa
- ❏ Retromandibular region

CHAPTER 24

ORBIT

Netter: 81–91, 120

McMinn: 64–67

Gray's Atlas: 460–471

Remove all soft tissues with a scalpel and expose the frontal and temporal bones. Reflect the temporalis muscle as laterally as possible.

With an electric saw or mallet and chisel, make a cut through the frontal bone, lateral to the supraorbital notch (Fig. 24-1). Extend this cut posteriorly through the roof of the orbit between the optic nerve and ethmoidal sinuses (Fig. 24-2).

With an electric saw or a mallet and chisel, make a second vertical cut through the squamous part of the temporal bone. Continue the cut horizontally toward the orbital process of the zygomatic bone at the infraorbital margin (see Fig. 24-1).

☝ *DISSECTION TIP:* Typically, the orbital roof is thin. In addition, the frontal nerve and extraocular muscles lie just underneath the orbital roof. Take care to keep the cuts through this bone as shallow as possible (Fig. 24-3).

☝ *DISSECTION TIP:* Once all bones are cut, the orbital roof and the orbital process of the zygomatic bone can be reflected en bloc, while the periorbita (periosteal covering of orbital bones) is left intact (Fig. 24-3). This is referred to as an *orbitozygomatic approach.*

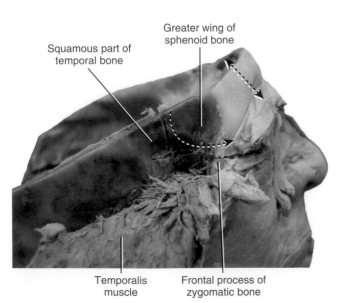

FIGURE 24-1. Anterolateral view of external orbit after craniotomy, with reflected temporalis muscle revealing bony landmarks; arrows indicate cuts through the frontal bone and orbital roof.

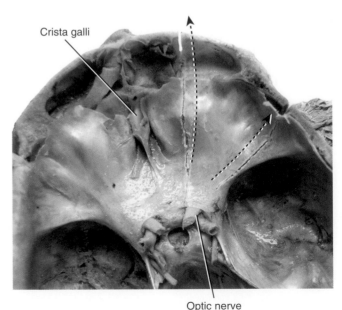

FIGURE 24-2. Craniotomy view of anterior cranial fossa, or superior roof of the orbit; arrows over dura represent osteotomy cuts.

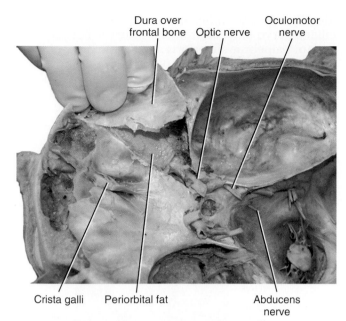

Dura over
frontal bone   Optic nerve   Oculomotor nerve

Crista galli   Periorbital fat   Abducens nerve

FIGURE 24-3. Craniotomy view highlighting anterior cranial fossa and dura mater, periorbital fat, crista galli, frontal bone, and nerves (optic, oculomotor, abducens).

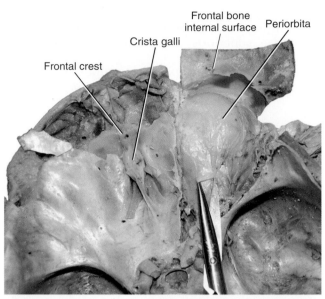

Frontal crest   Crista galli   Frontal bone internal surface   Periorbita

FIGURE 24-5. Craniotomy view of anterior cranial fossa with osteotomy to roof of right orbit, revealing scissors cutting periorbita.

Complete the reflection of the orbital roof anteriorly but do not detach it from the orbit (Fig. 24-4). With sharp scissors, make a small cut in the periorbital fascia (Fig. 24-5) Identify the frontal nerve and its two branches, the supraorbital and supratrochlear nerves (Fig. 24-6).

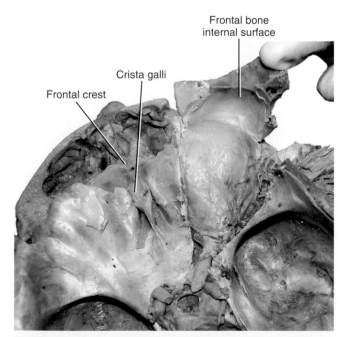

Frontal crest   Crista galli   Frontal bone internal surface

FIGURE 24-4. Craniotomy view of anterior cranial fossa with osteotomy performed to the roof of right orbit, revealing fat, frontal bone, frontal crest, and crista galli.

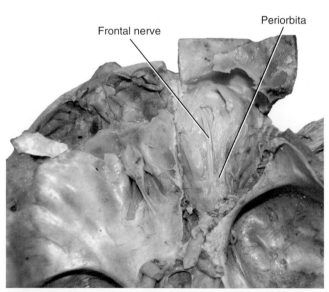

Frontal nerve   Periorbita

FIGURE 24-6. Craniotomy view of the anterior cranial fossa with osteotomy to orbital roof, highlighting periorbita and frontal nerve.

Clean and expose the frontal nerve and note the levator palpebrae superioris muscle lying underneath it (Fig. 24-7). Lateral and inferior to the levator palpebrae superioris, expose the superior rectus muscle (Fig. 24-8).

Medial to the levator palpebrae superioris muscle, remove a small portion of the periorbital fat and identify the *nasociliary nerve* (Fig. 24-9). The nasociliary nerve is located in the interval between the levator palpebrae superioris and the superior oblique muscles and crosses the optic nerve from lateral to medial (Fig. 24-10). Trace the terminal branches of the nasociliary nerve—the posterior ethmoidal, anterior ethmoidal, and infratrochlear nerves.

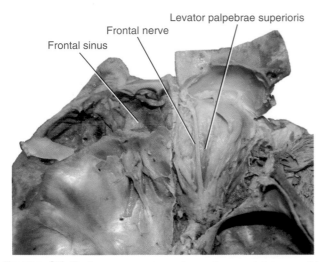

FIGURE 24-7. Craniotomy view of anterior cranial fossa with osteotomy to roof of orbit, revealing periorbita, frontal nerve/sinus, and levator palpebrae superioris muscle.

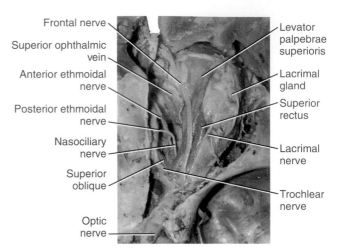

FIGURE 24-9. Craniotomy view of anterior cranial fossa with osteotomy to roof of orbit revealing nerves (optic, nasociliary, anterior/posterior ethmoidal, frontal, lacrimal), lacrimal gland, and key muscles (superior oblique, levator palpebrae superioris, superior rectus).

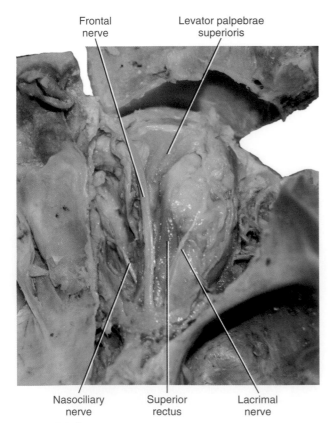

FIGURE 24-8. Craniotomy view of anterior cranial fossa with orbital roof osteotomy, revealing neurovascular landmarks.

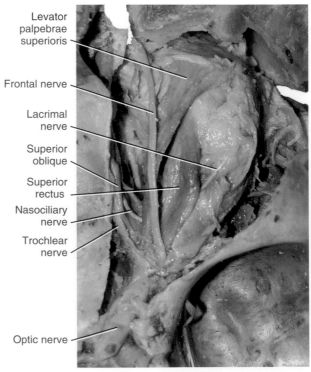

FIGURE 24-10. Craniotomy view of anterior cranial fossa with osteotomy to roof of orbit highlighting neurovascular musculature.

> ✋ *DISSECTION TIP:* The branches of the nasociliary nerve are small and delicate. The infratrochlear nerve is especially delicate and easily severed during dissection. The posterior ethmoidal nerve is often absent.

Clean the periorbital fat around the superior oblique muscle, and note the *trochlear nerve* entering the superior surface of the muscle proximally (Figs. 24-8 and 24-9).

> ✋ *DISSECTION TIP:* The superior oblique muscle is usually hidden from the orbital roof medially. Break away portions of the orbital roof to identify and clean the superior oblique muscle.

Distal to the interval between the superior oblique and levator palpebrae superioris muscles, look for a flat vessel, the superior ophthalmic vein. Remove all small tributaries of the ophthalmic veins (Figs. 24-8 and 24-9). On the lateral surface of the superior rectus muscle, trace and expose the lacrimal nerve and lacrimal gland (Fig. 24-10).

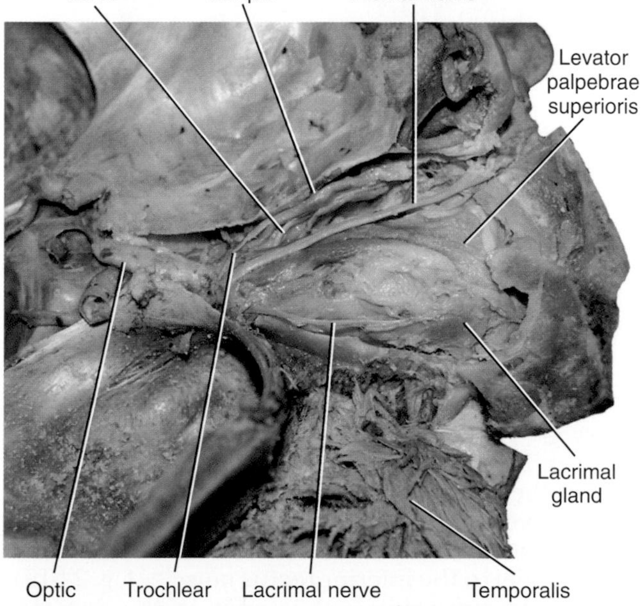

Deep to the lacrimal nerve, expose the lateral rectus muscle (Figs. 24-11 and 24-12). Pull the lateral rectus muscle laterally, and expose the *abducens nerve* on its medial side (Fig. 24-13). Look for the *superior ophthalmic vein* in the space between the superior rectus and lateral rectus muscles (Figs. 24-14 and 24-15).

> ✋ *DISSECTION TIP:* The lacrimal gland is located distally and is often confused with periorbital fat. Lift and pull up on the lacrimal nerve in order to trace it to the lacrimal gland.

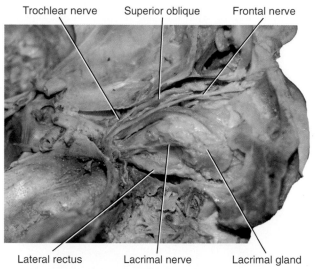

FIGURE 24-12. Craniotomy view of anterior cranial fossa with osteotomy to roof of orbit, revealing trochlear nerve, superior oblique muscle, frontal nerve, lacrimal nerve, lacrimal gland, and lateral rectus muscle.

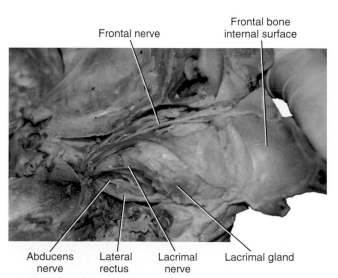

FIGURE 24-11. Craniotomy view of anterior cranial fossa with osteotomy to orbital roof, revealing neuromuscular landmarks and lacrimal gland.

FIGURE 24-13. Craniotomy view of anterior cranial fossa with orbital osteotomy, showing frontal nerve, internal surface of frontal bone, lacrimal nerve/gland, abducens nerve, and lateral rectus muscle.

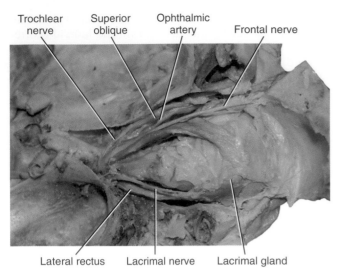

FIGURE **24-14.** Craniotomy view of anterior cranial fossa with osteotomy to roof of orbit, revealing trochlear nerve, superior oblique and lateral rectus muscles, ophthalmic artery, frontal nerve, lacrimal gland, and inferior ophthalmic vein.

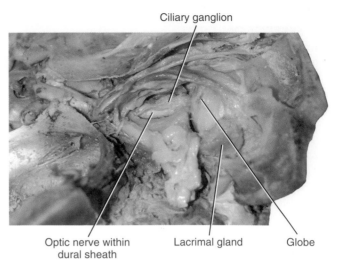

FIGURE **24-16.** Craniotomy view of anterior cranial fossa with osteotomy to roof of orbit, revealing long and short ciliary nerves with ciliary ganglion, optic nerve within dural sheath, globe (eyeball), and lacrimal gland.

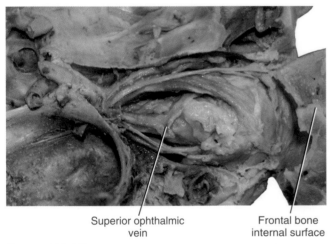

FIGURE **24-15.** Craniotomy view of anterior cranial fossa with osteotomy to orbital roof, highlighting superior ophthalmic vein.

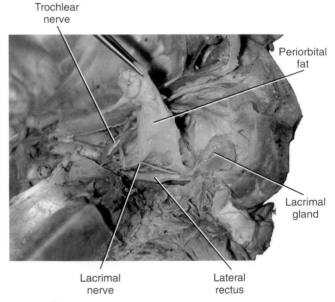

FIGURE **24-17.** Craniotomy view of anterior cranial fossa with orbital osteotomy showing key dissection landmarks.

After identifying the superior ophthalmic vein, remove the periorbital fat between the superior and lateral rectus muscles (Figs. 24-16 and 24-17). Observe the optic nerve, surrounded by short and long ciliary nerves (Fig. 24-18). Identify the *ciliary ganglion* on the lateral surface of the optic nerve and medial to the lateral rectus muscle (Figs. 24-16 and 24-18).

At the interval between the optic nerve and the lateral rectus muscle, identify the *ophthalmic artery* (Fig. 24-19). After entering the orbit, the ophthalmic artery gives off a central retinal branch to the optic nerve and usually crosses over the nerve and passes toward the medial wall of the orbit. Inferior to the optic nerve, remove the periorbital fat and identify the inferior division of the oculomotor nerve, which runs parallel to the inferior rectus muscle (Fig. 24-19).

Clean the periorbital fat inferior to the superior oblique muscle. Trace the anterior and posterior ethmoidal nerves to their entrance into the anterior and posterior ethmoidal foramina, respectively (Fig.

> ✋ *DISSECTION TIP:* Another important landmark is that the ciliary ganglion is connected by a small branch (motor root of ciliary ganglion) with the inferior division of the oculomotor nerve. The ganglion may be confused with periorbital fat.

Long ciliary nerves · Short ciliary nerves · Frontal nerve · Globe

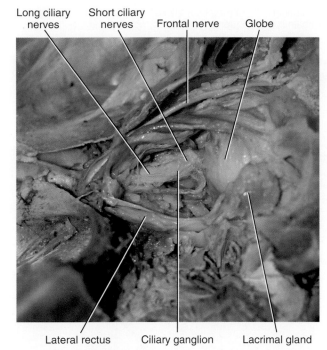

Lateral rectus · Ciliary ganglion · Lacrimal gland

FIGURE 24-18. Craniotomy view of anterior cranial fossa with osteotomy to orbital roof, revealing frontal nerve, reflected levator palpebrae superioris muscle, and highlighting long and short ciliary nerves and ciliary ganglion.

Posterior · Nasociliary ethmoidal · Superior · Anterior ethmoidal · Supratrochlear nerve · Supraorbital nerve

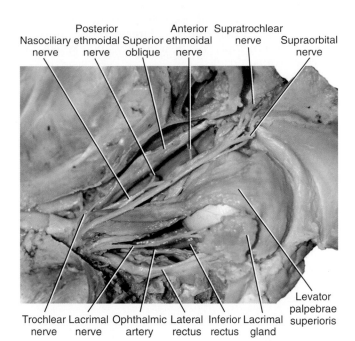

Trochlear nerve · Lacrimal nerve · Ophthalmic artery · Lateral rectus · Inferior rectus · Lacrimal gland · Levator palpebrae superioris

FIGURE 24-20. Craniotomy view of anterior cranial fossa with osteotomy to orbital roof, revealing orbital nerves (trochlear, nasociliary, posterior/anterior ethmoidal, supratrochlear, supraorbital, lacrimal), muscles (superior oblique, levator palpebrae superioris, lateral rectus), and lacrimal artery/gland.

24-20). The four recti muscles arise from a fibrous ring that encircles the optic foramen and a portion of the superior orbital fissure. The superior oblique and levator palpebrae muscles arise from points superior and medial to this anulus (annulus) tendineus communis (common tendinous ring, or anulus of Zinn) (Fig. 24-21).

Inferior division of oculomotor nerve · Optic nerve in dural sheath · Inferior rectus · Globe

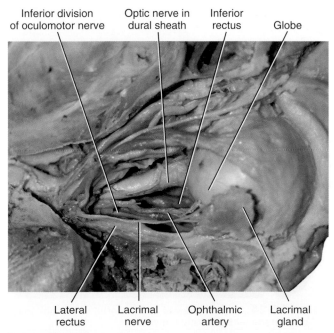

Lateral rectus · Lacrimal nerve · Ophthalmic artery · Lacrimal gland

FIGURE 24-19. Craniotomy view of anterior cranial fossa with osteotomy, highlighting optic nerve with dural sheath, inferior division of oculomotor nerve, ophthalmic artery, and lacrimal nerve/gland.

Supratrochlear nerve · Supraorbital nerve · Frontal nerve · Lacrimal gland

Trochlea · Superior ophthalmic vein · Ophthalmic artery · Anterior ethmoidal nerve · Posterior ethmoidal nerve · Nasociliary nerve · Superior oblique · Medial rectus · Frontal nerve

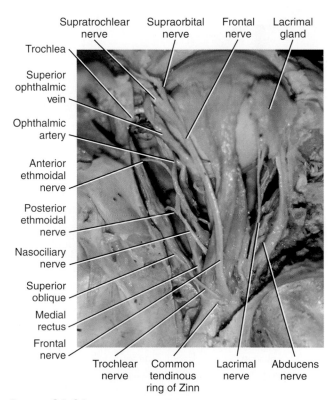

Trochlear nerve · Common tendinous ring of Zinn · Lacrimal nerve · Abducens nerve

FIGURE 24-21. Craniotomy view of anterior cranial fossa with osteotomy to roof of orbit, revealing orbital nerves (infratrochlear, frontal, lacrimal, abducens), superior ophthalmic vein, and lacrimal gland.

Reflect the nasociliary nerve and ophthalmic artery posteriorly and expose the medial rectus muscle (Fig. 24-22). Pull the lateral rectus muscle laterally and the optic nerve medially, and expose the inferior rectus muscle.

To trace the inferior oblique muscle, the inferior rectus muscle, and the nerve to the inferior oblique muscle, you need to dissect inferior to the globe (Fig. 24-23). Detach the orbital septum from the inferior orbital rim, and lift the orbit and periorbital fat superiorly (Fig. 24-24). Clean away the periorbital fat, and expose the inferior oblique muscle running obliquely from lateral to medial (Figs. 24-25 and 24-26). Remove all periorbital fat, and identify the inferior rectus muscle and the nerve to the inferior oblique muscle (Fig. 24-27).

Lift the orbicularis oculi muscle and identify the medial palpebral ligament (Fig. 24-28). Excess lacrimal fluid is drained by the *puncta* into *canaliculi,* which drain the fluid to the lacrimal sac. From this sac, the nasolacrimal duct passes into the nasal cavity.

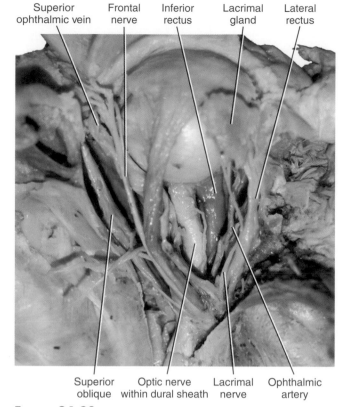

FIGURE 24-23. Craniotomy view of anterior cranial fossa with osteotomy to roof of orbit revealing musculature (superior oblique, inferior/lateral rectus), frontal nerve, ophthalmic vein, optic nerve within dural sheath, lacrimal nerve, and lacrimal gland.

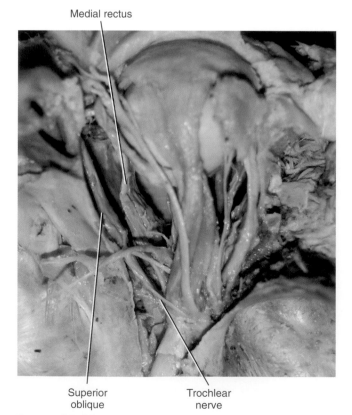

FIGURE 24-22. Craniotomy view revealing trochlear nerve and key muscles.

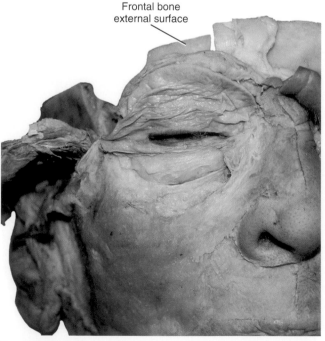

FIGURE 24-24. Anterior view of external orbit with craniotomy and vertical frontal bone osteotomy.

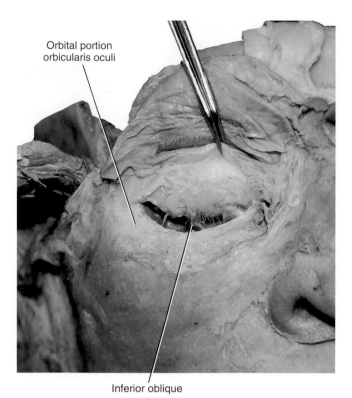

Orbital portion orbicularis oculi

Inferior oblique

FIGURE 24-25. Anterior view of external orbit with craniotomy using infraorbital approach, exposing orbital part of orbicularis oculi muscle, inferior oblique muscle, and floor of orbit.

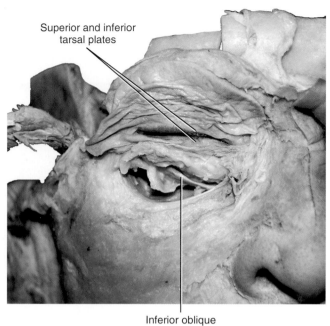

Superior and inferior tarsal plates

Inferior oblique

FIGURE 24-26. Anterior view of external orbit with craniotomy showing infraorbital approach, highlighting tarsal plates.

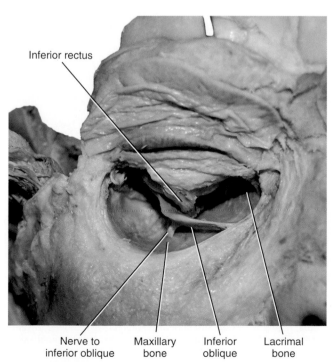

Inferior rectus

Nerve to inferior oblique   Maxillary bone   Inferior oblique   Lacrimal bone

FIGURE 24-27. Anterior view of orbit with eyeball removed, revealing maxilla, lacrimal bone, and nerve to inferior oblique muscle from inferior division of oculomotor.

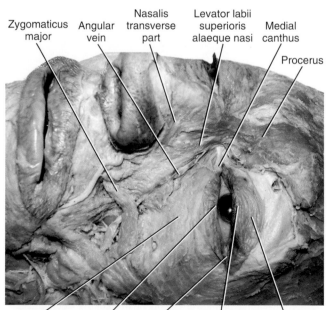

Zygomaticus major   Angular vein   Nasalis transverse part   Levator labii superioris alaeque nasi   Medial canthus   Procerus

Orbital region orbicularis oculi   Inferior tarsal plate   Lateral canthus   Superior tarsal plate   Palpebral portion orbicularis oculi

FIGURE 24-28. Anterior view of external orbit with skin reflected superiorly, revealing canthi, tarsal plates, angular vein, and key muscles (zygomaticus major, orbicularis oculi, levator labii superioris alaeque nasi, procerus, nasalis).

Reflect all musculature from the frontal process of the maxilla (Fig. 24-29). With an electric saw, cut the area inferior to the medial canthus and the inferomedial portion of the inferior orbital rim (Fig. 24-30). Identify the nasolacrimal duct within the lacrimal canal (Fig. 24-31).

If time permits, remove the eyeball en bloc with the surrounding extraocular muscles (Fig. 24-32).

> **✎ *DISSECTION TIP:*** The sclera is usually compressed and distorted. To restore its original shape, inject water into the eyeball with a hypodermic needle attached to a syringe (Fig. 24-33).

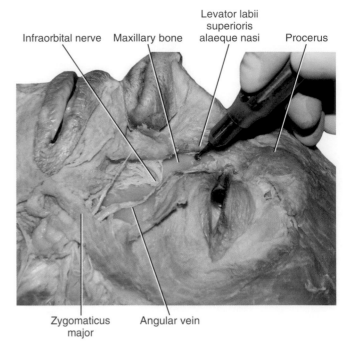

FIGURE 24-30. Anterolateral view of orbit with skin and subcutaneous tissue removed and orbital part of orbicularis oculi muscle reflected, revealing maxillary bone with osteotomy tool, infraorbital nerve, muscles (zygomaticus major, procerus, levator labii superioris alaeque nasi), and angular vein.

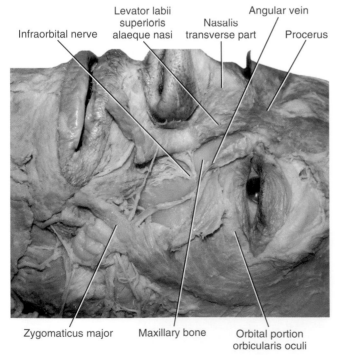

FIGURE 24-29. Anterior view of external orbit, nose, and maxilla, revealing palpebral region of orbicularis oculi muscle, procerus muscle, zygomaticus major muscle, orbital region of orbicularis oculi muscle, nasalis muscle, angular vein, levator labii superioris alaeque nasi muscle, infraorbital nerve, and maxilla.

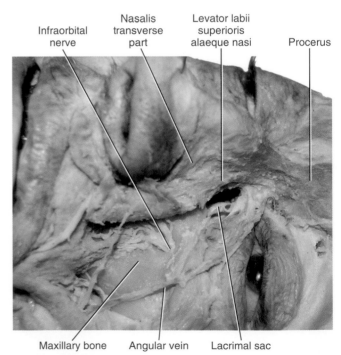

FIGURE 24-31. Anterior view of external orbit, highlighting medial region with skin and subcutaneous tissue removed, revealing maxillary bone, neuromuscular landmarks, and lacrimal sac.

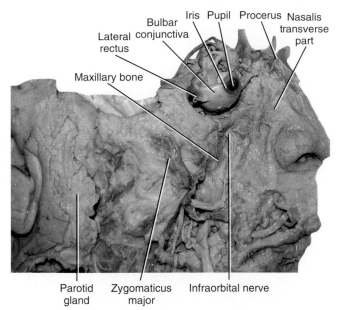

FIGURE 24-32. Lateral craniotomy view of orbit with skin and subcutaneous tissue removed, osteotomy to zygomatic bone, revealing globe, musculature (lateral rectus, nasalis, procerus, zygomaticus major), and parotid gland.

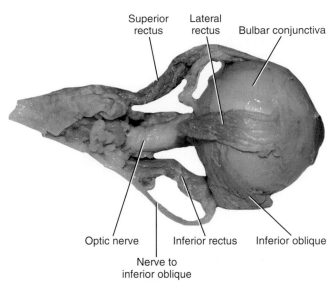

FIGURE 24-34. Superior view of globe with extraocular muscles removed from orbit, revealing superior rectus, superior oblique, lateral rectus, and inferior rectus muscles and bulbar conjunctiva.

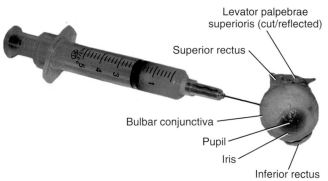

FIGURE 24-33. Anterosuperior view of globe removed from orbit, with fluid injected to maintain morphologic shape, showing muscles, bulbar conjunctiva, iris, and pupil.

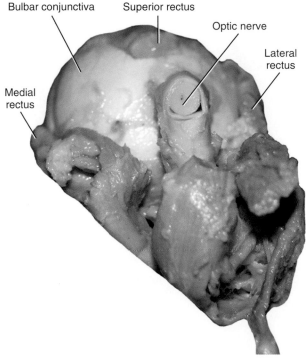

FIGURE 24-35. Posterior view of globe with extraocular muscles removed from orbit, revealing optic nerve and bulbar conjunctiva.

Once the shape of the *sclera* has been restored, observe its extraocular muscle attachments (Fig. 24-34). With a scalpel, cut the *optic nerve* and note the thick dura mater encircling it. At the middle of the cross section of the optic nerve, observe the small lumen that represents the central retinal artery (Fig. 24-35).

Have a classmate hold the sclera firmly with the fingers (Fig. 24-36) while you carefully incise the sclera with a scalpel (Fig. 24-37).

On the hemisected orbit, identify the *limbus,* which is the junction of the cornea and the sclera (Fig. 24-38). The space between the iris and cornea is the anterior chamber. This is usually filled with the aqueous humor, but in the cadaver it will be empty (Fig. 24-39).

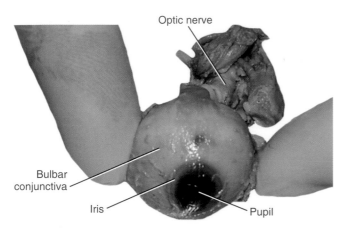

FIGURE 24-36. Anterosuperior view of globe with extraocular muscles cut and reflected, highlighting optic nerve, bulbar conjunctiva, iris, and pupil.

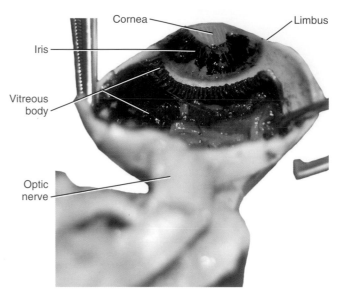

FIGURE 24-38. Sagittal section of globe with vitreous humor removed, revealing cornea, iris, and vitreous body.

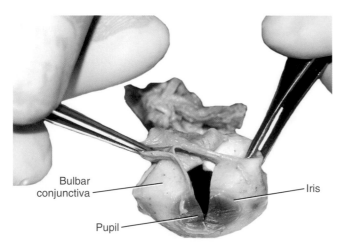

FIGURE 24-37. Anterosuperior view of globe removed from orbit, revealing vertical incision, superior rectus muscle, bulbar conjunctiva, iris, and pupil.

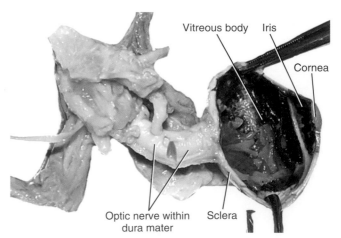

FIGURE 24-39. Sagittal section of globe removed from orbit, revealing optic nerve, extraocular muscles cut and reflected, vitreous body, iris, and cornea.

LABORATORY IDENTIFICATION CHECKLIST

Nerves
- ❏ Trochlear
- ❏ Frontal
  - ❏ Supratrochlear
  - ❏ Supraorbital
- ❏ Lacrimal
- ❏ Nasociliary
  - ❏ Posterior ethmoidal (inconstant)
  - ❏ Anterior ethmoidal
  - ❏ Infratrochlear
  - ❏ Long ciliary
- ❏ Oculomotor
- ❏ Superior division
- ❏ Inferior division
- ❏ Abducens
- ❏ Optic
- ❏ Short ciliary nerves (8-10)
- ❏ Infraorbital nerve

Ganglion/Fascia/Fat
- ❏ Ciliary ganglion
- ❏ Periorbita
- ❏ Periorbital fat
- ❏ Trochlea
- ❏ Annulus of Zinn

Arteries
- ❏ Ophthalmic
  - ❏ Anterior ethmoidal
  - ❏ Posterior ethmoidal
  - ❏ Retinal
  - ❏ Lacrimal

Veins
- ❏ Superior ophthalmic
- ❏ Inferior ophthalmic

Muscles
- ❏ Procerus
  - *Recti*
- ❏ Superior rectus
- ❏ Inferior rectus
- ❏ Medial rectus
- ❏ Lateral rectus
  - *Obliques*
- ❏ Superior oblique
- ❏ Inferior oblique
- ❏ Levator palpebrae superioris

Bones
- ❏ Frontal
- ❏ Lacrimal
- ❏ Maxilla
- ❏ Ethmoid
- ❏ Zygomatic

Gland
- ❏ Lacrimal

Sinuses
- ❏ Frontal
- ❏ Ethmoidal
  - ❏ Anterior air cells
  - ❏ Middle air cells
  - ❏ Posterior air cells

CHAPTER 25

EAR

Netter: 92–98

McMinn: 70–71

Gray's Atlas: 472–477

Identify the following bones in your atlas, text, and on a skull:

- Petrous part of temporal bone
- Squamous part of temporal bone
- Petrosquamous fissure (at junction of petrous and squamous parts)
- Arcuate eminence (overlies anterior semicircular canal)
- Internal acoustic meatus
- Hiatus of facial canal (greater petrosal nerve exits petrous bone from here)
- Groove for superior petrosal sinus

- Tegmen tympani (roof of middle ear between petrosquamous fissure and hiatus of facial canal)
- Jugular foramen
- Tympanic part of temporal bone (provides much of bony wall of external auditory canal)
- Mandibular fossa
- Petrotympanic fissure (for passage of chorda tympani nerve)
- Styloid process and stylomastoid foramen

Most anatomy courses do not dissect the ear because it is a time-consuming dissection. This chapter presents a new, time-efficient method for exposing the structures of the middle ear.

The ear, or *vestibulocochlear* organ, is subdivided into the external, the middle, and the internal ear. On the external ear of a classmate, identify the following structures (Fig. 25-1):

- Helix
- Antihelix and crura of antihelix
- Triangular fossa
- Concha
- Lobule
- Tragus
- Antitragus
- Intertragic notch
- External acoustic meatus

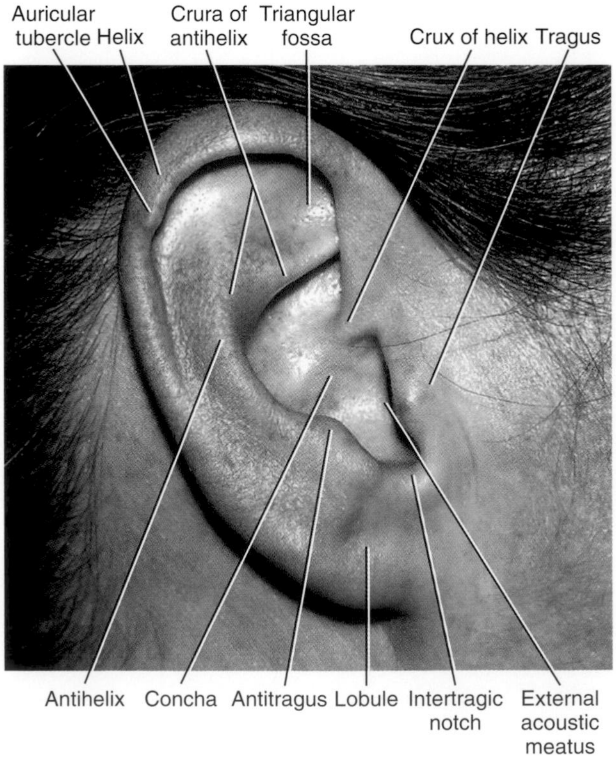

FIGURE 25-1. External view of external ear with several surface landmarks.

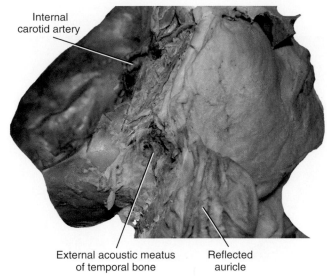

Internal
carotid artery

External acoustic meatus   Reflected
of temporal bone   auricle

FIGURE 25-2. Postcraniotomy horizontal section reveals lateral view of middle cranial fossa with external ear reflected, highlighting external auditory canal, external acoustic meatus of temporal bone, and internal carotid artery.

Internal carotid
artery

External auditory
canal

Reflected
auricle

Trigeminal
nerve

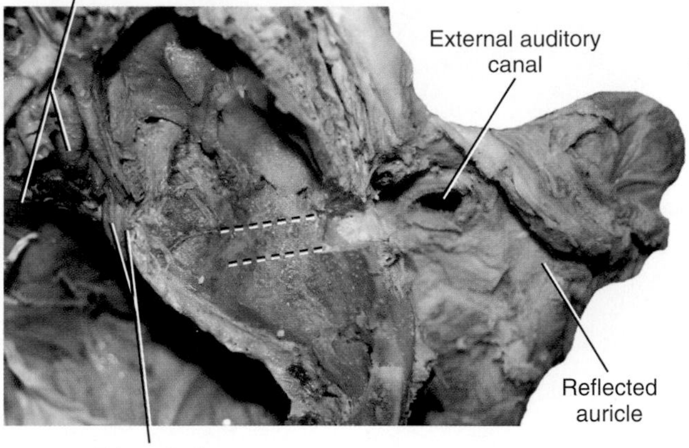

FIGURE 25-3. Horizontal section after craniotomy shows middle cranial fossa with external ear reflected, highlighting the external auditory canal, trigeminal nerve, and internal carotid artery. Dashed lines demarcate lateral borders of the external acoustic meatus on tegmen tympani (roof of tympanum).

OPTIONAL DISSECTION

If time permits, create a skin flap from the helix to expose part of the elastic fibrocartilage. Create a second skin flap at the lobule and note the dense, fibrous connective tissue.

With your scalpel, make an incision posterior to the auricle towards the neck. Dissect away most of the soft tissue and the external acoustic meatus (Fig. 25-2). Remove any debris present in the remaining part of the external canal.

> ☛ *DISSECTION TIP:* With the aid of an otoscope, attempt to inspect the tympanic membrane. Remove any wax (cerumen) that may obstruct your view.

Draw a line along the bony roof of the middle ear, the *tegmen tympani,* demarcating the length of the canal from the external acoustic meatus to the tympanic membrane. Draw two dashed lines at the outer borders of the canal (Fig. 25-3). With a chisel and a mallet, remove a small piece of bone, and expose the outer portion of the canal for inspection (Fig. 25-4).

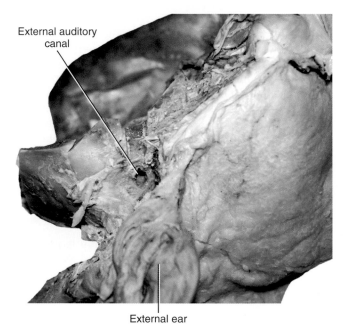

External auditory
canal

External ear

FIGURE 25-4. Postcraniotomy horizontal section reveals lateral view of middle cranial fossa with external ear reflected.

> ☛ *DISSECTION TIP:* With a cotton swab or forceps, clean the auditory canal of debris and cerumen (Fig. 25-4). Do not place the swab or forceps too deeply into the canal, to prevent damage to the tympanic membrane.

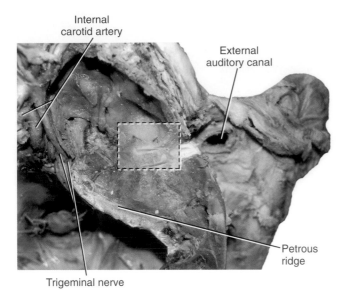

FIGURE 25-5. Horizontal section after craniotomy reveals middle cranial fossa with external ear reflected; highlighted on tegmen tympani, chisel marks and square in center indicates lateral borders of external acoustic meatus.

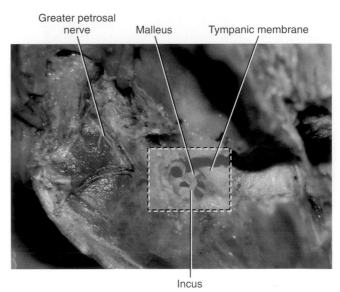

FIGURE 25-6. Tegmen tympani over external acoustic meatus (epitympanic recess) removed, exposing tympanic membrane and two ear ossicles. Note that connective tissue over external acoustic meatus is still intact.

Continue the removal of bone with the chisel and the mallet on the surface of the tegmen tympani (Fig. 25-5). The external acoustic meatus is about 3-4 cm long. Once the tegmen tympani is removed to the *epitympanic recess* (area superior to tympanic membrane), and using bone rongeurs, remove small pieces of bone and expose the tympanic membrane and three auditory ossicles (small bones)—malleus (hammer), incus (anvil), and stapes (stirrup) (Fig. 25-6).

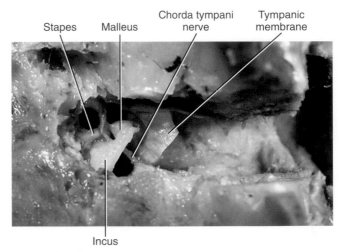

FIGURE 25-7. Magnified view of middle cranial fossa with auditory canal and middle ear exposed, revealing osseous auditory canal of external ear, tympanic membrane, ossicles (malleus, incus, stapes), and chorda tympani nerve.

> **DISSECTION TIP:** When exposing the tegmen tympani to reveal the malleus, incus, and stapes, grasp the outer part of the tympanic membrane, and pull it gently upward to maintain the position of the ossicles.

At the final stage of dissection, cut the connective tissue layer covering the canal, and appreciate the orientation of the tympanic membrane (Fig. 25-6). The membrane is positioned obliquely in spaces in the external meatus at an angle of about 55 degrees (Fig. 25-7). Note the following relationships:

- Stapedius muscle inserting onto the stapes.
- Tendon of the tensor tympani muscle inserting onto the malleus.
- Malleus attached to the tympanic membrane.

> **DISSECTION TIP:** Dissecting the internal ear cavity is time-consuming; more importantly, however, inspection requires a dissecting microscope to identify auricular structures clearly.

LABORATORY IDENTIFICATION CHECKLIST

Nerves
- ❏ Trigeminal
  - ❏ Mandibular (V3)
- ❏ Nervus intermedius
- ❏ Greater petrosal
- ❏ Facial
- ❏ Chorda tympani
- ❏ Vestibulocochlear
- ❏ Vagus

Ganglia
- ❏ Trigeminal
- ❏ Geniculate

Artery
- ❏ Internal carotid

Muscles
- ❏ Tensor tympani
- ❏ Stapedius
- ❏ Auricularis
  - ❏ Superior
  - ❏ Anterior
  - ❏ Posterior

Bones
- ❏ Petrous (ridge)
- ❏ Tegmen tympani (roof)

Auditory ossicles
- ❏ Malleus
- ❏ Incus
- ❏ Stapes

Other Structures
- ❏ External auditory meatus
- ❏ Tympanic membrane
- ❏ Oval window

Cartilage
- ❏ Helix
- ❏ Antihelix
- ❏ Tragus
- ❏ Antitragus
- ❏ Auricular tubercle

CHAPTER 26

NASAL CAVITY

Netter: 36–50, 63–65

McMinn: 54, 62, 68–69

Gray's Atlas: 486–487, 518–523, 529

Exposure of the contents of the nasal cavity requires a midsagittal transection through the head (Fig. 26-1). Place the saw as close as possible to the midline. Begin the cut externally from the face toward the midportion of the head (Figs. 26-2 and 26-3). Split the head in half, and choose one of the two halves to decapitate (Figs. 26-4 and 26-5).

> ☞ *DISSECTION TIP:* Electric saws are usually too small for transection of the head. Make sure that one of your classmates holds the cadaver head firmly as you cut with the saw.

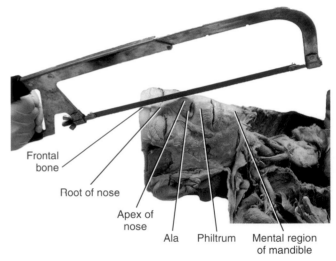

FIGURE 26-2. Anterior view of face with previous craniotomy, preparing for a sagittal section of nasal cavity.

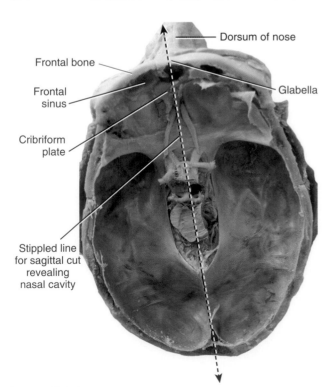

FIGURE 26-1. Craniotomy view with dashed line for sagittal section.

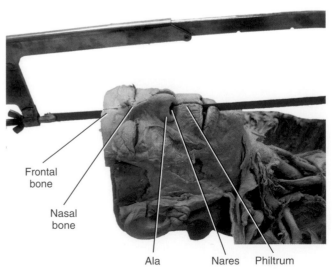

FIGURE 26-3. Anterolateral view of face with previous craniotomy, demonstrating sagittal cut of nasal cavity.

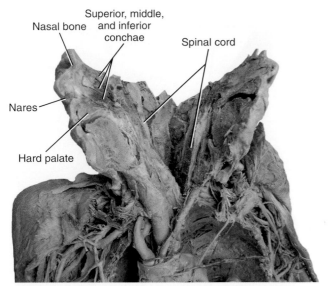

FIGURE 26-4. Anterior view of sagittal cut of nasal and oral cavities revealing nasal septum with left and concha on right.

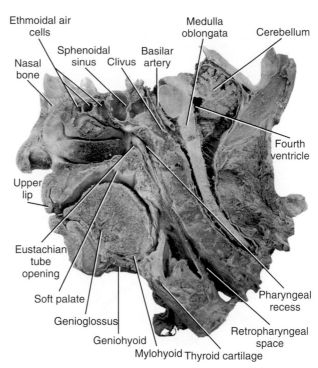

FIGURE 26-6. Sagittal view of nasal and oral regions. Nasal region structures include sphenoidal sinus, ethmoidal sinus (anterior, middle, and posterior air cells), nasal concha, and eustachian tube opening. Oral structures include lips, hard and soft palate, tongue, oral floor muscles (genioglossus, geniohyoid, mylohyoid), epiglottis, pharyngeal recess, and retropharyngeal space.

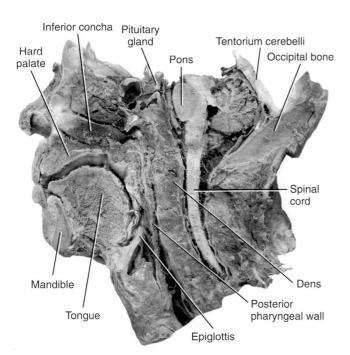

FIGURE 26-5. Sagittal view of nasal and oral cavities revealing nasal bone, cartilage, concha, and openings. Structures of mouth and pharynx include hard palate, soft palate, tongue, mandible, epiglottis, and posterior pharyngeal wall.

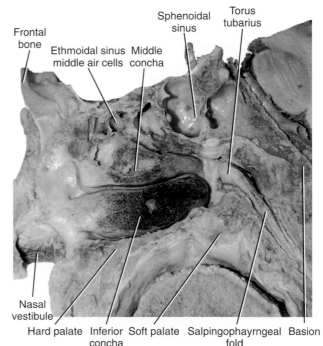

FIGURE 26-7. Sagittal view of nasal cavity, revealing sphenoidal, ethmoidal, and frontal sinuses; concha; nasal bone; torus tubarius; and salpingopharyngeal fold.

Clean away soft tissues or any bony fragments after the hemisection (compare Fig. 26-5 with Fig. 26-6). Identify several landmarks as indicated on the dissection photographs of the hemisected head. The nasal cavities extend from the nares anteriorly to the choanae posteriorly, constituting the *nasal cavity proper*. Identify the superior, middle, and inferior nasal *conchae,* which are located within the nasal cavity proper (Fig. 26-7).

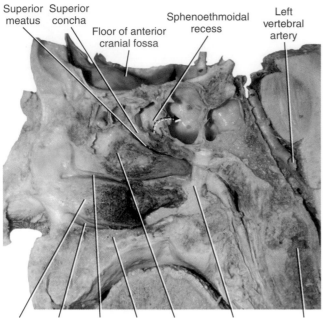

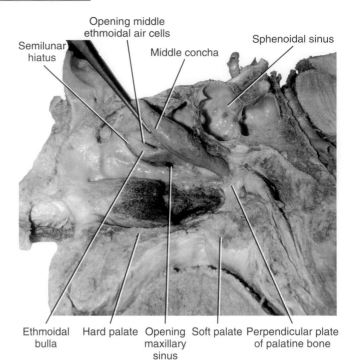

FIGURE 26-8. Sagittal view of nasal cavity, revealing sphenoidal and ethmoid sinuses and nasal concha, highlighting drainage pathways that include sphenoethmoidal recess and meatus associated with superior, middle, and inferior conchae.

FIGURE 26-9. Sagittal view of nasal cavity with middle concha reflected revealing opening of ethmoidal air cells, ethmoidal bulla, semilunar hiatus, and maxillary sinus opening.

Identify the *superior meatus,* the space between the superior and middle conchae. Continue inferiorly and identify the space between the middle and inferior conchae, the *middle meatus.* Finally, identify the space between the inferior concha and the hard palate, the *inferior meatus* (Fig. 26-8).

Posterior to the superior concha is a space referred to as the *sphenoethmoidal recess.* Identify the opening for the sphenoidal sinus into this recess (Fig. 26-8). Identify the anterior, middle, and posterior *ethmoidal air cells.* In the superior meatus, find the ostia of the posterior ethmoidal air cells (see Fig. 26-10).

> ☞ *DISSECTION TIP:* In most cadavers it is necessary to break away part of the thin, medial wall of the sphenoidal sinus to gain access to its interior. Some specimens may also have a "supreme" concha.

With a scalpel, scrape off the posterior one third of the mucosa covering the middle and inferior conchae, and identify the underlying bone.

> ☞ *DISSECTION TIP:* Some specimens will have an increased thickness of the nasal mucosa (see Figs. 26-7 and 26-8).

With forceps, lift the middle meatus upward and identify the ethmoidal bulla; locate the opening of the ethmoidal infundibulum into the semilunar hiatus (Fig. 26-9). With scissors or a scalpel, cut the middle concha away from its junction with the lateral wall of the nasal cavity, and completely expose the middle meatus (Fig. 26-10). The *hiatus semilunaris* is the long, semicircular groove into which the frontonasal duct drains (drainage of frontal sinus through infundibulum), as well as the anterior ethmoidal air cells. Identify the opening of the maxillary sinus. Pass a probe into this opening.

> ☞ *DISSECTION TIP:* Inspect the area of the middle meatus to determine whether there may be accessory openings for the maxillary sinus.

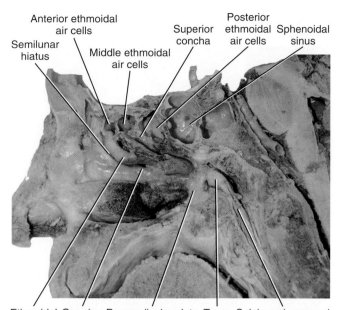

Anterior ethmoidal air cells — Middle ethmoidal air cells — Superior concha — Posterior ethmoidal air cells — Sphenoidal sinus — Semilunar hiatus

Ethmoidal bulla — Opening maxillary sinus — Perpendicular plate of palatine bone — Torus tubarius — Salpingopharyngeal fold

FIGURE 26-10. Sagittal view of nasal cavity with superior concha cut and middle concha removed revealing sphenoidal sinus and posterior, middle, and anterior ethmoidal air cells. Middle concha removed, highlighting ethmoidal bulla, semilunar hiatus, and maxillary sinus opening.

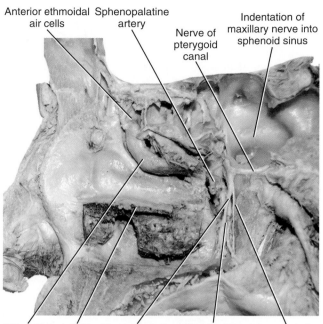

Anterior ethmoidal air cells — Sphenopalatine artery — Nerve of pterygoid canal — Indentation of maxillary nerve into sphenoid sinus

Ethmoidal bulla — Inferior concha cut — Greater palatine nerve — Descending palatine artery — Lesser palatine nerve

FIGURE 26-11. Sagittal view of nasal cavity with middle concha removed and inferior concha cut and partially removed revealing drainage pathways of superior, middle, and inferior conchae (nasolacrimal duct) and osteotomy to pterygopalatine fossa. Pterygopalatine fossa includes ganglion, nerve of pterygoid canal, greater and lesser palatine nerves, and sphenopalatine and descending palatine arteries.

The *ethmoidal bulla* is formed by the bulging of ethmoidal air cells into the middle meatus (Fig. 26-10). The ethmoidal bulla can be oversized from hypertrophy of the ethmoidal air cells. Remove the anterior half of the inferior nasal concha and identify the opening of the nasolacrimal duct (Fig. 26-11). Place a probe in the nasolacrimal duct.

Before dissection of the pterygopalatine fossa, identify the opening to the auditory or pharyngotympanic tube *(eustachian tube)* and place a probe into it (Fig. 26-12). Identify the elevation of the auditory tube and its muscular ridge, the *salpingopharyngeal fold.* At the opening of the eustachian tube, dissect away the mucous membrane (Fig. 26-13), and identify the *levator* veli palatini muscle (Fig. 26-14). Anterior to the levator veli palatini, dissect out fat and other connective tissues (Fig. 26-15) and identify the *tensor* veli palatini muscle (Fig. 26-16).

✋ *DISSECTION TIP:* The tensor veli palatini and levator veli palatini muscles are easy to distinguish because of the white, *tendinous* fibers of the *tensor* veli palatini (Fig. 26-16).

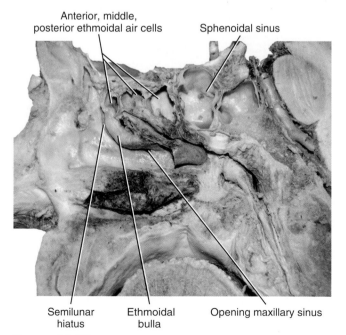

Anterior, middle, posterior ethmoidal air cells — Sphenoidal sinus

Semilunar hiatus — Ethmoidal bulla — Opening maxillary sinus

FIGURE 26-12. Sagittal view of nasal cavity revealing sphenoidal, posterior middle, and anterior ethmoidal air cells. Middle concha removed, revealing semilunar hiatus, ethmoidal bulla, and maxillary sinus opening.

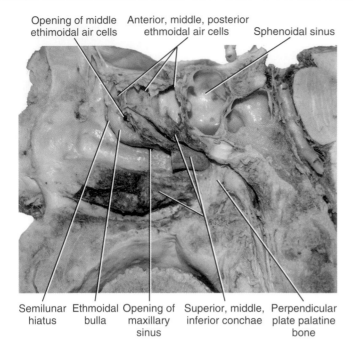

FIGURE 26-13. Sagittal view of nasal cavity revealing sphenoidal, posterior middle, and anterior ethmoidal air cells. Middle concha removed, revealing semilunar hiatus, ethmoid bulla, maxillary sinus opening, and superior, middle, and inferior conchae, as well as the perpendicular plate of palatine bone.

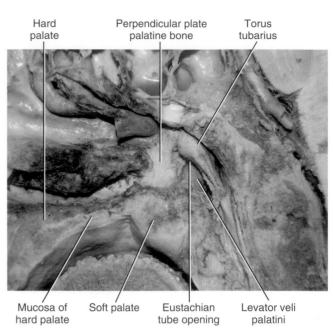

FIGURE 26-14. Sagittal view of nasal cavity revealing hard and soft palate, torus tubarius, salpingopharyngeal fold, opening of eustachian tube, and levator veli palatini muscle.

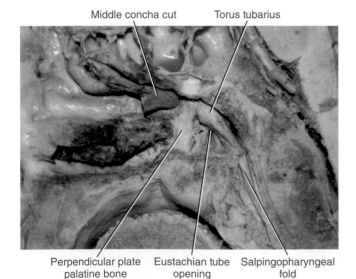

FIGURE 26-15. Sagittal view of nasal cavity, revealing middle concha cut, torus tubarius, salpingopharyngeal fold, perpendicular plate of palatine bone, and eustachian opening.

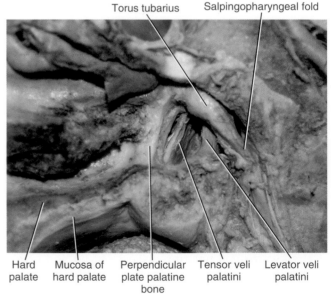

FIGURE 26-16. Sagittal view of nasal cavity, highlighting hard palate and revealing tensor and levator veli palatini muscles, torus tubarius, and salpingopharyngeal fold.

Lift the soft tissues and mucous membranes at the space posterior to the nasal conchae and the tensor veli palatini (in essence, the posterior plate of the pterygoid process of the sphenoid bone) (Fig. 26-17). Cut the posterior one third of the middle and superior conchae, and remove the mucosa and soft tissues to expose the palatine bone (Fig. 26-18).

> ✋ *DISSECTION TIP:* The palatine bone is thin, and you can identify the course of the greater and lesser palatine nerves and vessels before removing it.

With a small electric drill, cut away the palatine bone, making a vertical cut from the sphenoidal sinus to the hard palate and posteriorly to the middle concha (Figs. 26-19 and 26-20). First, expose the greater and lesser palatine nerves, as well as the descending palatine artery and the greater and lesser palatine arteries (Figs. 26-21 and 26-22).

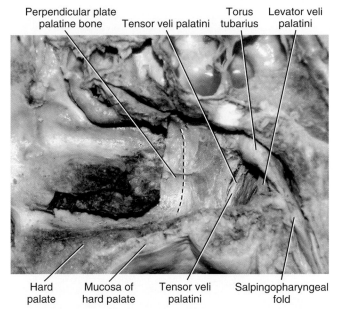

FIGURE 26-18. Sagittal view of nasal cavity, highlighting perpendicular plate of palatine bone, tensor and levator veli palatini muscles, torus tubarius, and mucosa of hard palate.

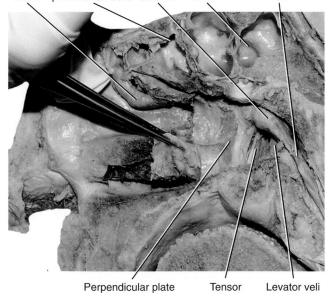

FIGURE 26-17. Sagittal view of nasal cavity with superior, middle, and inferior conchae cut, revealing perpendicular plate of palatine bone, tensor and levator veli palatini, torus tubarius, and salpingopharyngeal fold.

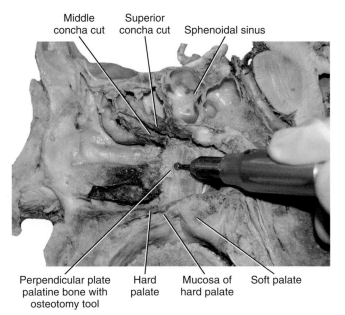

FIGURE 26-19. Sagittal view of nasal cavity, highlighting middle and superior conchae cut and perpendicular plate of palatine bone with small osteotomy to reveal pterygopalatine fossa structures.

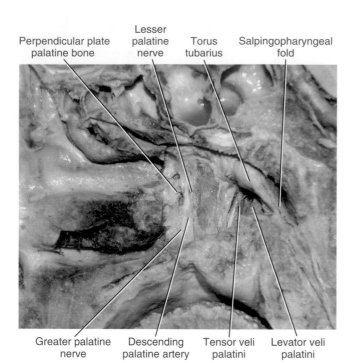

FIGURE 26-20. Sagittal view of nasal cavity highlighting perpendicular plate of palatine bone with partial osteotomy to reveal greater and lesser palatine nerves and descending palatine artery.

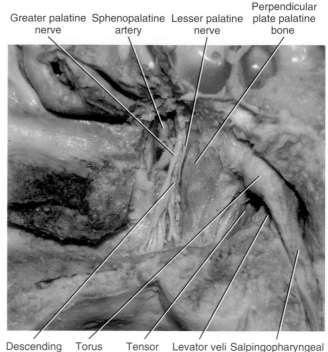

FIGURE 26-22. Sagittal view of nasal cavity highlighting osteotomy of perpendicular plate of palatine bone to reveal sphenopalatine artery, greater and lesser palatine nerves, and descending palatine artery.

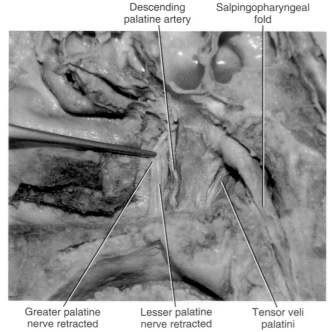

FIGURE 26-21. Sagittal view of nasal cavity with greater and lesser palatine nerves retracted revealing descending palatine artery.

Continue drilling upward to the sphenoidal sinus. Identify the sphenopalatine artery and the pterygopalatine ganglion (Fig. 26-23).

> **DISSECTION TIP:** In this part of dissection, use fine forceps and scissors to separate the delicate nerves and arteries.

Continue drilling posteriorly to the pterygopalatine ganglion and inferior to the sphenoidal sinus. Expose the *vidian nerve* (nerve to pterygoid canal) (Fig. 26-24). The greater and deep petrosal nerves unite and form the nerve of the pterygoid canal. This nerve passes through the pterygoid canal of the sphenoid bone and then into the pterygopalatine fossa.

If time permits, drill away the sphenoidal sinus, and expose the connection of the pterygopalatine ganglion with the maxillary nerve (Fig. 26-25). With scissors, reflect the oral mucosa from the hard palate, and identify the distribution of the greater and lesser palatine nerves (Fig. 26-26).

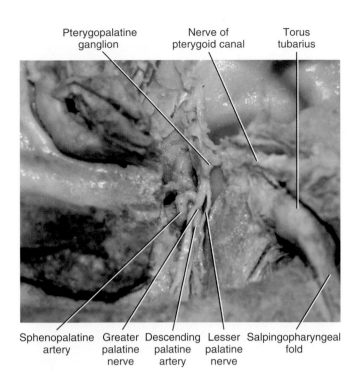

Pterygopalatine ganglion · Nerve of pterygoid canal · Torus tubarius

Sphenopalatine artery · Greater palatine nerve · Descending palatine artery · Lesser palatine nerve · Salpingopharyngeal fold

FIGURE 26-23. Sagittal view of nasal cavity with osteotomy of perpendicular plate of palatine bone revealing sphenopalatine artery, pterygopalatine ganglion, nerve of pterygoid canal, greater and lesser palatine nerves, and descending palatine artery.

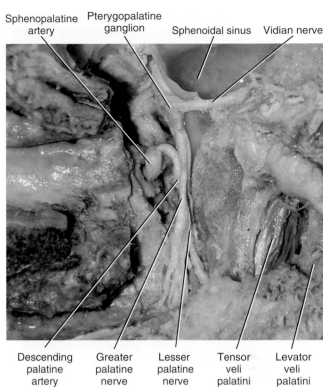

Sphenopalatine artery · Pterygopalatine ganglion · Sphenoidal sinus · Vidian nerve

Descending palatine artery · Greater palatine nerve · Lesser palatine nerve · Tensor veli palatini · Levator veli palatini

FIGURE 26-24. Sagittal view of nasal cavity with osteotomy of perpendicular plate of palatine bone revealing pterygopalatine ganglion, nerve of pterygoid canal, greater and lesser palatine nerves, and descending palatine artery.

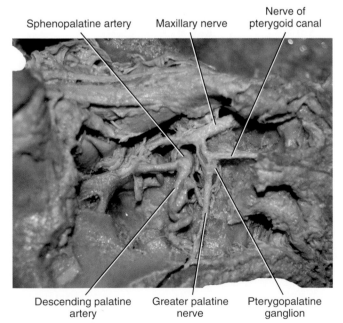

Sphenopalatine artery · Maxillary nerve · Nerve of pterygoid canal

Descending palatine artery · Greater palatine nerve · Pterygopalatine ganglion

FIGURE 26-25. Sagittal view of nasal cavity highlighting osteotomy of perpendicular plate of palatine bone and the sphenoidal sinus and revealing pterygopalatine fossa with pterygopalatine ganglion, nerve of pterygoid canal, greater palatine nerve, descending palatine artery and maxillary nerve.

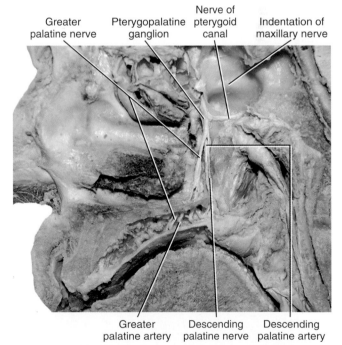

Greater palatine nerve · Pterygopalatine ganglion · Nerve of pterygoid canal · Indentation of maxillary nerve

Greater palatine artery · Descending palatine nerve · Descending palatine artery

FIGURE 26-26. Sagittal view of nasal cavity highlighting osteotomy of perpendicular plate of palatine bone, to show pterygopalatine fossa with pterygopalatine ganglion, nerve of pterygoid canal, greater and lesser palatine nerves and arteries, and descending palatine artery.

The lateral wall of the nasal cavity is dissected on one side of the head, as well as the pterygopalatine fossa. Dissect the nasal septum on the opposite side, i.e., the other hemisected head (Fig. 26-27). Remove the mucous membranes from the exposed surface of the nasal septum (Fig. 26-28). Identify the septal cartilage, perpendicular plate of the ethmoid bone, and the vomer bone (Fig. 26-29).

> ☞ *DISSECTION TIP:* Usually, it is difficult and time-consuming to find any of the nerves or vessels on the nasal mucosa, because of drying and shrinkage from fixation.

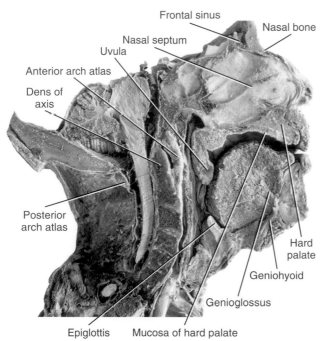

FIGURE 26-27. Sagittal view of nasal and oral cavities revealing nasal septum and sphenoidal/frontal sinuses. Oral cavity reveals hard palate, soft palate, uvula, pharynx, floor of tongue muscles (genioglossus, geniohyoid), and epiglottis.

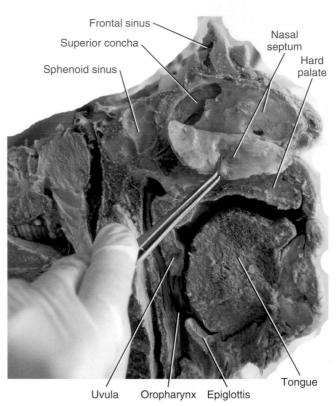

FIGURE 26-28. Sagittal view of nasal and oral cavities with nasal septum reflected, revealing superior concha, vomer bone, sphenoidal sinus, and frontal sinus. Oral cavity reveals tongue, floor of tongue muscles, uvula, epiglottis, and pharynx.

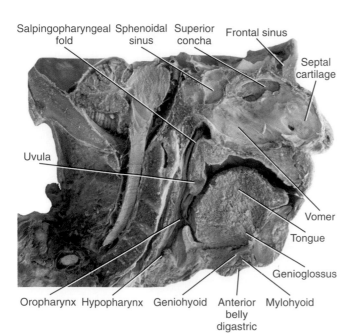

FIGURE 26-29. Sagittal view of nasal and oral cavities, revealing sphenoidal and frontal sinuses, septal cartilage, vomer bone, superior concha, and nasal pharynx. Oral cavity reveals uvula, tongue, and genioglossus, geniohyoid, mylohyoid, and anterior belly of digastric muscles.

Identify the following:
- *Sphenoethmoidal recess,* posterior to the superior concha, the location of the opening for the sphenoidal sinus.
- *Superior nasal meatus,* beneath the superior concha, the opening for the posterior ethmoidal air cells.
- *Middle nasal meatus,* the ethmoidal bulla, with openings for middle ethmoid air cells and the maxillary sinus.

- *Inferior nasal meatus,* the opening of the nasolacrimal duct.
- *Ethmoidal infundibulum,* for the opening of the frontonasal duct from the frontal sinus.
- *Hiatus semilunaris,* the semilunar hiatus, the long, crescent-shaped opening for the anterior ethmoidal air cells.

LABORATORY IDENTIFICATION CHECKLIST

Nerves
❐ Nerve of pterygoid canal
❐ Greater palatine
❐ Lesser palatine
❐ Maxillary

Arteries
❐ Sphenopalatine
   ❐ Descending palatine
      ❐ Greater palatine
      ❐ Lesser palatine

Muscles
❐ Tensor veli palatini
❐ Levator veli palatini
❐ Salpingopharyngeus

Bones
❐ Nasal
❐ Frontal
❐ Ethmoid
   ❐ Cribriform plate
   ❐ Perpendicular plate
❐ Sphenoid
❐ Palatine
   ❐ Horizontal plate
   ❐ Perpendicular plate
❐ Palatine process of maxilla
❐ Vomer
❐ Conchae
   ❐ Superior
   ❐ Middle
   ❐ Inferior

Sinuses
❐ Sphenoidal
❐ Ethmoidal
   ❐ Posterior air cells
   ❐ Middle air cells
   ❐ Anterior air cells
❐ Frontal
❐ Maxillary

Drainage Pathways
❐ Sphenoethmoidal recess
❐ Superior meatus
❐ Middle meatus
❐ Inferior meatus
❐ Ethmoidal bulla
❐ Semilunar hiatus
❐ Nasolacrimal duct
❐ Sphenopalatine foramen
❐ Maxillary sinus ostium
❐ Nares (nostrils)
   ❐ Choanae
❐ Vestibule

Ganglion
❐ Pterygopalatine

Other Structures
❐ Basion
❐ Clivus
❐ Dens
❐ Epiglottis
❐ Torus tubarius
❐ Uvula
❐ Septal cartilage

CHAPTER 27

PHARYNX AND ORAL CAVITY

Netter: 51–55, 58–65

McMinn: 69

Gray's Atlas: 529–535

Identify the borders of the nasopharynx, oropharynx, and laryngopharynx on the cadaver.

The tensor veli palatini and the levator veli palatini muscles have been identified during the dissection of the pterygopalatine fossa (Fig. 27-1; see Chapter 26). Identify the *torus tubarius,* a cartilaginous elevation of the auditory tube (see Figs. 26-7 and 27-3), and locate the pharyngeal tonsil superior to it. Lateral to the pharyngeal tonsil, look for the tubal tonsil. Posterior to the torus tubarius, note the pharyngeal recess (Fig. 27-1). Extending inferiorly from the torus tubarius is the *salpingopharyngeal fold,* formed by the underlying salpingopharyngeus muscle (see Fig. 27-6).

Locate the borders of the tonsillar fossa in the oropharynx and identify the palatine tonsil bounded by two arches. Anteriorly, observe the *palatoglossal arch,* a mucosal fold formed by the palatoglossus muscle (Fig. 27-2). In the tonsillar fossa, use your forceps to lift the mucous membrane and pull it off of the underlying musculature (Figs. 27-3 to 27-5). Posteriorly, a second arch, the *palatopharyngeal arch,* is formed by a mucosal fold from the underlying palatopharyngeus muscle. Similarly, remove the mucous membrane and expose the palatopharyngeus muscle (Fig. 27-6).

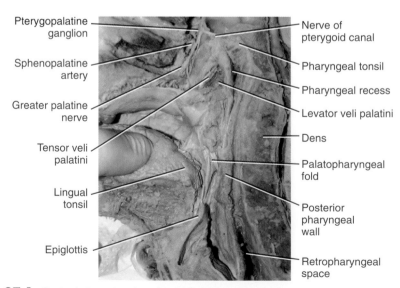

FIGURE 27-1. Sagittal view of oral cavity, including nasal and pharyngeal regions revealing nerve of pterygoid canal, sphenopalatine artery, greater and lesser palatine nerves, pterygopalatine ganglion, tensor and levator veli palatini muscles, lingual tonsil, epiglottis, dens, posterior pharyngeal wall, retropharyngeal space, and palatopharyngeal fold.

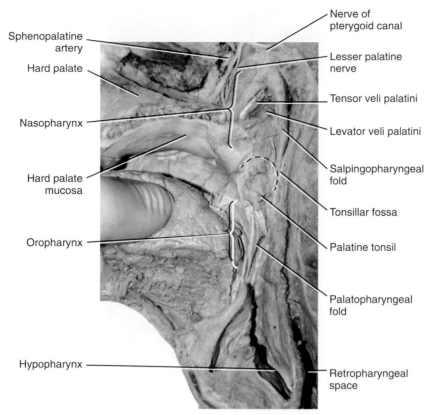

FIGURE 27-2. Sagittal view of oral cavity, including nasal and pharyngeal regions revealing hard palate, nasopharynx region, hard palate mucosa, oral pharynx region, hypopharynx region, retropharyngeal space, and salpingopharyngeal fold.

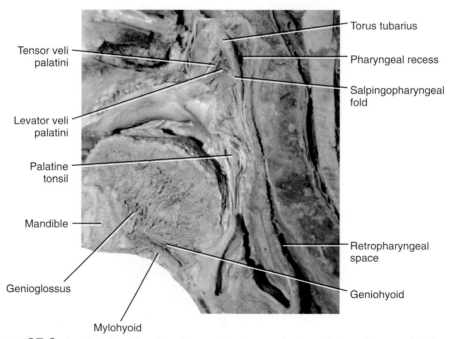

FIGURE 27-3. Sagittal view of oral cavity revealing torus tubarius, salpingopharyngeal fold, palatine tonsil, mandible, muscles (genioglossus, geniohyoid, mylohyoid), retropharyngeal space, and posterior pharyngeal wall.

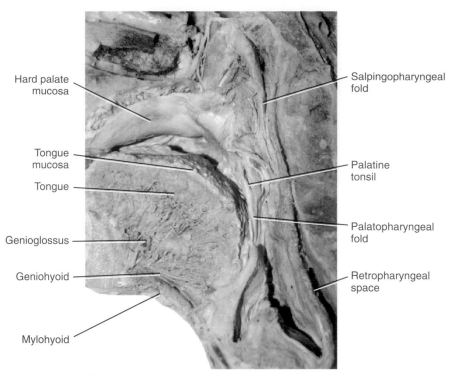

FIGURE 27-4. Appreciate the palatine tonsil and palatopharyngeal fold.

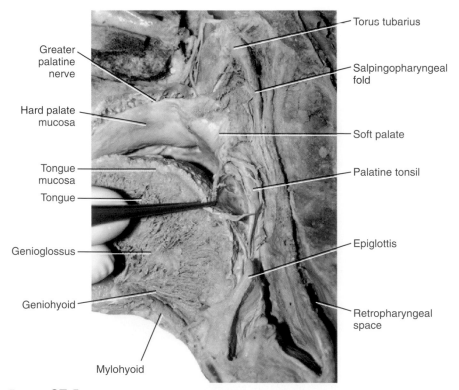

FIGURE 27-5. Removal of mucous membranes and exposure of underlying musculature.

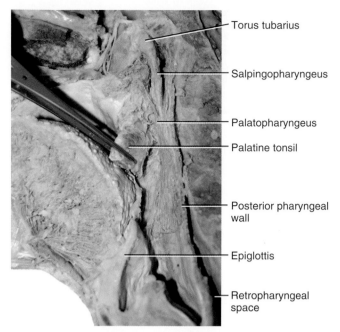

FIGURE 27-6. Musculature of palatine tonsil reflected anteriorly, exposing the salpingopharyngeus, palatopharyngeus, and posterior pharyngeal wall.

FIGURE 27-7. Musculature of palatine tonsil reflected posteriorly exposing the palatoglossal fold and palatoglossus muscle.

✋ DISSECTION TIP: In the laryngopharynx, at the level of the epiglottis, the palatopharyngeus, salpingopharyngeus, and stylopharyngeus muscles give the impression that they blend and fuse with the posterior pharyngeal constrictor muscles (Fig. 27-6). However, the posterior pharyngeal constrictors are separated from these muscles by a thin fascia, the *buccopharyngeal fascia.* In some specimens, this fascia may appear as a white vertical line.

Continue the dissection by removing the mucous membranes from the tonsillar fossa and the palatoglossal arch, and expose the palatoglossus muscle (Fig. 27-7). Because this muscle is located deep and lateral to the tongue, pull the tongue forward and the palatine tonsil backward to expose it fully. Pull the palatine tonsil forward, and expose the palatopharyngeus muscle (Fig. 27-8).

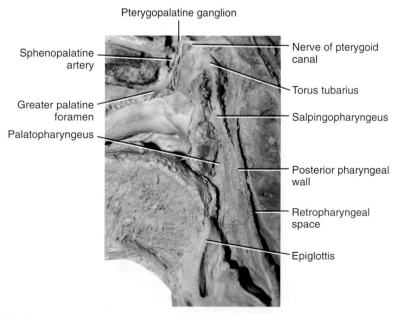

FIGURE 27-8. Sagittal view of oral cavity, including nasal and pharyngeal regions, revealing pterygopalatine ganglion, greater palatine foramen, palatopharyngeus muscle, epiglottis, salpingopharyngeus muscle, torus tubarius, tensor veli palatini muscle, and nerve of pterygoid canal.

Identify the space between the epiglottis and the tongue. Look for a membranous ridge, the *median glossoepiglottic fold,* connecting the posterior surface of the tongue to the epiglottis (Fig. 27-9). This fold divides the area between the epiglottis and the tongue into two spaces, the *valleculae* (Fig. 27-10). Divide the palatoglossus muscle, and identify the glossopharyngeal nerve (Fig. 27-11). Lastly, at the base of the tongue, identify the *lingual tonsil.*

> ✋ *DISSECTION TIP:* To find the glossopharyngeal nerve, place your thumb at the lateral border of the epiglottis, between the palatine tonsil and the epiglottis. Split the palatoglossus muscle lateral to your thumb (Fig. 27-11).

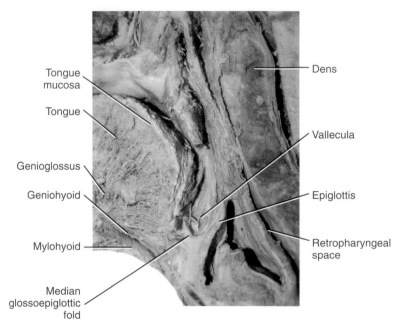

FIGURE 27-9. Appreciate the connection between the tongue and epiglottis, the *median glosso-epiglottic fold,* and spaces lateral to it (valleculae)

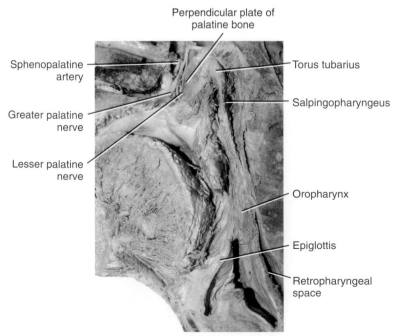

FIGURE 27-10. Sagittal view of the oral cavity revealing the sphenopalatine artery, greater and lesser palatine nerves, epiglottis, uvula, salpingopharyngeus muscle, and torus tubarius.

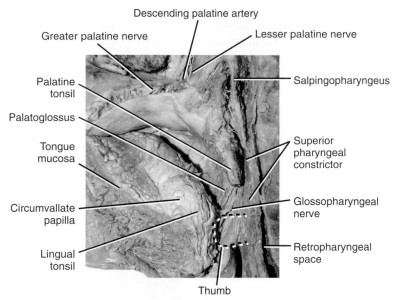

Descending palatine artery

Greater palatine nerve

Lesser palatine nerve

Palatine tonsil

Salpingopharyngeus

Palatoglossus

Tongue mucosa

Superior pharyngeal constrictor

Circumvallate papilla

Glossopharyngeal nerve

Lingual tonsil

Retropharyngeal space

Thumb

FIGURE 27-11. To find the glossopharyngeal nerve, the thumb is placed *(dashed area)* lateral to the epiglottis between it and the palatine tonsil.

INSPECTION

The oral cavity occupies the space between the lips anteriorly and the palatoglossal folds posteriorly. For descriptive purposes, the oral cavity is also divided into the vestibule and the oral cavity proper. The *vestibule* includes the area between the external surfaces of the teeth and the internal surface of cheeks. The *oral cavity proper* is the space filled by the tongue.

Pull the tongue toward the midline and note the *vestibule.* Identify the mucous membrane, the *frenulum,* between the inferior aspect of the tongue and the floor of the mouth (Fig. 27-12). Lateral to the frenulum, identify multiple tributaries of the lingual veins and orifices of the submandibular glands, the *sublingual* papilla (sublingual *caruncle*).

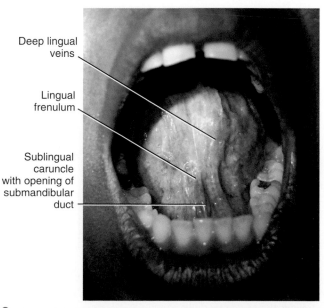

Deep lingual veins

Lingual frenulum

Sublingual caruncle with opening of submandibular duct

FIGURE 27-12. Appreciate the lingual frenulum, deep lingual vein, and submandibular duct.

Continue the inspection of the anterior surface of the tongue, and identify the *filiform* papillae. Appreciate the much larger and sometimes reddish *fungiform* papillae. At the posterior surface of the tongue, identify the sulcus terminalis and *vallate* papillae. At the midpoint of the sulcus terminalis, attempt to visualize the *foramen cecum* (Fig. 27-13).

Pull the tongue medially and make a shallow incision through the mucous membranes lateral to the tongue alongside the mandible (Fig. 27-14). Extend the incision toward the palatoglossus but do not sever this muscle (Fig. 27-15).

Lift the mucous membranes of the vestibule and expose the mylohyoid muscle (Figs. 27-16 and 27-17). In the space between the palatoglossus and mylohyoid muscles, identify the *lingual nerve* descending from the infratemporal fossa into the floor of the mouth (Fig. 27-18). Clean the soft tissues and mucous membranes around the lingual nerve (Fig. 27-19).

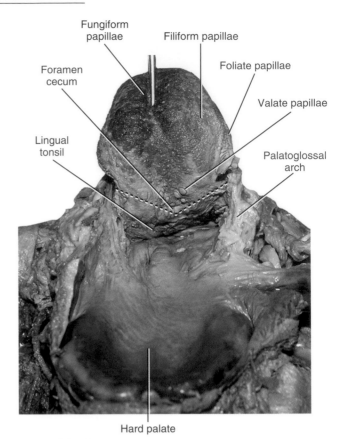

FIGURE 27-13. Hard palate reflected posteriorly with view from above revealing filiform, fungiform, and foliate papillae, and at the posterior third of the tongue, the sulcus terminalis *(dashed line)* and 10 to 12 vallate papillae.

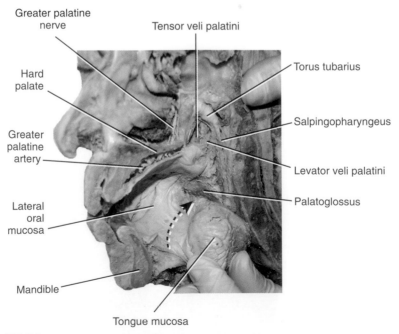

FIGURE 27-14. Tongue pulled medially with shallow incision *(arrow)* through mucous membranes lateral to tongue alongside mandible.

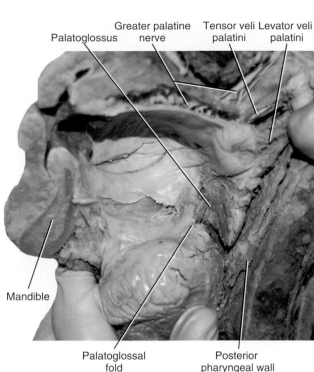

FIGURE 27-15. Incision extended toward palatoglossus muscle.

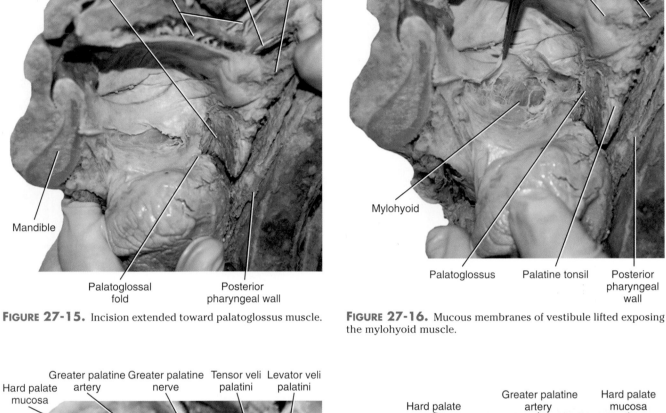

FIGURE 27-16. Mucous membranes of vestibule lifted exposing the mylohyoid muscle.

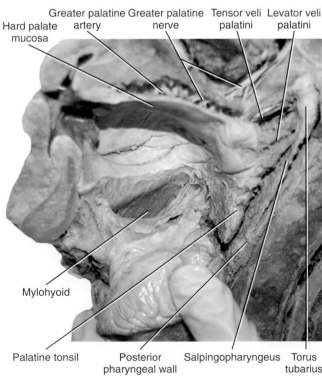

FIGURE 27-17. Appreciate neuromuscular structures with the mylohyoid muscle exposed.

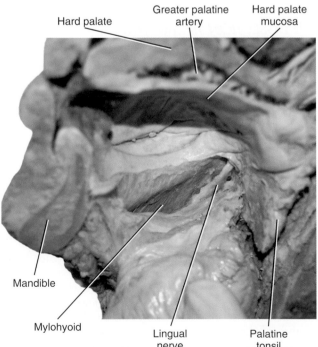

FIGURE 27-18. Appreciate the lingual nerve descending from the infratemporal fossa into the floor of the mouth, between palatoglossus and mylohyoid muscles.

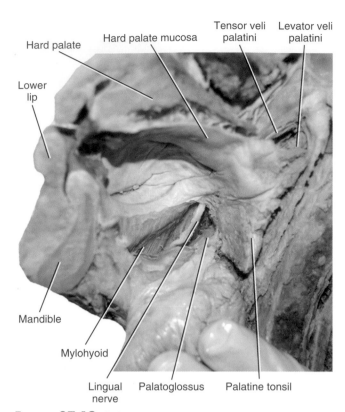

FIGURE 27-19. Soft tissues and mucous membranes cleaned around lingual nerve.

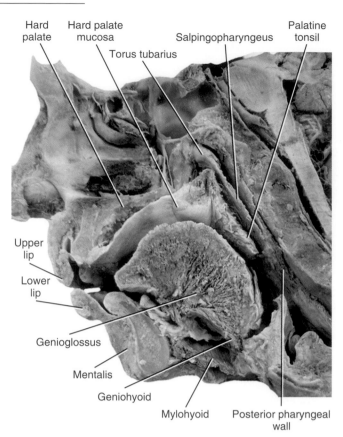

FIGURE 27-20. Sagittal view of oral cavity, including nasal and pharyngeal regions, revealing hard palate mucosa, upper/lower lips, uvula, and mentalis, genioglossus, geniohyoid, mylohyoid, and salpingopharyngeus muscles.

👆 *DISSECTION TIP:* The dissection of the lingual nerve will also continue from the floor of the mouth. Therefore, do not attempt to dissect the nerve too deeply.

Make an incision through the mucous membrane of the floor of the mouth between the geniohyoid and mylohyoid muscles (Fig. 27-20), and identify the *lingual artery* (Figs. 27-21 and 27-22).

👆 *DISSECTION TIP:* Between the geniohyoid and mylohyoid muscles, a plane of loose connective tissue is found. Lift the geniohyoid muscle upward and clean the soft tissue. Note the lingual artery, which is tortuous in some specimens (Figs. 27-21 and 27-22).

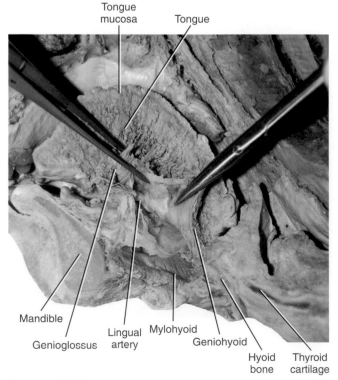

FIGURE 27-21. Geniohyoid muscle lifted upward to clean soft tissue.

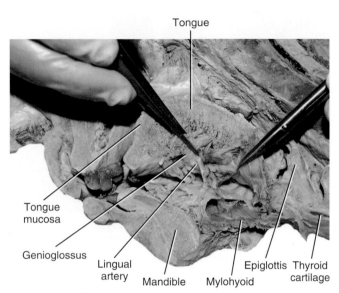

FIGURE 27-22. Sagittal view of oral cavity revealing mucosa of tongue, tongue, genioglossus muscle, lingual artery, mandible, mylohyoid muscle, hyoid bone, and epiglottis.

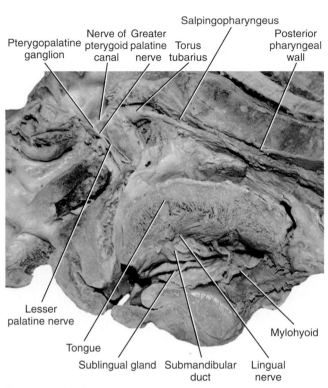

FIGURE 27-23. Submandibular duct exposed posteriorly from origin at submandibular gland around posterior edge of the mylohyoid muscle.

As the mucous membranes are reflected laterally from the midline, identify the *submandibular duct* (Wharton's duct) and the *sublingual gland.* Expose the submandibular duct posteriorly to its origin from the submandibular gland, around the posterior edge of the mylohyoid muscle (Fig. 27-23). Distal to the tortuous lingual artery identify the lingual nerve. The lingual nerve passes medially toward the tongue as it crosses over the submandibular duct (Fig. 27-24). Posterior to the tongue expose the hypoglossal nerve.

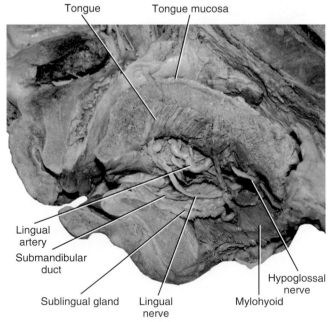

FIGURE 27-24. Appreciate lingual nerve distal to tortuous lingual artery, passing medially toward tongue and crossing over submandibular duct, and hypoglossal nerve posteriorly.

Pull the tongue posteriorly and expose the mylohyoid muscle (Fig. 27-25). Trace the lingual nerve as it descends from the infratemporal fossa between the palatoglossus and mylohyoid muscles. Note the submandibular duct crossing the lingual nerve (Fig. 27-26).

With the tongue pulled posteriorly, dissect between the lingual nerve and submandibular gland, and expose the *submandibular ganglion* (Fig. 27-26).

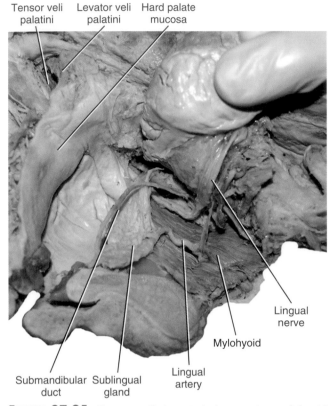

FIGURE 27-25. Tongue pulled posteriorly exposing mylohyoid muscle.

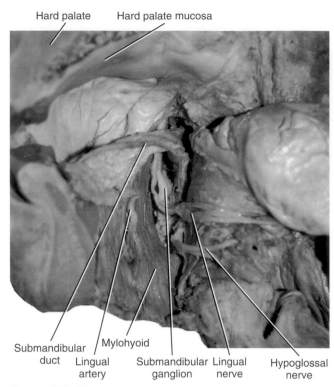

FIGURE 27-26. Appreciate lingual nerve descending from infratemporal fossa and submandibular duct crossing over it.

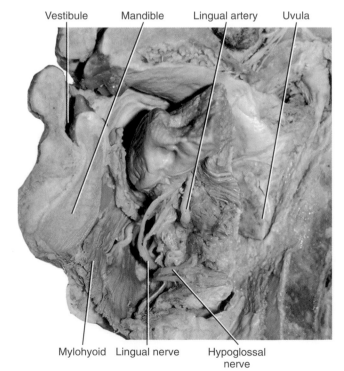

FIGURE 27-27. Sagittal view of oral cavity, including nasal and pharyngeal regions, revealing vestibule, lingual artery, hypoglossal nerve, lingual nerve, mylohyoid muscle, uvula, and hyoid bone.

🖝 *DISSECTION TIP:* The following landmarks help to identify the different structures in the floor of the mouth (Figs. 27-27 and 27-28):
- The *lingual artery* passes deep to the hyoglossus muscle and is often tortuous.
- The *hypoglossal nerve* passes superficial to the hyoglossus muscle and is seen at the posterior part of the tongue.
- Seen from the midline with the tongue in situ, the *lingual nerve* passes medially toward the tongue as it crosses over the submandibular duct (Fig. 27-24).
- With the tongue reflected posteriorly, note the *submandibular duct* crossing over the lingual nerve (see also Figs. 27-25 and 27-26).

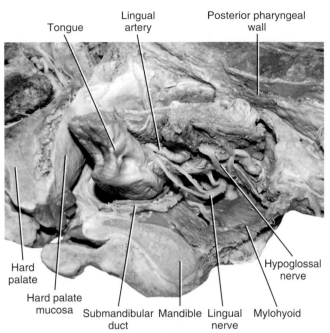

FIGURE 27-28. Sagittal view of the oral cavity, highlighting hard palate and mucosa, tongue, hypoglossal nerve, lingual artery and nerve, mylohyoid muscle, and posterior pharyngeal wall.

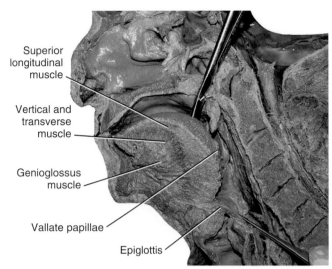

FIGURE 27-29. Midsagittal section of cadaveric head reveals intrinsic muscle of tongue.

👆 *DISSECTION TIP:* To identify the following muscles, note their course:
The *genioglossus* muscle runs from the mandible to the tongue.
The *geniohyoid* runs from the mandible to the hyoid bone.
The *hyoglossus* runs from the tongue to the hyoid bone.
The *styloglossus* arises from the styloid process and enters the tongue posteriorly and passes under the palatoglossus to fuse with the hyoglossus muscle.

👆 *DISSECTION TIP:* In some cadavers, you may find some bony outgrowths in the oral cavity the torus palatinus and torus mandibularis.

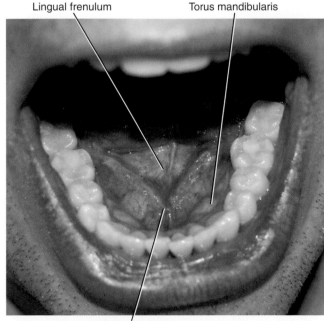

FIGURE 27-30. Torus mandibularis is a benign, bony outgrowth of the lateral side of the mandible.

If time permits, separate and expose the hyoglossus, genioglossus, geniohyoid, styloglossus, and mylohyoid muscles.

After you identify these muscles, make a small vertical cut near the tip of the tongue, and expose the vertical muscle fibers and intrinsic transverse muscle fibers. Make another incision in the superficial tissue from the dorsum of the tongue, and expose the intrinsic longitudinal fibers (Fig. 27-29).

The *torus palatinus* and *torus mandibularis* are variant benign excrescences of the hard palate and mandible, respectively (Fig. 27-30).

LABORATORY IDENTIFICATION CHECKLIST

Nerves
- ❐ Lingual
- ❐ Hypoglossal
- ❐ Nerve to mylohyoid
- ❐ Glossopharyngeal

Ganglion
- ❐ Submandibular

Artery
- ❐ Lingual

Vein
- ❐ Lingual

Muscles
- ❐ Digastric
  - ❐ Anterior belly
  - ❐ Posterior belly
- ❐ Mylohyoid
- ❐ Geniohyoid
- ❐ Genioglossus
- ❐ Tongue
  - ❐ Superior longitudinal fibers
  - ❐ Inferior longitudinal fibers
  - ❐ Horizontal fibers
  - ❐ Vertical fibers
  - ❐ Hyoglossus
  - ❐ Styloglossus

Bones
- ❐ Mandible
- ❐ Hyoid bone
- ❐ Styloid process
- ❐ Mastoid process

Glands
- ❐ Submandibular
  - ❐ Superficial and deep lobes
  - ❐ Submandibular duct (Wharton's duct)
- ❐ Sublingual

CHAPTER 28

LARYNX

Netter: 76–80

McMinn: 58–60

Gray's Atlas: 504, 510–517

INSPECTION

Technique 1

The larynx occupies the space between the epiglottis superiorly and the inferior border of the cricoid cartilage. The inspection begins by examining the larynx in a hemisected head.

In a hemisected specimen, identify the epiglottis, laryngopharynx, thyroid cartilage, vallecula, uvula, posterior pharyngeal wall, cervical vertebrae, and trachea (Figs. 28-1 and 28-2). If the thyroid and cricoid cartilages are not hemisected, complete the hemisection and expose the contents of the larynx using scissors (Fig. 28-3).

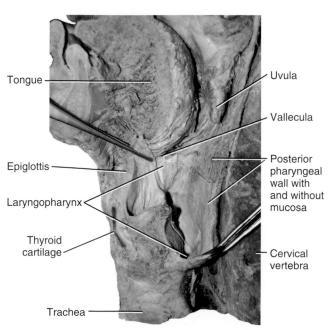

FIGURE 28-1. Sagittal view of mouth and larynx, revealing tongue, epiglottis, laryngopharynx, thyroid cartilage, vallecula, uvula, posterior pharyngeal wall, cervical vertebrae, and trachea.

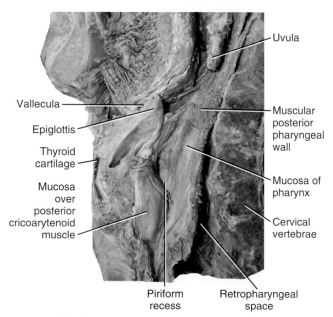

FIGURE 28-2. Sagittal orolaryngeal section, demonstrating uvula, vallecula, epiglottis, thyroid cartilage, mucosa covering posterior cricoarytenoid muscle, piriform recess, retropharyngeal space, cervical vertebrae, mucosa of pharynx, and muscular posterior pharyngeal wall.

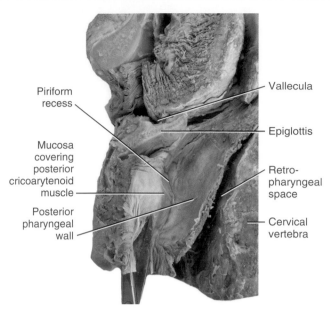

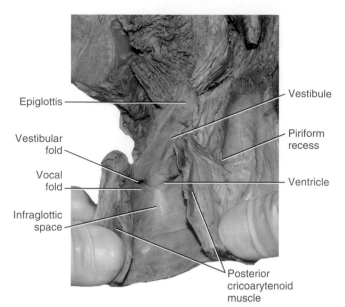

FIGURE 28-3. Sagittal view of mouth and larynx with posterior pharyngeal wall reflected from vertebral column, revealing vallecula, epiglottis, piriform recess, posterior wall of pharyngeal muscle and mucosa (inferior constrictor), retropharyngeal space, and cervical vertebrae.

FIGURE 28-4. Sagittal view of mouth with open posterior view of larynx, highlighting epiglottis, vestibule/laryngeal inlet, vocal fold, vestibular fold, ventricle, posterior cricoarytenoid muscle, and piriform recess.

✋ *DISSECTION TIP:* Do not cut directly in the midline of the cricoid and thyroid cartilages. Try to perform the cut as laterally as possible.

With your fingertips, keep the larynx open, and identify the supraglottic space, or *vestibule,* extending from the epiglottis to the vestibular folds (Fig. 28-4). The *ventricle* is the space between the false vocal (vestibular) folds and the true vocal folds. Note the space between the true vocal folds, the *rima glottidis* (Fig. 28-5). Identify the infraglottic space between the true vocal fold and the first tracheal ring.

With scissors, cut the remaining part of the larynx in the midsagittal plane (Fig. 28-5). Identify the *aryepiglottic fold,* the mucous membrane stretched between the epiglottis to the apex of the arytenoid cartilages.

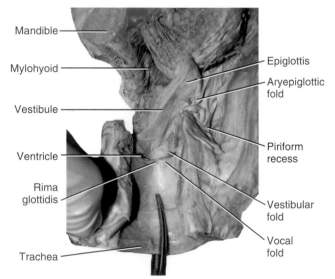

FIGURE 28-5. Sagittal oral view with open posterior laryngeal view, revealing mandible, mylohyoid muscle, epiglottis, vestibule/laryngeal inlet, piriform recess, vestibular fold, vocal fold, ventricle, and trachea.

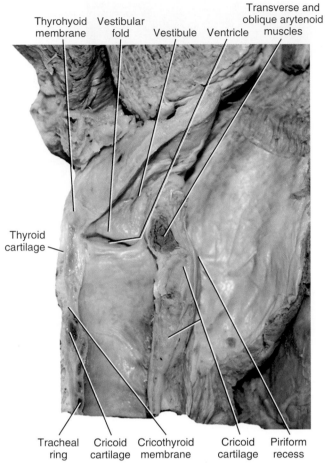

Thyrohyoid membrane   Vestibular fold   Vestibule   Ventricle   Transverse and oblique arytenoid muscles

Thyroid cartilage

Tracheal ring   Cricoid cartilage   Cricothyroid membrane   Cricoid cartilage   Piriform recess

FIGURE 28-6. Sagittal orolaryngeal view with vestibule/laryngeal inlet, vestibular fold, vocal fold, ventricle, thyroid and cricoid cartilages, tracheal ring, transverse arytenoid muscle, and piriform recess.

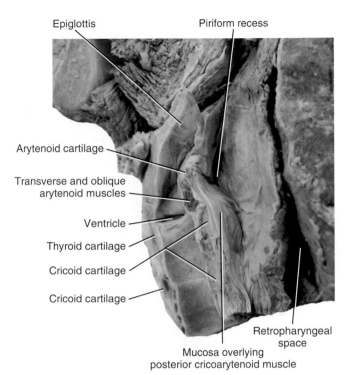

Epiglottis   Piriform recess

Arytenoid cartilage

Transverse and oblique arytenoid muscles

Ventricle

Thyroid cartilage

Cricoid cartilage

Cricoid cartilage

Retropharyngeal space

Mucosa overlying posterior cricoarytenoid muscle

FIGURE 28-7. Sagittal view of mouth and larynx with posterior wall of pharynx reflected from cervical vertebrae, revealing epiglottis, transverse arytenoid muscle, ventricle, thyroid cartilage, anterior and posterior regions of cricoid cartilage, posterior cricoarytenoid mucosa, retropharyngeal space, and piriform recess.

Identify the epiglottis, thyroid, and cricoid cartilages (Fig. 28-6). Note the thyroid cartilage and its attachment to the hyoid bone through the thyrohyoid membrane. Identify the attachment of the thyroid cartilage to the cricoid cartilage by the cricothyroid membrane.

Palpate the arytenoid cartilages (Fig. 28-7) and at their free edge in the aryepiglottic fold, feel the corniculate and cuneiform cartilages (see Fig. 28-11).

Palpate the cricoid cartilage and make a midline incision along its posterior surface through the mucous membrane exposing the posterior cricoarytenoid muscle (Fig. 28-7). Superior to the posterior cricoarytenoid muscle, identify the transverse and oblique arytenoid muscles (Figs. 28-8 and 28-9). Reflect the mucous membrane over the aryepiglottic fold, and expose the corniculate and cuneiform cartilages (Figs. 28-10 and 28-11).

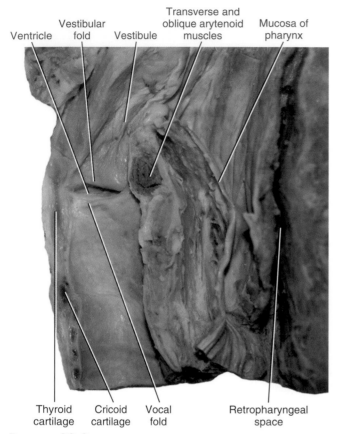

FIGURE 28-8. Sagittal view of laryngeal region, revealing vestibule/laryngeal inlet, arytenoid muscle, vestibular fold, vocal fold, ventricle, cricoid cartilage, thyroid cartilage, mucosa of the pharynx, and retropharyngeal space.

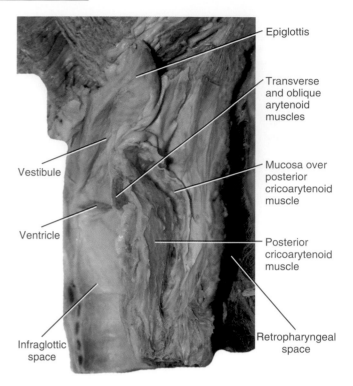

FIGURE 28-9. Sagittal laryngeal view, highlighting epiglottis hypopharynx, and retropharyngeal space.

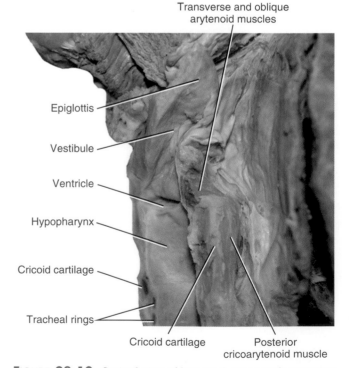

FIGURE 28-10. Sagittal view of laryngeal region with posterior wall of pharynx reflected from cervical vertebrae, revealing epiglottis, vestibule/laryngeal inlet, ventricle, hypopharynx, cricoid cartilage, tracheal rings, posterior cricoarytenoid, mucosa of pharynx, and transverse arytenoid muscle.

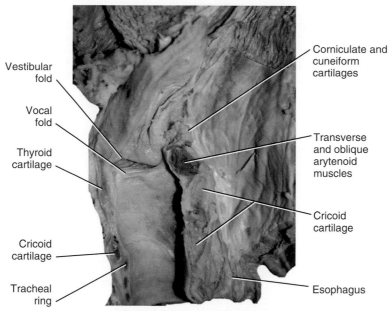

FIGURE 28-11. Sagittal view of laryngeal region, highlighting corniculate and cuneiform cartilages, pharyngeal mucosa, and esophagus.

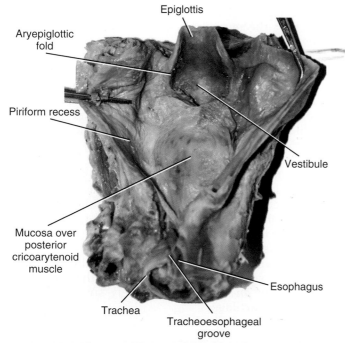

FIGURE 28-12. Posterior view of larynx with posterior pharyngeal wall reflected from midline, revealing epiglottis, aryepiglottic fold, vestibule/laryngeal inlet, piriform recess, and tracheal-esophageal groove.

Technique 2

Another technique for exposing the structures of the larynx is to remove the laryngopharynx and larynx en bloc from the cadaver and examine it.

Remove the laryngopharynx en bloc from the cadaver, and identify the aryepiglottic fold, piriform recess, and epiglottis (Fig. 28-12).

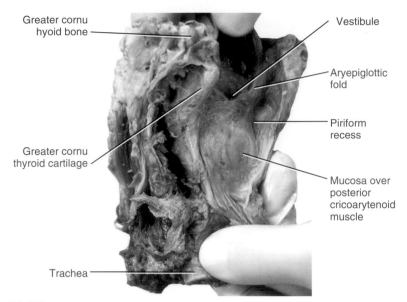

FIGURE 28-13. Posterior view of larynx with posterior pharyngeal wall reflected from midline, highlighting horns (cornu) of hyoid and thyroid cartilage, mucosa over posterior cricoarytenoid muscle, aryepiglottic fold, and piriform recess.

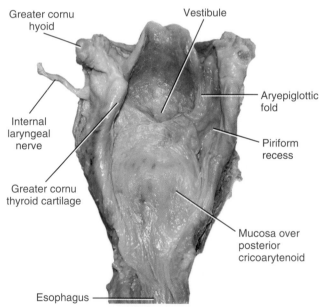

FIGURE 28-14. Posterior view of larynx with posterior pharyngeal wall reflected, revealing vestibule/laryngeal inlet, greater cornu of hyoid and thyroid cartilage, and internal laryngeal nerve.

Palpate the greater horns (cornu) of the hyoid bone and thyroid cartilage, and remove the soft tissues around the larynx (Fig. 28-13). Just inferior to the greater cornu of the hyoid bone, notice the internal laryngeal nerve penetrating the thyrohyoid membrane (Fig. 28-14).

Reflect the mucosa over the posterior portion of the cricoid cartilage, and expose the posterior cricoarytenoid muscle (Fig. 28-15). Identify the posterior cricoarytenoid and transverse and oblique arytenoid muscles (Fig. 28-16). Make a midline incision through the cricoid cartilage, and identify the true and false vocal cords (Fig. 28-17). Pull the lateral edges of the cartilages open, to fully expose the space between the vocal cords (Fig. 28-18).

Turn the specimen anteriorly and identify the *cricothyroid muscle.* Reflect the cricothyroid muscle anteriorly from the cricoid cartilage, and identify the median cricothyroid ligament in the midline between the thyroid and cricoid cartilages. Identify the *thyroarytenoid muscle* lateral to the transverse and oblique arytenoids, ascending posteriorly from the midline to the arytenoid cartilage. Inferior to the thyroarytenoid muscle, a small muscle strip, the *lateral cricoarytenoid muscle,* runs obliquely superior to the arytenoid cartilage.

✔ DISSECTION TIP: If time permits, reflect the thyrohyoid membrane, and trace the course of the internal laryngeal nerve to the piriform recess.

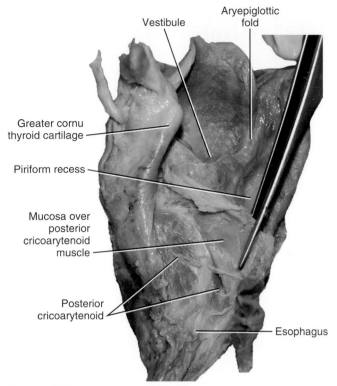

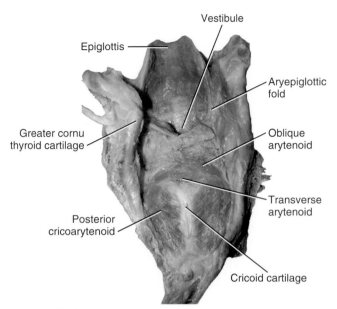

FIGURE 28-15. Posterior view of larynx with pharyngeal wall cut from midline, revealing vestibule/laryngeal inlet, greater cornu of thyroid cartilage, posterior cricoarytenoid, esophagus, mucosa over posterior cricoarytenoid muscle, aryepiglottic fold, and piriform recess.

FIGURE 28-16. Posterior view of larynx with posterior pharyngeal wall reflected, revealing epiglottis, vestibule/laryngeal inlet, posterior cricoarytenoid muscle, posterior cricoid cartilage, transverse and oblique arytenoids, and aryepiglottic fold.

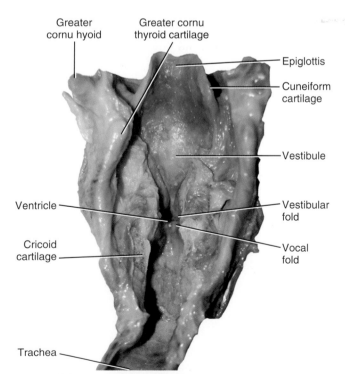

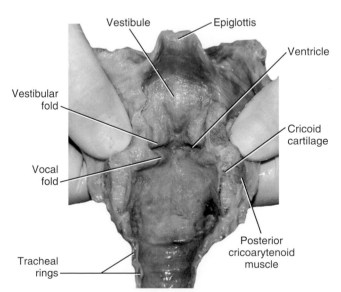

FIGURE 28-17. Posterior midline view of larynx with cricoid cartilage reflected from midline, highlighting epiglottis, greater cornu (hyoid, thyroid cartilage), vocal and vestibular folds, cuneiform cartilage, ventricle, posterior region of cricoid cartilage, and trachea.

FIGURE 28-18. Posterior view of larynx with cricoid cartilage reflected from midline, revealing epiglottis, vestibule/laryngeal inlet, vestibular fold, vocal fold, ventricle, posterior region of cricoid cartilage, posterior cricoarytenoid muscle, and tracheal rings.

LABORATORY IDENTIFICATION CHECKLIST

Nerves
- ❏ Superior laryngeal
- ❏ External laryngeal
- ❏ Internal laryngeal
- ❏ Recurrent laryngeal
- ❏ Inferior laryngeal

Arteries
- ❏ Superior laryngeal
- ❏ Inferior laryngeal

Muscles
- ❏ Uvula
- ❏ Posterior pharyngeal (with/without mucosa)

External side of larynx
- ❏ Cricothyroid

Internal larynx
- ❏ Posterior cricoarytenoid
- ❏ Transverse cricoarytenoid
- ❏ Oblique cricoarytenoid
- ❏ Vocalis
- ❏ Lateral cricoarytenoid
- ❏ Thyroarytenoid

Bones
- ❏ Hyoid
  - ❏ Greater cornu

Cartilages
- ❏ Epiglottic
- ❏ Thyroid
  - ❏ Greater cornu
- ❏ Cricoid
- ❏ Arytenoid
- ❏ Corniculate
- ❏ Cuneiform
- ❏ Tracheal ring

Membranes
- ❏ Thyrohyoid
- ❏ Cricothyroid

Ligament
- ❏ Cricothyroid

Spaces/Recess/Folds
- ❏ Piriform recess
- ❏ Vestibule
- ❏ Vocal folds
- ❏ Ventricle
- ❏ Vestibular folds
- ❏ Aryepiglottic folds
- ❏ Hypopharynx

CHAPTER 29

RETROPHARYNGEAL REGION AND PHARYNX

Netter: 66–76, 129–130

McMinn: 55–57

Gray's Atlas: 504–509

Place the cadaver in the supine position, and identify the following landmarks in the postcraniotomy skull (Fig. 29-1):
• Anterior, middle, and posterior cranial fossae
• Transverse and sigmoid sinuses
• Confluence of sinuses
With toothed forceps and a scalpel, remove the dura mater from the posterior cranial fossa (Fig. 29-2).

With a mallet and chisel, make an inverted-V–shaped cut (*dashed line* in Fig. 29-2) in the posterior cranial fossa. Place the chisel 1 to 2 cm in the front of the foramen magnum at the midportion of the clivus, and make a deep cut. Continue this cut laterally and posteriorly between the jugular foramen and the hypoglossal canal toward the edge of the occipital bone (Fig. 29-3).

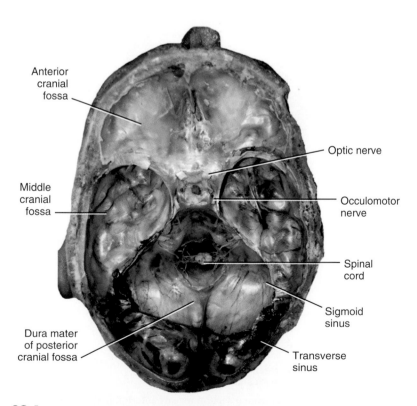

FIGURE 29-1. Horizontal section after craniotomy shows anterior, middle, and posterior cranial fossae, highlighting dura mater, dural venous sinuses (transverse, sigmoid), spinal cord, and cranial nerves (optic, oculomotor).

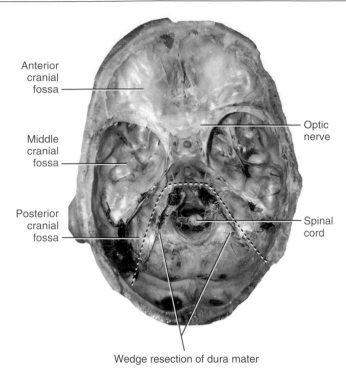

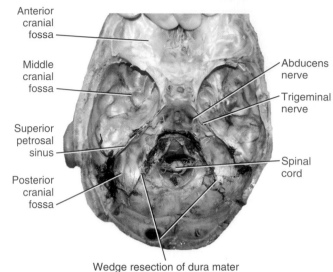

Once the incisions are complete, pull the occipital bone backward to separate it from the skull base. Use a scalpel to cut the soft tissues between the bone fragments. In addition, have a laboratory partner keep the head stable by holding it as shown in Figure 29-4.

FIGURE 29-2. Postcraniotomy horizontal section reveals anterior, middle, and posterior cranial fossae, with inverted-V–shaped section of dura mater removed from posterior cranial fossa, highlighting dural venous sinuses, spinal cord, and cranial nerves.

FIGURE 29-3. Horizontal section after craniotomy reveals anterior, middle, and posterior cranial fossae, with section of dura mater removed from posterior cranial fossae, and a cut from clivus to occipital bone, highlighting dura mater, dural venous sinuses (superior petrosal), spinal cord, and cranial nerves (abducens, trigeminal).

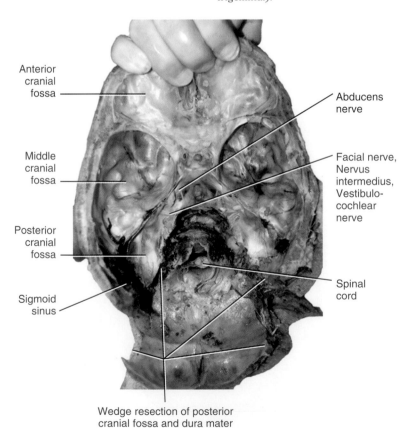

FIGURE 29-4. Postcraniotomy horizontal section reveals anterior, middle, and posterior cranial fossa, with wedge resection from posterior cranial fossa reflected, highlighting dural venous sinuses (sigmoid sinus), spinal cord, and cranial nerves (abducens, facial, nervus intermedius, vestibulocochlear).

Retropharyngeal space   Clivus

Posterior longitudinal ligament   Occipital condyle

FIGURE 29-5. Horizontal section after craniotomy, magnifying clival region of posterior cranial fossa and revealing small opening at retropharyngeal space.

✋ *DISSECTION TIP:* Be careful in making the separation in the region posterior to the jugular foramen. This is where the carotid sheath emerges, and aggressive dissection can damage its contents. As you pull the posterior cranial fossa backward (Fig. 29-5), place your finger in the opening you created at the clivus, and pull backward (Fig. 29-6).

Complete the separation of the posterior cranial fossa and musculature from the retropharyngeal space (Fig. 29-7). Carefully cut any soft tissues obstructing the separation. Once the separation is complete, stabilize the head in the upright position, and fully expose the retropharyngeal space (Fig. 29-8). Identify the sternocleidomastoid muscle laterally.

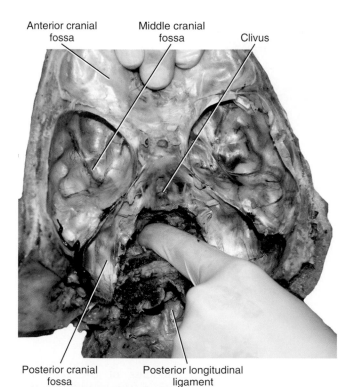

Anterior cranial   Middle cranial
fossa   fossa   Clivus

Posterior cranial   Posterior longitudinal
fossa   ligament

FIGURE 29-6. Postcraniotomy horizontal section highlighting anterior, middle, and posterior cranial fossae, with wedge osteotomy resection of the posterior cranial fossa and finger in retropharyngeal space, pulling posterior cranial fossa posteriorly.

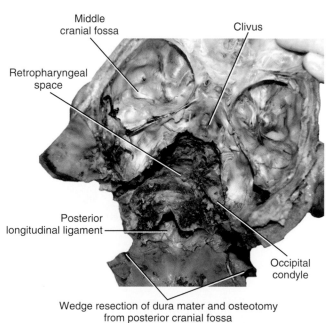

Middle
cranial fossa   Clivus

Retropharyngeal
space

Posterior
longitudinal ligament

Occipital
condyle

Wedge resection of dura mater and osteotomy
from posterior cranial fossa

FIGURE 29-7. Horizontal section after craniotomy of middle and posterior cranial fossae, with wedge osteotomy resection of posterior cranial fossa, revealing a large opening, the *retropharyngeal space.*

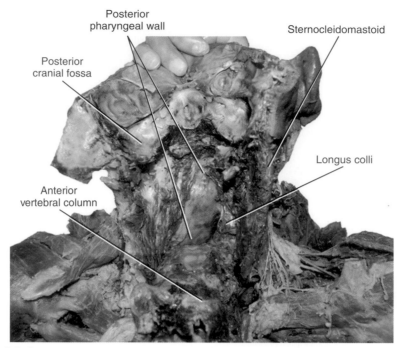

FIGURE 29-8. Posterior view of pharynx after retropharyngeal dissection. Anterior view of vertebral column reveals fascia, sternocleidomastoid and longus colli muscles, and posterior cranial fossa.

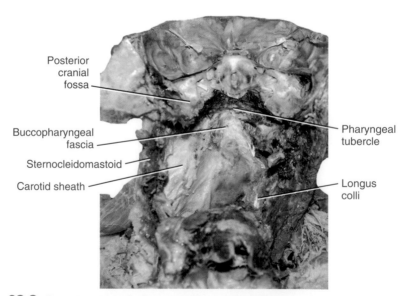

FIGURE 29-9. Posterior view of pharynx with wedge osteotomy resection of posterior cranial fossa, highlighting buccopharyngeal fascia and pharyngeal tubercle.

Palpate the *pharyngeal tubercle,* which provides attachment to the fibrous raphe (seam) of the pharynx and is the point of attachment for the superior pharyngeal constrictor muscle (Fig. 29-9). Beneath the tubercle, the *buccopharyngeal fascia* invests the constrictor muscles of the pharynx. Lateral to this fascia, note a thickened, whitish condensed fascia, the *carotid sheath.* With forceps, lift up the carotid sheath and expose its contents (Figs. 29-10 and 29-11).

Superior
cervical ganglion   Buccopharyngeal
fascia

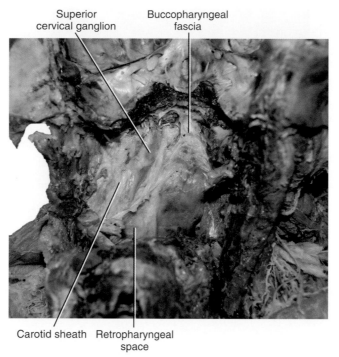

Carotid sheath   Retropharyngeal
space

FIGURE 29-10. Posterior view of pharynx with wedge osteotomy resection of posterior cranial fossa, revealing buccopharyngeal fascia, sternocleidomastoid muscle, and base of skull. Note beginning of dissection of carotid sheath and exposure of superior cervical ganglion behind sheath.

Internal   Common   Superior
jugular   carotid   cervical   Buccopharyngeal
vein   artery   ganglion   fascia

Contents
of carotid
sheath

Vagus
nerve

Cervical
sympathetic
trunk

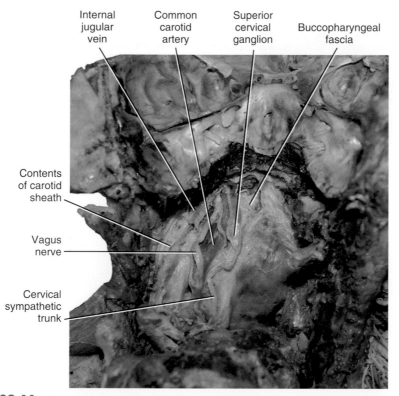

FIGURE 29-11. Posterior view of pharynx with wedge osteotomy resection of posterior cranial fossa, revealing buccopharyngeal fascia, cervical sympathetic trunk, superior cervical ganglion, common carotid artery, internal jugular vein, and vagus nerve.

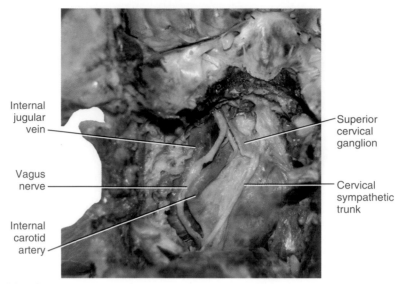

Internal jugular vein

Vagus nerve

Internal carotid artery

Superior cervical ganglion

Cervical sympathetic trunk

FIGURE 29-12. Posterior view of pharynx with wedge osteotomy resection of posterior cranial fossa, highlighting contents of carotid sheath—internal jugular vein, common carotid artery, and vagus nerve—as well as superior cervical ganglion and cervical sympathetic trunk.

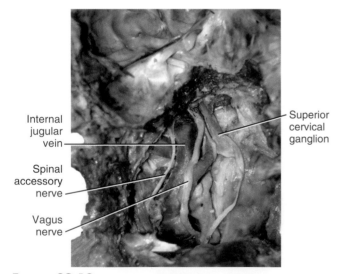

Internal jugular vein

Spinal accessory nerve

Vagus nerve

Superior cervical ganglion

FIGURE 29-13. Posterior view of pharynx with wedge osteotomy resection of posterior cranial fossa, revealing internal jugular vein, common carotid artery, inferior vagal ganglion (nodose ganglion), vagus nerve, superior cervical ganglion, and cervical sympathetic trunk.

Identify and clean the internal jugular vein, common carotid artery, superior cervical ganglion, and vagus nerve (Fig. 29-12). Dissect the internal jugular vein, and identify the spinal accessory nerve at its entrance into the sternocleidomastoid muscle (Fig. 29-13). Trace the vagus nerve toward the base of the skull, and identify its inferior (nodose) ganglion and the jugular ganglion.

> ✍ *DISSECTION TIP:* The jugular ganglion of the vagus nerve is located superior to the nodose ganglion.

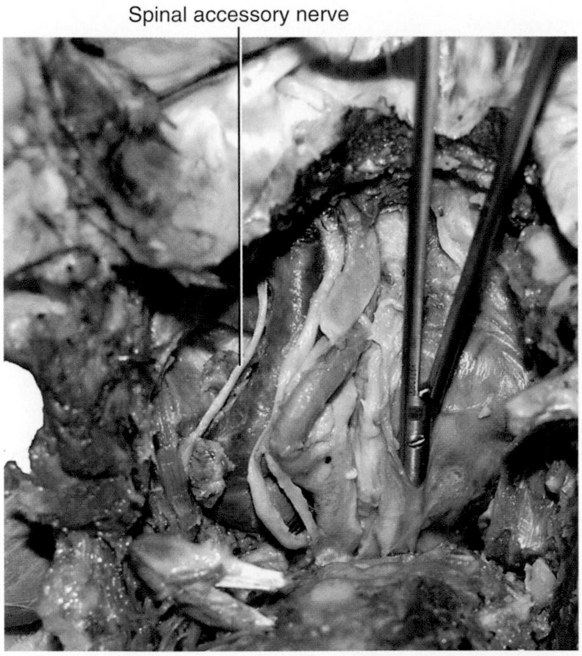

Spinal accessory nerve

FIGURE 29-14. Scissors removing remnants of carotid sheath and buccopharyngeal fascia, further exposing neurovascular structures and superior, middle, and inferior pharyngeal muscles.

Continue cleaning the carotid sheath and the buccopharyngeal fascia inferiorly (Fig. 29-14), and fully expose its contents (Fig. 29-15). Identify the superior laryngeal nerve from its origin from the vagus nerve. Trace the hypoglossal nerve from its emergence from the hypoglossal canal (Fig. 29-16). Lift the internal carotid artery and trace the pathway of the internal laryngeal artery and its division into internal and external branches (Fig. 29-17).

> ☝ *DISSECTION TIP:* Medial to the internal carotid artery, identify the *superior laryngeal nerve.* Its internal branch will travel near the gap between the middle and inferior constrictor muscles of the pharynx or the space between the external carotid artery and cornu of the hyoid bone. The *hypoglossal nerve* passes lateral to the internal carotid artery (Fig. 29-16). You may encounter multiple lymph nodes around the internal jugular vein. After you identify these, remove them from the field of dissection (Fig. 29-17).

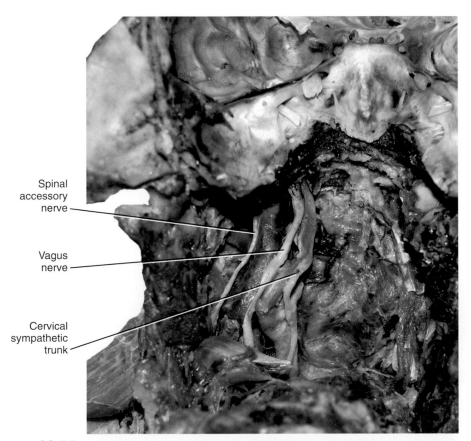

Spinal accessory nerve

Vagus nerve

Cervical sympathetic trunk

FIGURE 29-15. Posterior view of pharynx with wedge osteotomy resection of posterior cranial fossa, highlighting spinal accessory and vagus nerves and cervical sympathetic trunk, as well as internal jugular vein, common carotid artery, inferior (nodose) ganglion, vagus nerve, and superior cervical ganglion.

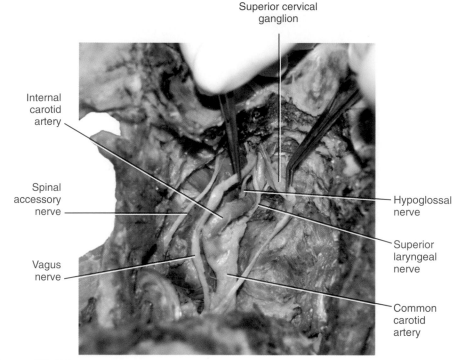

FIGURE 29-16. Forceps retracting superior cervical ganglion medially, further exposing internal jugular vein, common carotid artery, inferior (nodose) ganglion, vagus nerve, superior laryngeal nerve, and hypoglossal nerve.

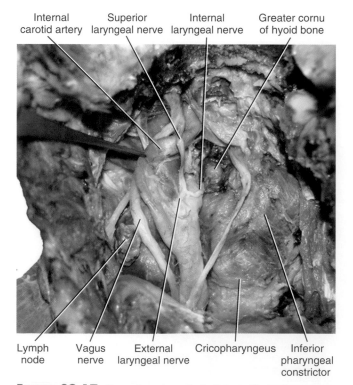

FIGURE 29-17. Posterior view of pharynx with wedge osteotomy resection of posterior cranial fossa, revealing inferior pharyngeal constrictor (cricopharyngeus) and division of superior laryngeal nerve into internal and external branches.

Identify the superior, middle, and inferior pharyngeal constrictor muscles, and carefully clean the buccopharyngeal fascia and adipose tissue (Fig. 29-17). Make a midsagittal incision at the midline of the pharyngeal constrictor muscles to expose the internal aspect of the pharynx and to visualize such structures as the cervical sympathetic trunk and the epiglottis (Figs. 29-18 and 29-19).

DISSECTION OF UNDIVIDED SPECIMEN

A different method of dissection of the retropharyngeal space is through the suboccipital region. In this approach, all the musculature of the back as well as the cervical vertebrae and spinal cord are removed, exposing the retropharyngeal space (Fig. 29-20).

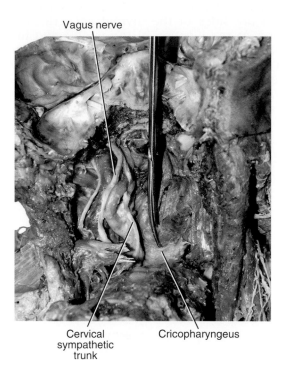

Vagus nerve

Cervical sympathetic trunk   Cricopharyngeus

FIGURE 29-18. Midsagittal incision at midline of superior middle and inferior pharyngeal constrictors, exposing internal aspect of pharynx.

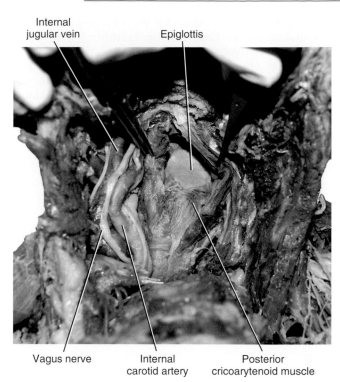

Internal jugular vein   Epiglottis

Vagus nerve   Internal carotid artery   Posterior cricoarytenoid muscle

FIGURE 29-19. Vertical incision of pharynx with pharyngeal wall reflected, revealing epiglottis and posterior cricoarytenoid muscle.

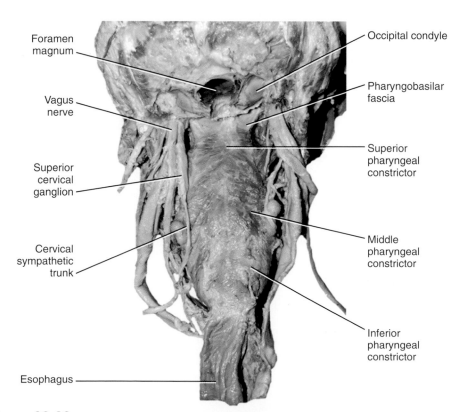

Foramen magnum

Vagus nerve

Superior cervical ganglion

Cervical sympathetic trunk

Esophagus

Occipital condyle

Pharyngobasilar fascia

Superior pharyngeal constrictor

Middle pharyngeal constrictor

Inferior pharyngeal constrictor

FIGURE 29-20. Posterior view of pharynx and base of skull, revealing foramen magnum, occipital condyle, pharyngobasilar fascia, and superior, middle, and inferior pharyngeal constrictors, as well as superior cervical ganglion and cervical sympathetic trunk.

The pharyngeal constrictor muscles are especially useful landmarks that can be identified with both dissecting methods as follows:

- *Superior pharyngeal constrictor:* Identify the gap between the upper border of the superior pharyngeal constrictor muscle and the base of the skull. Clean the pharyngobasilar fascia that occupies this space, and expose the levator veli palatini muscle, auditory tube, and ascending palatine artery (Fig. 29-21).

- *Middle pharyngeal constrictor:* This muscle attaches to the greater cornu of the hyoid bone. At the junction of the superior and middle pharyngeal constrictors, identify the stylopharyngeus muscle and the glossopharyngeal nerve (Fig. 29-21).

- *Inferior pharyngeal constrictor:* This muscle arises from the sides of the thyroid and cricoid cartilages. At the junction of the middle and inferior pharyngeal constrictors, identify the internal laryngeal nerve and the superior laryngeal artery (Fig. 29-21). The inferior part of the inferior constrictor is also known as the *cricopharyngeus* muscle.

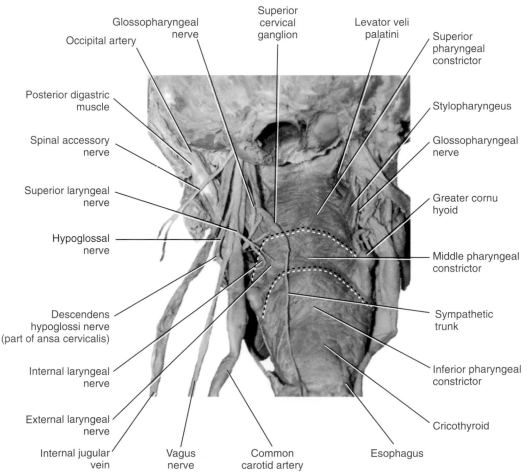

FIGURE 29-21. View of retropharyngeal space, with vast majority of neurovascular structures and muscles exposed; dashed lines demarcate borders of superior, middle, and inferior pharyngeal constrictor muscles.

LABORATORY IDENTIFICATION CHECKLIST

Nerves
- ❑ Sympathetic trunk/chain
- ❑ Vagus
- ❑ Recurrent laryngeal
- ❑ Inferior laryngeal
- ❑ Spinal accessory
- ❑ Hypoglossal
- ❑ Glossopharyngeal
  - ❑ Carotid sinus branch

Ganglia
- ❑ Superior cervical
- ❑ Middle cervical

Arteries
- ❑ Common carotid
- ❑ Internal carotid
- ❑ External carotid
- ❑ Vertebral

Vein
- ❑ Internal jugular

Muscles
- ❑ Sternocleidomastoid
- ❑ Stylopharyngeus
- ❑ Superior constrictor
- ❑ Middle constrictor
- ❑ Inferior constrictor
- ❑ Longus colli

Bones
- ❑ Occipital
- ❑ Mastoid process
- ❑ Styloid process
- ❑ Hyoid
- ❑ Atlas (C1)
- ❑ Axis (C2)
- ❑ C3 to C7

Cartilages
- ❑ Thyroid
- ❑ Cricoid

Ligaments
- ❑ Transverse, of atlas
- ❑ Alar

Glands
- ❑ Thyroid
- ❑ Parathyroid

Fasciae
- ❑ Buccopharyngeal
- ❑ Retropharyngeal
- ❑ Prevertebral

CRICOTHYROTOMY

Gray's Anatomy for Students: 806, 1001

Netter: 28, 77

Clinical Application

Procedure creates an emergent airway through the cricothyroid membrane.

Anatomic Landmarks (Figs. VIII-1 and VIII-2)

Palpation of midline structures
- Hyoid cartilage
- Thyroid cartilage
- Cricoid cartilage

Skin/subcutaneous tissue
- Cricothyroid arteries and small veins (may traverse the cricothyroid membrane)
- Cricothyroid membrane

TRACHEAL INTUBATION

Gray's Anatomy for Students: 992, 1004

Netter: 63, 66, 77–78

Clinical Application

Procedure maintains and controls definitive airway by introducing a tube orally that passes down through the larynx between the vocal cords, stopping before the tracheal bifurcation.

Anatomic Landmarks (Fig. VIII-3)

- Mouth
  Incisor teeth
  Anterior arch: palatoglossus muscle
  Palatine tonsil
  Posterior arch: palatopharyngeus muscle
- Oral pharynx
- Epiglottis
- Vallecula
- Piriform recess
- Vocal cords
- Trachea

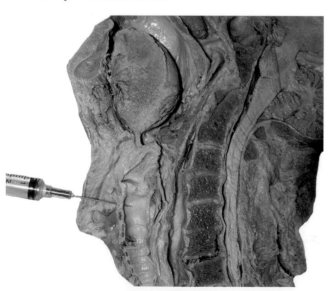

FIGURE VIII-1.

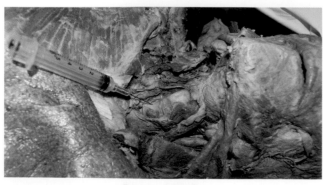

FIGURE VIII-2.

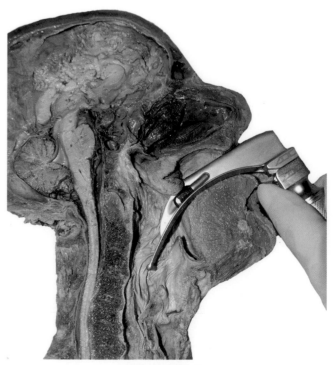

FIGURE VIII-3.

NASOTRACHEAL INTUBATION

Gray's Anatomy for Students: 992, 1004

Netter: 63, 66, 77–78

Clinical Application

Procedure maintains and controls an airway by introducing a tube nasally that passes down through the oral pharynx and larynx between the vocal cords, stopping short of the tracheal bifurcation.

Anatomic Landmarks

- Right or left nostril
- Concha or turbinates
- Nasopharynx
- Oropharynx
- Laryngopharynx
- Trachea

BURR HOLES FOR CRANIOTOMY

Gray's Anatomy for Students: 815

Netter: 15

Clinical Application

Procedure creates a hole in the skull to evacuate blood from an epidural or subdural hemorrhage.

Anatomic Landmarks

- Scalp
- Skin
- Connective tissue
- Aponeurosis
- Loose areolar tissue
- Periosteum
- Bones of the calvaria
- Dura mater

AKINOSI TECHNIQUE: TRIGEMINAL-MANDIBULAR NERVE BLOCK

Gray's Anatomy for Students: 932, 934

Netter: 121

Clinical Application

Procedure allows a local anesthetic to be deposited near the mandibular division of the trigeminal nerve, when opening the mouth is prohibited.

Anatomic Landmarks

- Oral vestibule
- Mucosa medial to ramus
- Maxillary bone and mucosa
- Trigeminal nerve–mandibular nerve branches

INDEX

Page numbers followed by "f" indicate figures.